Lecture Notes in Computational Vision and Biomechanics

Volume 15

For further volumes:
http://www.springer.com/series/8910

The research related to the analysis of living structures (Biomechanics) has been a source of recent research in several distinct areas of science, for example, Mathematics, Mechanical Engineering, Physics, Informatics, Medicine and Sport. However, for its successful achievement, numerous research topics should be considered, such as image processing and analysis, geometric and numerical modelling, biomechanics, experimental analysis, mechanobiology and enhanced visualization, and their application to real cases must be developed and more investigation is needed. Additionally, enhanced hardware solutions and less invasive devices are demanded.

On the other hand, Image Analysis (Computational Vision) is used for the extraction of high level information from static images or dynamic image sequences. Examples of applications involving image analysis can be the study of motion of structures from image sequences, shape reconstruction from images and medical diagnosis. As a multidisciplinary area, Computational Vision considers techniques and methods from other disciplines, such as Artificial Intelligence, Signal Processing, Mathematics, Physics and Informatics. Despite the many research projects in this area, more robust and efficient methods of Computational Imaging are still demanded in many application domains in Medicine, and their validation in real scenarios is matter of urgency.

These two important and predominant branches of Science are increasingly considered to be strongly connected and related. Hence, the main goal of the LNCV&B book series consists of the provision of a comprehensive forum for discussion on the current state-of-the-art in these fields by emphasizing their connection. The book series covers (but is not limited to):

- Applications of Computational Vision and Biomechanics
- Biometrics and Biomedical Pattern Analysis
- Cellular Imaging and Cellular Mechanics
- Clinical Biomechanics
- Computational Bioimaging and Visualization
- Computational Biology in Biomedical Imaging
- Development of Biomechanical Devices
- Device and Technique Development for Biomedical Imaging
- Digital Geometry Algorithms for Computational Vision and Visualization
- Experimental Biomechanics
- Gait & Posture Mechanics
- Multiscale Analysis in Biomechanics
- Neuromuscular Biomechanics
- Numerical Methods for Living Tissues
- Numerical Simulation
- Software Development on Computational Vision and Biomechanics
- Grid and High Performance Computing for Computational Vision and Biomechanics
- Image-based Geometric Modeling and Mesh Generation
- Image Processing and Analysis
- Image Processing and Visualization in Biofluids
- Image Understanding
- Material Models
- Mechanobiology
- Medical Image Analysis
- Molecular Mechanics
- Multi-Modal Image Systems
- Multiscale Biosensors in Biomedical Imaging
- Multiscale Devices and Biomems for Biomedical Imaging
- Musculoskeletal Biomechanics
- Sport Biomechanics
- Virtual Reality in Biomechanics
- Vision Systems

Paolo Di Giamberardino · Daniela Iacoviello
Renato Natal Jorge · João Manuel R. S. Tavares
Editors

Computational Modeling of Objects Presented in Images

Fundamentals, Methods and Applications

Springer

Editors
Paolo Di Giamberardino
Daniela Iacoviello
Department of Computer, Control and Management Engineering Antonio Ruberti
Sapienza Università di Roma
Rome
Italy

Renato Natal Jorge
João Manuel R. S. Tavares
Department of Mechanical Engineering
Universidade do Porto
Porto
Portugal

ISSN 2212-9391 ISSN 2212-9413 (electronic)
ISBN 978-3-319-38018-6 ISBN 978-3-319-04039-4 (eBook)
DOI 10.1007/978-3-319-04039-4
Springer Cham Heidelberg New York Dordrecht London

Printed on acid-free paper

Springer is part of Springer Science+Business Media (www.springer.com)

Preface

Computational vision domain presents a multidisciplinary nature involving different applications in society. Medicine, material science, surveillance, biometric, robotics, defence, satellite data, traffic analysis, and architecture, among other areas, use signal and image processing and analysis, arousing interest in methodological and applicative aspects.

Due to its intrinsic interdisciplinary aspects, different approaches, such as optimization methods, geometry, principal component analysis, stochastic methods, neural networks, and fuzzy logic, are currently discussed by the Researchers.

Several research fields related to the acquisition, the use and the analysis of images are involved in the areas of image processing and analysis, image segmentation, 2D and 3D reconstruction, data acquisition, interpolation and registration, scientific data visualization, remote sensing, modeling and simulation, biometric recognition, medical imaging, motion and deformation analysis, material science, computer vision in robotics and automation, and architecture.

This book contains extended versions of selected papers presented at the third edition of the *International Symposium CompIMAGE 2012: Computational Modeling of Object Presented in Images: Fundamentals, Methods and Applications*, that was held in Rome, at the Department of Computer, Control, and Management Engineering Antonio Ruberti of Sapienza University of Rome, September 2012. *CompIMAGE 2012* brought together researchers representing several fields such as Biomechanics, Engineering, Medicine, Mathematics, Physics, Statistic, and Architecture, presenting new trends in these fields. In particular, the latter topic, which was addressed for the first time in this edition, due to the particularity of the hosting Country for what concerns the Historical, Architectural, Cultural, and urban heritages resources, puts in evidence the important role that images also have in such less technical fields.

The Editors wish to thank all the *CompIMAGE 2012* Authors, Invited Lecturers, and members of the Scientific Committee for sharing their expertise, and also to the Department of Computer, Control, and Management Engineering Antonio Ruberti, the University of Rome La Sapienza, The Italian Group of Fracture (IGF), the Consorzio Interuniversitario Nazionale per l'Informatica (CINI), Sapienza Innovazione, Zètema Progetto Cultura S.r.l, the Universidade do Porto (UP), the Faculdade de Engenharia da Universidade do Porto (FEUP), the Fundação para a Ciência e a Tecnologia (FCT), the Instituto de Engenharia Mecânica (IDMEC-

Polo FEUP), and the Instituto de Engenharia Mecânica e Gestão Industrial (INEGI), for the help and the support given in the organization of this Roman third Edition of the *Symposium CompIMAGE 2012*.

Paolo Di Giamberardino
Daniela Iacoviello
Renato Natal Jorge
João Manuel R. S. Tavares

Contents

The Surveying and Representation Process Applied to Archaeology: A Quest for Invariants in a Highly Variable Context

Carlo Bianchini, Francesco Borgogni, Alfonso Ippolito and Luca J. Senatore

Abstract The study and analysis of archaeological elements often swings from large sites to small objects. This variability in dimensions and typology actually determines an equal variability of problems encountered during the surveying and representation process so that it is hard to retrieve a reliable common theoretical and operational background able to guide the researcher through the various steps. The problems connected with the interpretation of data (and their lack of clarity) disturb in fact considerably the final goal of surveying: achieve the most profound knowledge of the object analyzed. Taking into consideration numerous survey campaigns carried out for years, this chapter seeks to present a *modus operandi* that seems to be indispensable for standardizing and regulating procedures of data collecting, elaborating and representing applied by our research team from the Department of History, Drawing and Restoration of Architecture (Sapienza—University of Rome), the aim being to make the final result *scientific*, i.e. more objective and correct. Together with a general methodological framing, we shall describe a number of research

Even if present study has been developed together by all authors, different authorships can be recognized within the chapter. In particular Sects. 2 and 3 have been written by Carlo Bianchini, Sect. 4 by Alonso Ippolito, Sect. 5 by Luca. J. Senatore and finally Sect. 6 by Francesco Borgogni. All other parts have instead been written in common.

C. Bianchini (✉) · F. Borgogni · A. Ippolito · L. J. Senatore
Department of History, Drawing and Restoration of Architecture, Sapienza—University of Rome, Rome, Italy
e-mail: Carlo.bianchini@uniroma1.it

F. Borgogni
e-mail: Francesco_borgogni@yahoo.it

A. Ippolito
e-mail: Alfonso.Ippolito@uniroma1.it

L. J. Senatore
e-mail: Luca.senatore@uniroma1.it

P. Di Giamberardino et al. (eds.), *Computational Modeling of Objects Presented in Images*, Lecture Notes in Computational Vision and Biomechanics 15,
DOI: 10.1007/978-3-319-04039-4_1,

projects spanning from large sites (Petra), single buildings/architectural structures (The Temple of Divus Claudio, Rome) and small objects (Tombs and artifacts in Crustumerium – Rome).

Keywords Archaeological survey · 3D modelling · Integrated survey · Knowledge system

1 Introduction

The study and analysis of archaeological elements often swings from large sites to small objects. This variability in dimensions and typology actually determines an equal variability of problems encountered during the surveying and representation process so that it is hard to retrieve a reliable common theoretical and operational background able to guide the researcher through the various steps.

Nevertheless worthwhile to make an effort and attempt to outline a general framework in this field, especially relying on the great possibilities offered by the massive capturing and digital representation technologies.

In the past, in fact, field workers had to deal with several problems related to the "intrinsic" limits both of the equipment used for data acquisition and of the graphic models used to communicate the information registered and elaborated. As a result: the surveying process was highly time-consuming; the amount of information collected was often inadequate for most research and practical purposes; the high subjectivity of representations (i.e. graphic models) often produced "reinterpretations" too little corresponding to the surveyed object; any graphic model was produced in a unique sample difficult to be reproduced and shared with the scientific community.

The technological development we've experimented with in the last 20 years has actually provided a number of possible solutions for the above mentioned problems: surveying operation can be presently carried out through semi-automatic processes, with a low level of uncertainty and above all acquiring points in millions instead of dozens; this feature produces very detailed models that on one side ensures an extended coverage of the surveyed object while on the other minimizes the possibility of subjective reinterpretation; finally the whole representation process has become "digital" so that the "raw" data as well as any model (2D or 3D) can be reproduced and shared in a potentially infinite number of copies completely identical to the original [1, 6, 10, 12].

This chapter discusses the interrelations between the issues listed in the previous paragraph and aims at proposing some possible guidelines derived from the activities carried out in the last years by our research group within the Department of History, Drawing and Restoration of Architecture of Sapienza—University of Rome. Together with a general methodological framing, we shall describe a number of research projects spanning from large sites (Petra—Fig. 1), single buildings/architectural

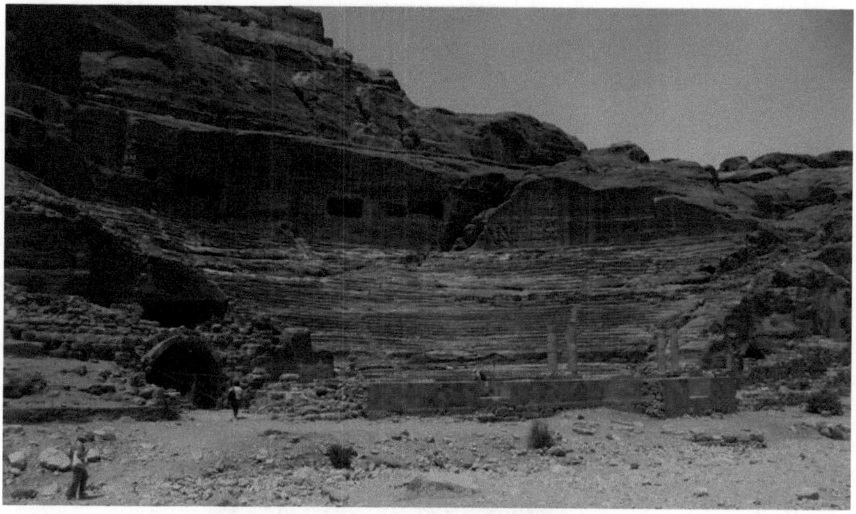

Fig. 1 Archaeological site of Petra

structures (Temple of Divus Claudio, Rome—Fig. 2) and small objects (Tombs and artifacts in Crustumerium site, Rome—Fig. 3).

2 Survey, Modeling, Interpretation as Multidisciplinary Components of a Knowledge System

There can be no doubt that the first step in approaching the study of any archaeological element is constructing a Knowledge System that will enable us to collect, interpret and store information about it.

The components making up this system, however, are of various types: quantitative, first and foremost (essentially resulting from surveying operations), but also qualitative. While the former can and have to be channeled through a rigorous scientific approach, the latter draw on the investigator's sensitivity and interpretative flair, that show themselves, at times even intuitively and extemporaneously, capable of attaining levels of understanding that are denied to simple "measurement".

In studies of archaeological elements (both on the large and the small scale), this process is particularly marked: not only is it necessary to construct a multidisciplinary database that is as consistent and rigorous as possible, but many different skills must be integrated in order to suggest interpretations that transcend the sectorial.

While the qualitative component lies in the reign of irrefutability (in the sense proposed by Popper), to the quantitative one belongs the Survey, one of the most powerful and reliable tools developed over the years by researchers (archaeologist, architects,

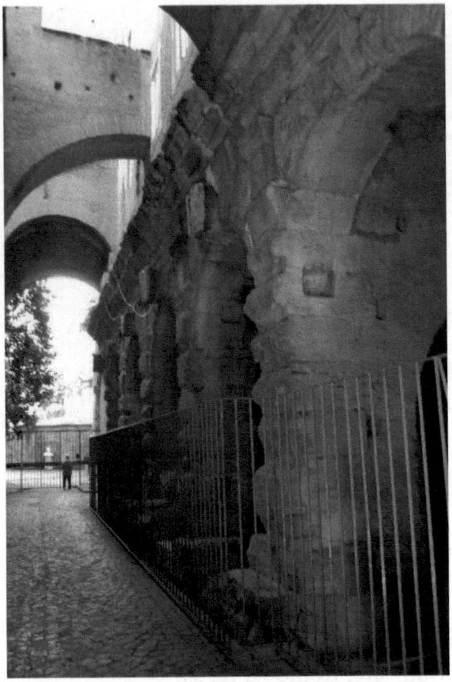

Fig. 2 The Temple of Divus Claudio, Rome

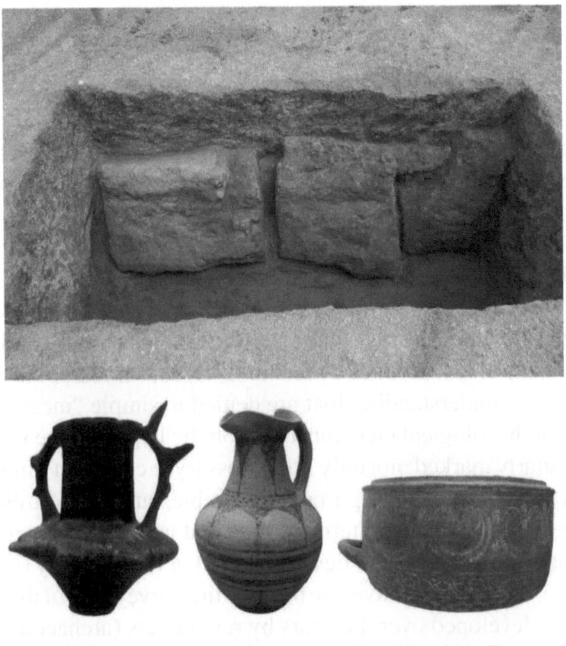

Fig. 3 Tombs and artifacts in the archaeological site of Crustumerium, Rome

historians, etc.) to achieve what Descartes used to define "profound knowledge".[1] It actually implies the idea of measurement, that is the possibility of turning into quantity some qualities of the studied phenomenon (in this case an artifact, a building, a site, etc.) by using the ratio between the measured quantity and an appropriate unit of measure.

Thanks to this method, that operationally implies the measurements of a certain number of points, we build a simplified *model* of the complex phenomenon we are investigating. Quite apart from the theoretical framework, it's paramount how in practical terms the implementation of this strategy depends on the available measurement technologies. As for centuries the limited amount of measurable points implied a preliminary attentive design of the survey operations in order to capture the really significant ones (*selection* before *acquisition*), in the last decades this order has been somehow turned upside down thanks to new massive measurement technologies in which selection often follows acquisition [4, 5].

Let's try then to clarify this fundamental point, firstly from a linguistic point of view: the term *Survey* refers in fact to a very structured process that leads to the construction of 2D or 3D models starting from a real object. The whole workflow can be broken-down into several different tasks of which, certainly, the *acquisition of data* (*surveying*) represents the first step. All following tasks (in the survey process) dealing with *selection*, *interpretation* and *representation* of acquired data actually lead to models (3D, 2D-drawings, etc.) that somehow concur in enlightening the investigated phenomenon. The traditional survey approach implied (and obviously still implies) a strict dependence of the surveying phase on a preliminary deep investigation able to guide the limited measurement possibilities (Fig. 4).

This intrinsic limit obliges somehow to an as accurate as possible design of the surveying operations in which selection, interpretation and representation of data come even before the measurement, as if the survey existed in the surveyor mind before the physical set up of the operations and expected somehow only a verification. The Survey's workflow is in this framework potentially defined right from the start.

Massive acquisition technologies have actually separated all different steps: site preliminary study is only oriented to the position and number of stations (scans, shots, etc.) while the topographic support is reduced to the minimum when even no more necessary in the surveying phase. Selection, interpretation, and representation of data are instead carried out in a second phase.

Together, these considerations thus establish the horizon of research, putting the Survey process in the more general framework of a Knowledge System as the non-additive result of single sectorial contributions, where there is a clear boundary between the procedures for acquiring and organizing data (which strive for the maximum objectivity) and the criteria for selecting and processing the database itself (critical expressions invariably subjective).

[1] Whenever human beings have had to deal with complex phenomena during their evolutive journey, they always tried to develop learning strategies that would allow them to overcome the limits of their own senses. Descartes well explained how this approach involves two different kind of knowledge: *common sense* (that we acquire through experience) and *profound* which instead can be attained only through study methods and techniques that can reveal to the mind what our senses cannot.

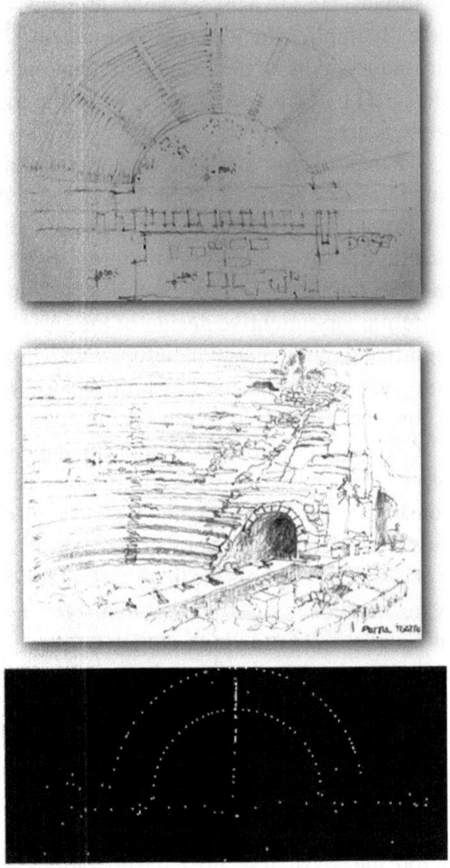

Fig. 4 Selection of data: form perception to measurement

3 Towards a "Scientific" Surveying

It is precisely by establishing this boundary, this demarcation, that we can view the entire question in the light of the Scientific Method consolidated among the various communities of researchers, putting it to the test of Karl Popper's "principle of falsifiability", still the benchmark for evaluating scientific theories.[2]

[2] With this principle, Popper sought to resolve the impasse that arose between Russell's fruitless attempts to construct "complete" logical deductive systems, and the cataclysm that swept through epistemological thinking following Kurt Gödel's proof of the Incompleteness Theorem. Popper, well aware of the inherent inadequacy of the tools that human beings have for cognizing reality and that, in the final analysis, it is substantially impossible to provide "positive" proof that any given statement is true, shifts the centre of gravity of knowledge from proving that something is true to showing that it is false: for Popper, a theory is scientific only if it is possible to devise experiments that demonstrate its inadequacy, i.e., that refute it as false. This approach has revealed as highly profitable in terms of advancing knowledge: if a theory withstands an attempt to falsify it, it will be

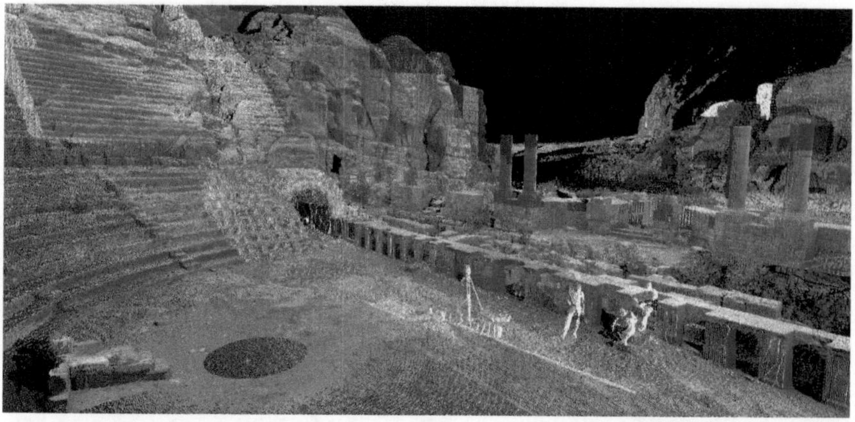

Fig. 5 Archaeological site of Petra—the data acquired using scanning techniques

The Surveying phase, in fact, seems to be highly compatible with the strict scientific methodological assessment that is commonly utilized by other research areas (physics, biology, etc.) [4, 5, 13].

It's unfortunately impossible in this occasion to provide an exhaustive discussion concerning the Scientific Method adopted by the general scientific community. Nevertheless we cannot proceed without listing at least the crucial points of this Method: currently considered scientific is (1) *the investigation of a phenomenon developed using a set of techniques*; (2) *based on the gathering of observable, empiric and measureable data affected by a controlled and declared level of uncertainty*; (3) *those data will have to be archived, shared and independently assessed*; (4) *all used procedures have to be replicable in order to eventually acquire a comparable set of data*.

These four main points can be substantially respected during the Acquisition phase:

1. *The investigation of the phenomenon has to be developed using a set of techniques* (Fig. 5)—Being the "phenomenon" in our case the object to be surveyed, this prescription is clearly respected because any survey uses methods and techniques able to guide the surveyor during the measurement phase. As already discussed, only metric information complies with this criterion being instead excluded all that, perceived or even intuited by the surveyor, cannot be codified in quantitative terms thanks to measure operations.
2. *Based on the gathering of observable, empiric and measurable data affected by a controlled and declared level of uncertainty* (Figs. 6 and 7)—All data are actually observable (they represent the "material" points of the object), empiric (they

(Footnote 2 continued)
stronger, more general and thus closer to the truth; if, conversely, the attempt succeeds, an aspect will be revealed that the theory was unable to explain, and a new and stimulating line of research will thus be opened up.

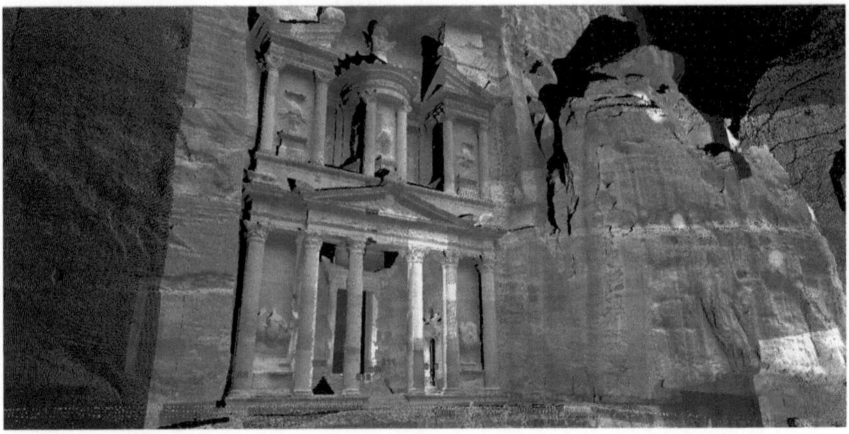

Fig. 6 Archaeological site of Petra—the observable, empiric data acquired on site

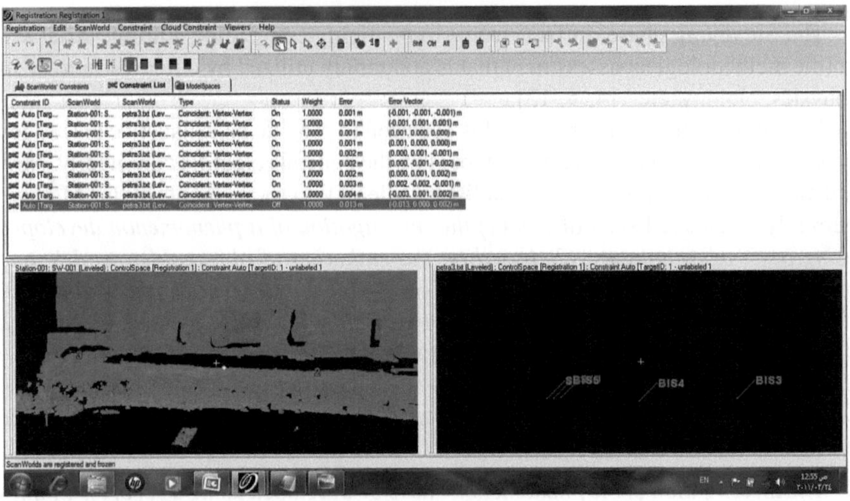

Fig. 7 Archaeological site of Petra—the measurable data acquired on site

result from experimental activities), measurable (they are acquired using measure equipment and techniques) and affected by a controlled and declared level of uncertainty (resulting from the instruments, the systematic errors, etc.). The actual compliance with this prescription can be assured provided that all steps (from the survey project to the measurement and assessment process) are documented with accuracy and attached to the data themselves, so to create a unique set composed by data (the measures) and metadata (the process information). Unfortunately this procedure is too seldom adopted in the survey activities.

3. *Data will have to be archived, shared and independently assessed*—The so-called "digital revolution" has affected this aspect very deeply. In the specific field of

architectural Survey it wasn't at all a consolidated habit to arrange and archive systematically both the final deliverables and the metadata describing the procedure used during the experiment called "survey" (survey project, field notebook, measured points monograph, instrumental features, etc.). The quick and sudden switch to new equipment for massive point acquisition (3D scanning, photomodeling, etc.) has actually mitigated a lot this problem as many metadata are already archived in a database form by the instruments themselves. Furthermore, archives are "born digital" with clear advantages in terms of transmission, sharing and duplicability, features that in the recent past were impossible being each archive a single, original set of data. The sharing and independent assessment seems to be a more critical aspect: differently from other research areas that show more consolidated traditions in immediately online sharing of experimental data, the archaeological (and in general the cultural heritage) sector is still too affected by high confidentiality levels. We should thus all work to catch up with other research areas so that the archived data could more easily circulate within our scientific community and any researcher could develop its activity on high quality data. In this framework some attempts are being carried out but much work has still to be done.[3]

4. *All used procedures have to be replicable in order to eventually acquire a comparable set of data*—This last point actually comes up as a sort of corollary form the previous three. Nevertheless, it can produce very significant effects involving the definition of procedures suitable in "diachronically" integrating data acquired in different time segments and with different technologies. In this way all information connected with a certain object would find a compatible space in a single database that, in case of new investigations, would not start from scratch but simply be updated and improved with the new surveyed data.

4 From Acquisition to Selection and Interpretation of Data: From Surveying to the Models

Selection and interpretation complete the proposed path for Survey. It has been already widely discussed how both phases concur not secondarily to the construction of the *geometric model* of the surveyed object, that is to that reduction process of the objective multi-dimensional complexity to its geometric essence made of points, lines, surfaces. A biunique correspondence is set in this way between the object and its virtual substitute which can be used to simulate different operations as they were made directly on the object itself.

From a strictly epistemological point of view such a model can be considered the result of a selection operation carried on by a subject on an object aiming at extracting some of the potentially infinite available information. The selected data, though, are not the result of a random or automatic reading: on the contrary they strictly comply

[3] In this framework we would like to cite *500 Initiative* promoted by CyArk (www.cyark.org).

with rules set, even if with different level of consciousness, in advance by the subject himself. In this way a stable relationship real object/model is crated: a relationship that intrinsically already represents an interpretation of the selected data. In other words, starting from the selected set of data, we always tend to demonstrate an hypothesis we have beforehand formulated.

This particular process has been traditionally rooted in the following principles:

- Human beings have an ability, innate or acquired, to conceive the qualities of physical space.
- Of the *n* qualities of physical space, the geometrical qualities optimize the operations of control and manipulation.
- Space can be concretely manipulated and modified thanks to the correspondence between the real object and its geometric abstraction (Geometric Model).
- The Geometric Model, through the process of Representation becomes a Two Dimensional Geometric Model.
- The tool that ensures that the mechanisms for controlling and manipulating the graphic model are effective is Drawing.

This procedure establishes a biunique correspondence between the Object and its Graphical Representation which can more appropriately be considered a Two-Dimensional Graphical Model, or in other words a virtual substitute on which the most widely varied operations can be simulated as if they were actually performed in reality.[4]

Since digital media burst on the scene and modeling software came into common use, however, this scheme has changed in a number of significant ways. First, the correspondence between physical space and representation has become practically perfect in the case of the latter development (Fig. 8): each material point P_r identified by its coordinates x_r, y_r, z_r in real space corresponds immediately to a virtual point P_v, likewise identified by a unique set of three Cartesian coordinates x_v, y_v, z_v, essentially freeing itself from any and all constraints associated with the size of the support or with projection and sectioning.

The computer screen becomes the *de facto* interface between these two parallel universes, a window from which we can look out onto the space of these truly three-dimensional models. Nevertheless, it is also the definite limit of our exploration that keeps us firmly and forever *on this side of the glass*, so that the only opportunities for interaction with the virtual space are provided by the tools that enable us to explore, model and manipulate virtual entities.

[4] From an epistemological standpoint, we can say that the *model* is the product of the selection operation that a subject carries out on an object (real or imaginary) in order to extract some of the infinite information available from the object. It can thus be the product of a discretization, or in other words, of reading and recording certain parameters (which may be metric, angular, color parameters or other types) by an operator or an instrument which actively explores the object to identify singular points (this is the approach employed in direct and indirect surveying, as well as the procedure used by three-dimensional scanner), or, conversely, the model can be the result of the passive and uniform recording of information from the object (the photogrammetric approach).

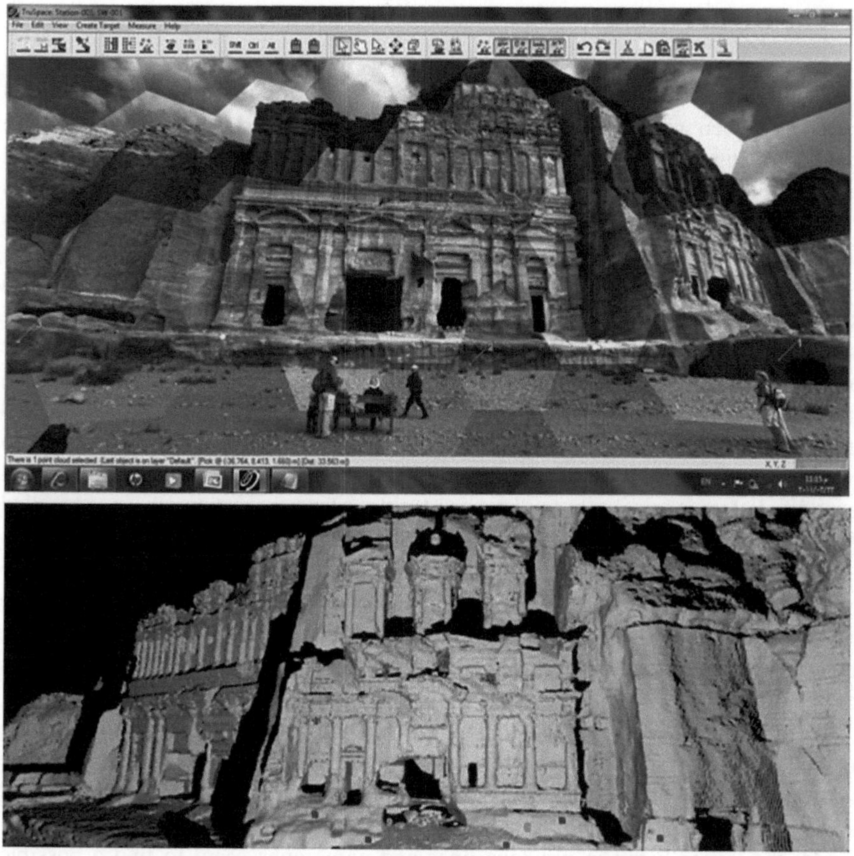

Fig. 8 Archaeological site of Petra—the correspondence between reality and model

Important though it is, however, this new technology has not brought about any kind of practical simplification: indeed, it has significantly thinned the ranks of those who are capable of making full use of the new opportunities. If with conventional systems it was enough to know the "language" of the object to be studied (architecture or archaeology, in our case) and master the tool of "drawing", the advent of digital systems has added the need to develop far from inconsiderable skills with the hardware and software used for data capturing, processing, modeling and CAD drawing.

Currently, this problem has opened a wide gulf between the true beneficiaries of this technological innovation (archaeologists, especially) and hardware and software developers and specialists. The challenge, then, is two-fold: envisioning ways of using digital media that are better suited to the abilities of entry level users, and making efforts to increase "digital literacy" that can add to the pool of experts who are able to use these profitable technologies [8, 11, 14, 17].

5 The Digital Model

Interaction between new surveying methods has become something of a required procedure when working on large archaeological sites [3, 8, 15, 16, 18, 20]. Modern methods using non-contact 3D data acquisition equipment now allow us to obtain a large number of points providing a wealth of data and enable us to handle surveys on any scale. We are able to work on any element, no matter its dimensions, its geometrical complexity or the level of detail required.

However, one issue that is not quite so simple is the representation of the acquired surfaces, even more so if these involve complex surfaces and geometries, and subsequent processing. These operations are not altogether immediate, especially if the aim is not to stray too far from the topology of the initial form. In fact, as the geometric complexity of the model increases, there is also an increase in processing and editing operations. These digital geometry procedures are fundamental especially in relation to the topology of the surface to be represented and described. Our experience has led us increasingly to distance ourselves from operations that are handled fully automatically by the software and to favor conceptual mediation resulting from the combination of historical and geometric knowledge and experience, where the operator's role is to recognize and select the surfaces to reconstruct. Managing the passage from point clouds—used as primitives—to complex surfaces is an evolving field, where operational and management procedures still provide for wide margins of exploration.

It is practically indispensable to choose a method based on the principle that the model and its representation must be constructed while expressly communicating the cultural positions, objectives and operational procedures of those who built, designed and created it.

All the issues listed in previous lines and paragraphs seem to find a possible solution thanks to the *digital model*, i.e. a computer-based model, which enables the analysis, reading, knowledge and an intense, rapid and controlled interaction, with perception and navigation facilities between user and model which are often not available from the object itself (Fig. 9).

These digital models use a single representation system to cover the entire range of possible models, thus providing the same performance as traditional iconic models on one hand, as well as non-iconic models on the other (diagrammatic and mathematical models) [1, 7]. In other words, they present themselves as the synthesis of the most varied forms of modeling practiced and defined by: geometry (the description of the coordinates of the vertices—Fig. 10); topology (the description of the connection relationships between geometric components and the study of forms—Fig. 11); texture (that characteristic which, when applied to geometry and topology determines the unique properties of the surface rendering it totally recognizable and linked to the original—Fig. 12). So, on one side geometry and topology define the two-dimensional and three-dimensional geometric qualities of the object and, on the other, texture characterizes the two previous patterns. Once the characteristics

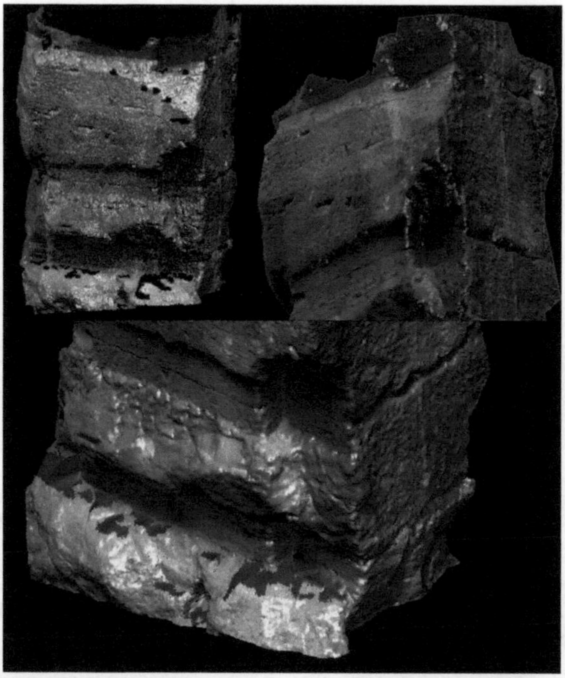

Fig. 9 Temple of Divus Claudio, Rome—digital model of a pillar

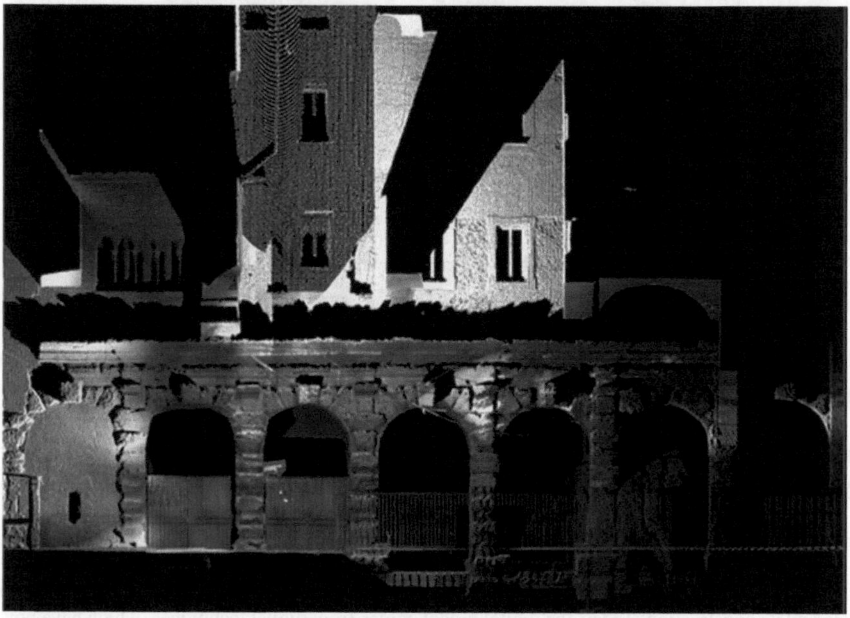

Fig. 10 Temple of Divus Claudio, Rome—digital representation of vertices (geometry)

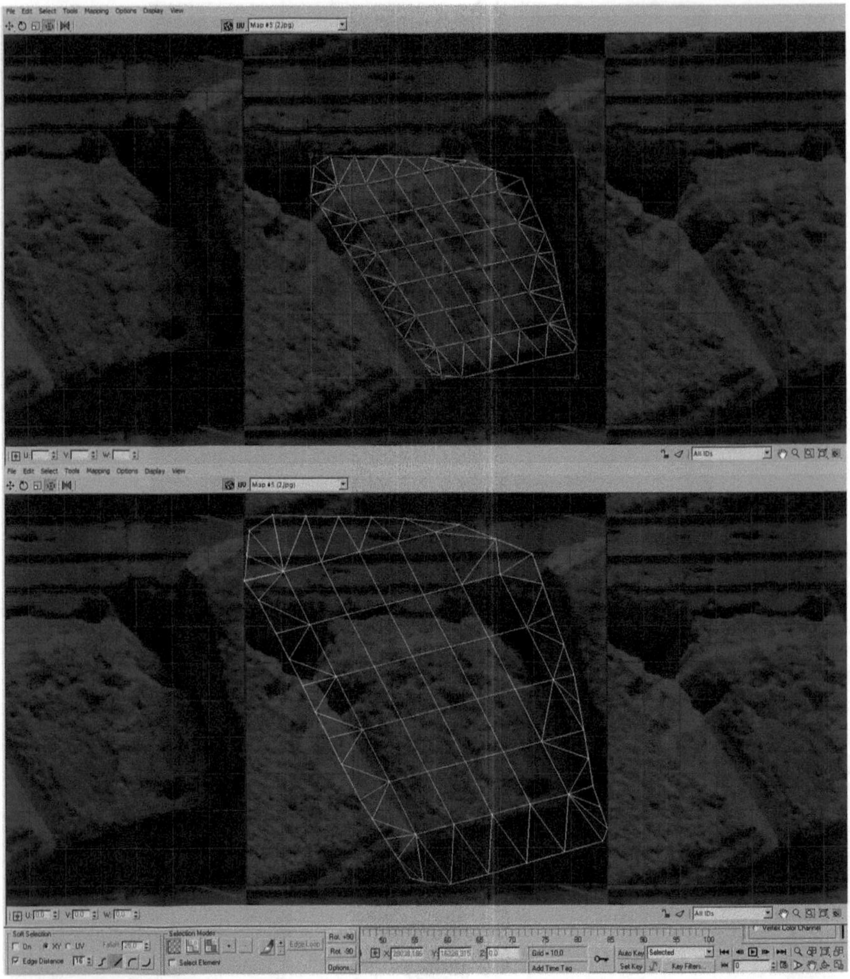

Fig. 11 Temple of Divus Claudio, Rome—digital model and topology

defining the object have been identified, the procedures for the models which are to represent the same object can be outlined.[5]

The possibility of building a digital model through three-dimensional representations, albeit only experienced via the flat screen of a computer, has created a new type of model which is no longer static but dynamic, interactive and able to rep-

[5] For the sake of full understanding, we can consider for its similarities the development of the *architectural model* in its historical sense, conceptually defined as the stage between the design idea and its construction. Today, the digital model comes from digital techniques, which have now spread to all instruments of representation and have finally reached full relevance at the same time of surveying.

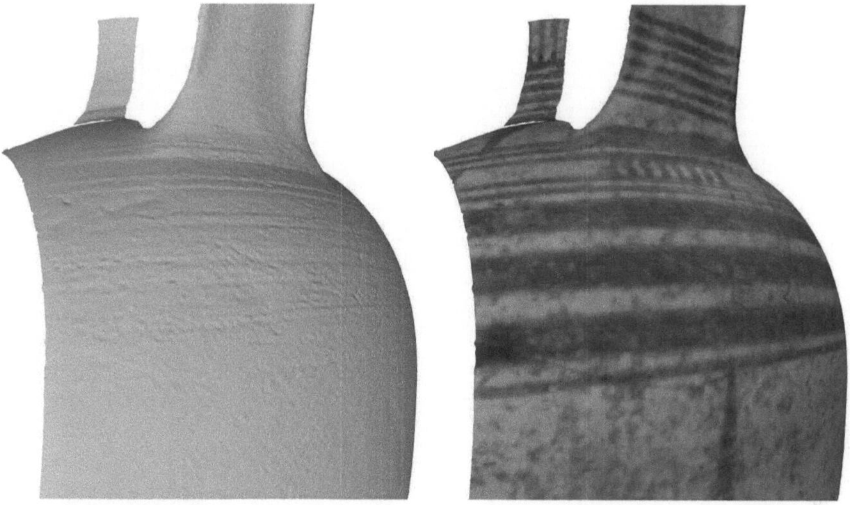

Fig. 12 Crustumerium, Rome—digital model and texture

resent, process and change sequentially the various stages in its development and travel around it and pass from the outside to the inside. Ultimately, it is an interaction between the temporal and the spatial. A full and complex level of interactivity has thus developed between real object and virtual digital model, thanks also to the possibility of producing lifelike surfaces by mapping digital images. An extraordinary opportunity for interaction between the real and the virtual (between plastic models and digital models) has been provided by computer systems designed for industrial production.

We can also say that, at least in science and technology, models have acquired "simulative" functions, and not in relation to the object itself, but in terms of the functions the object is intended for and the consequences of these functions. It is even more important to specify that not only are these models produced using computer tools, but also that their functions are also *managed* by computer. In other words, a complex and total interactivity has now developed between the real plastic model, the virtual digital model and the management of functions. This interactivity, or at least complementarity, also applies to the architectural/archaeological digital model where a special relationship has now been established with the new technologies of computerized graphic representation. The simultaneous presence of the architectural/archaeological digital model and digital three-dimensional graphics has become established practice. The two representation methods coexist with their ability to relate to each other in a way that is complementary to the project.

This methodological approach has made it possible to develop a "critical operational method" gradually optimized on the basis of on-site experiments carried out in recent years. For several years now, in fact, our research team has worked alongside research groups of archaeologists with the aim of establishing such a method

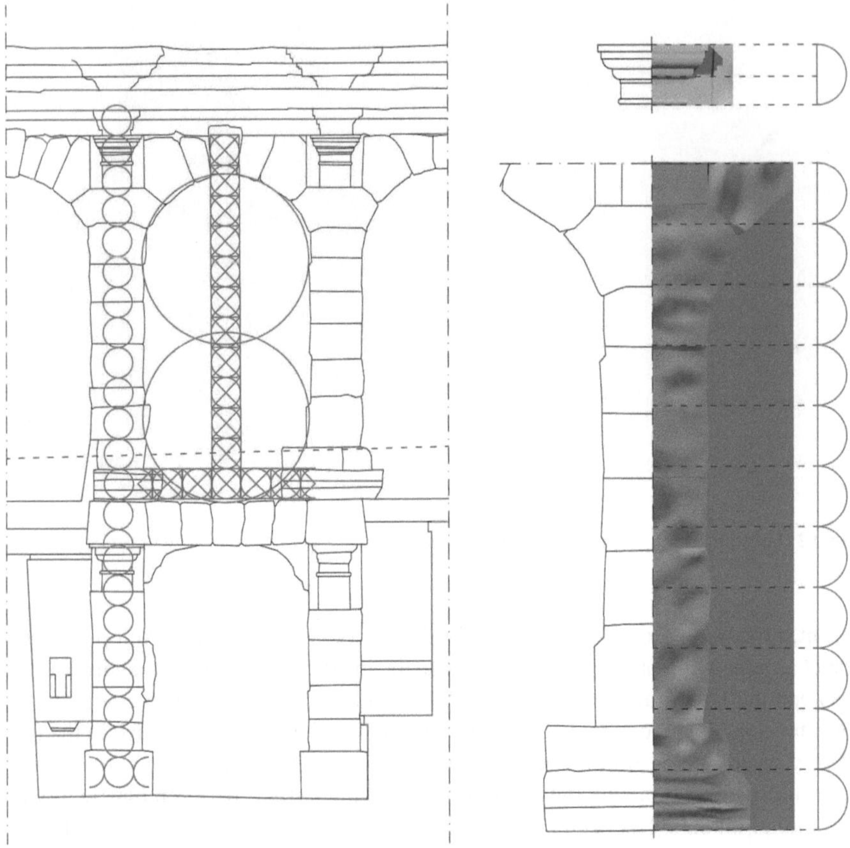

Fig. 13 Temple of Divus Claudio, Rome—the proportional study

that, according to the scientific criterion recalled in previous paragraphs, is standard, repeatable and verifiable, which begins at the acquisition stage, through the selection and interpretation stage and ends with survey output and the creation of digital models.

A proper definition of a "critical operational method" for the construction of three-dimensional models requires, first of all, a precise outlining of the intended purpose and also an identification of two integrated stages: *critical survey*, which leads to the definition of the object from its geometrical and morphological characteristics; *objective survey*, which consists in ensuring that data is free of criticalities to enable a detailed specialist reading.

The representations that are to become the digital model for an archaeological representation will be defined by: geometric representation identifying the three-dimensional position of points; proportioning which enables a metric reading of the ancient to seek the original units used by the designers (Fig. 13); texture which

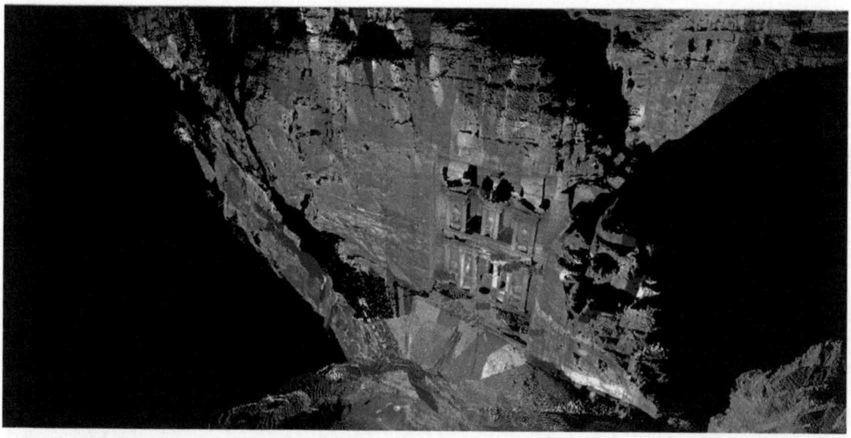

Fig. 14 Texturized model of Petra treasure

uses photographic mapping or the reflectance data from the scan (Fig. 14). The construction of three-dimensional models may follow different paths, but never in a way that defers automatic creation of surfaces to the software. In addition, these models may or may not be characterized by high-resolution digital photographs in order to provide more information about the appearance of materials and their level of conservation (Fig. 15). Each element of the virtual model must be displayed with an image of the real model in order to achieve coherence with reality.

Another important element for defining the digital model is multi-level analytical documentation represented by architectural details which in turn consists of a layout that is designed to aid a profound understanding of the object of study. It is important to emphasize that the construction of these details must be established before the surveying phase since it is absolutely essential to acquire a large amount of information. The layout describing them consists of a schedule identifying the characteristics to be acquired and the scales of representation of the models to be built. This schedule contains: raw data for acquisition to allow each researcher to use it as he or she will; 3D models up to a scale of 1:1 physical prototypes resulting from acquisition (short-range 3D laser scanner) which may feature textures, which ensure the portability of the survey data (e.g. inscriptions and engravings); the publisher which allows the user to view and examine high-definition panoramic images of the point cloud, even online, and presents the positions of the scanner during acquisition and also provides the possibility to extract the coordinates of the selected points and measure distances.

This method, along with 3D surveying leading to the creation of models, enables us to construct an interactive analogue model of the relationship between design and representation, which provides a continuous interaction between the representation of the object and the user, leaving constant the relationship between the scale of representation and the actual object.

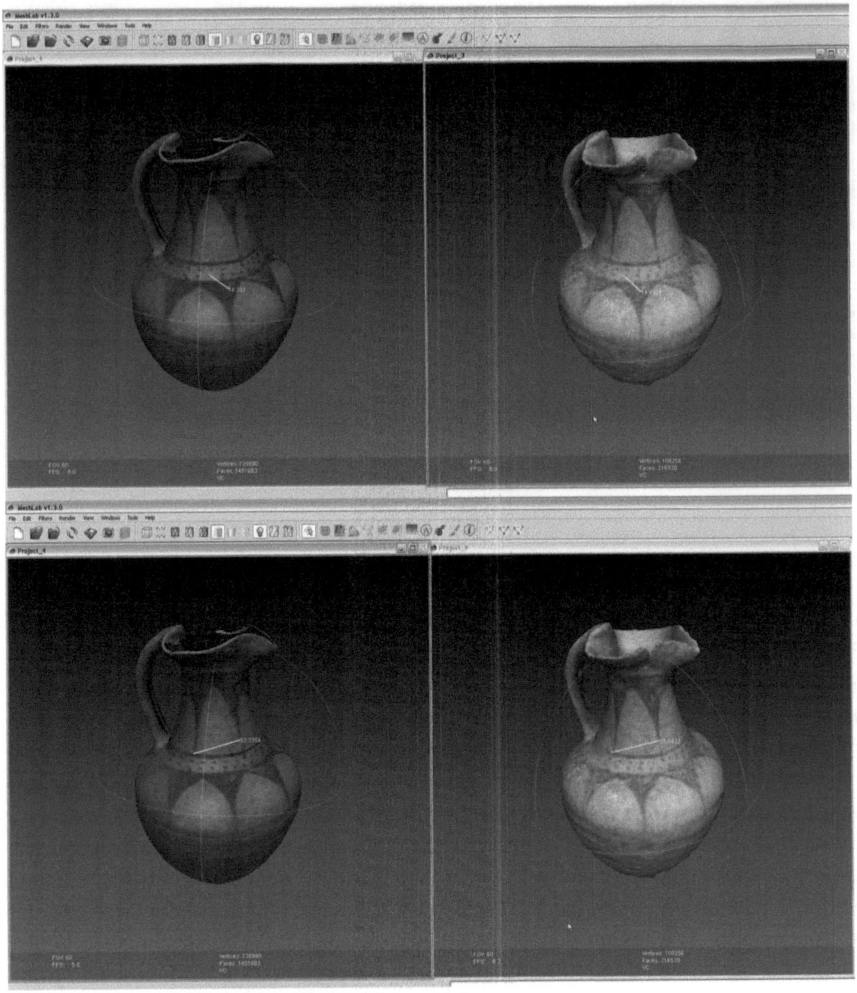

Fig. 15 Texturized model of one of the artifacts found in Crustumerium

We are dealing with the constant relationship between iconicity and virtualization of the object under survey and study by means of digital tools. In this relationship the actual model is static, but is also self-referential, whereas the digital model is dynamic and totally depends on the object/image it represents: it is no longer a metaphor, but rather an allegory, a narrative.

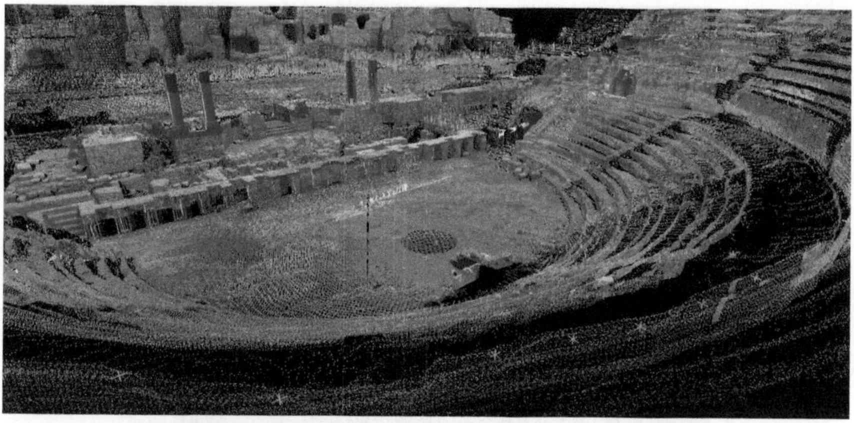

Fig. 16 Archaeological site of Petra: the theatre

6 From the Large to the Small Scale: Three Examples

For a few years now a number of researchers from the Department of History, Drawing and Restoration of Architecture—Sapienza University of Rome have been focusing on these issues while developing survey projects, especially in the archaeological field. Although many works and papers have been already devoted to this same topic, nevertheless we want to present our "critical operational method" that, far from establishing an actual general operative protocol nevertheless we hope would concur in enhancing the methodology of surveying and representing archaeological piece of heritage.

Our operative guidelines are obviously dynamic and constantly evolving. They have been tested and refined during numerous surveying campaigns [3, 4]. They were conceived—and this point must be emphasized—in order to preserve the surveying process from becoming completely mechanical. The idea has always been to provide aid and reliable references to the technician without demoting his critical role. Furthermore, an intense collaboration with some teams of specialized archaeologists made it possible to fully understand their aims and expectations connected with each surveying campaign.

We present here three examples representing the territorial/urban, the building and the small object scale. Belong to the territorial/urban dimension the surveying campaigns of the sites of Petra that starting from the ancient theatre extended to a great part of the entire site (Figs. 16, 17 and 18); to the building scale, instead, the Temple of Divus Claudio (Rome—Fig. 19); to the smaller scale, finally, the survey of the excavation campaign developed in Crustumerium (Rome—Fig. 20).

As already underlined, in all these campaigns the cooperative work between architects and archaeologists played an effective role. Indeed, it enabled the whole group to balance accuracy in acquisition, sound documentation, multi-level models (for archi-

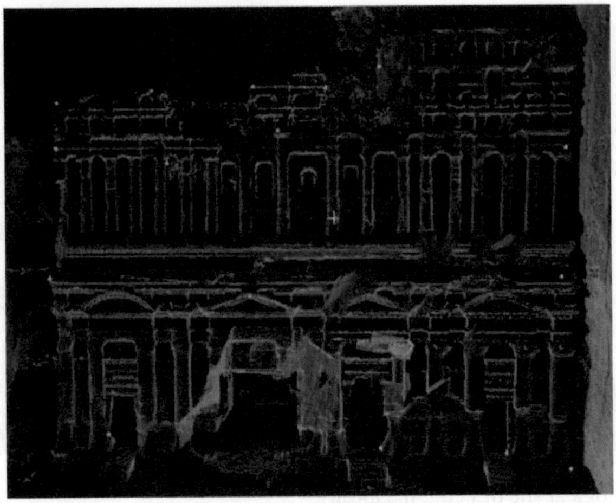

Fig. 17 Archaeological site of Petra: the Royal Tomb

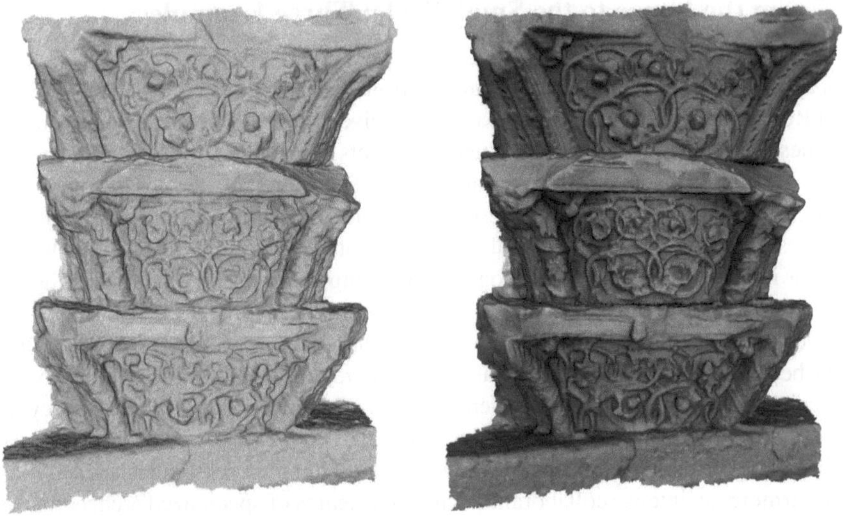

Fig. 18 Archaeological site of Petra: a capital

tects, archaeologists, etc., powerful communication and managing tools for various stakeholders).

Quite apart from the preliminary activities dealing essentially with the collection of all information able to recreate a synthetic picture of the studied object or site, the conceiving and testing of an adequate Project of Survey appears to be a crucial step. This document (extemporary or structured) will describe as much in detail as possible the sequence of successive works to be conducted, the choice of one or more

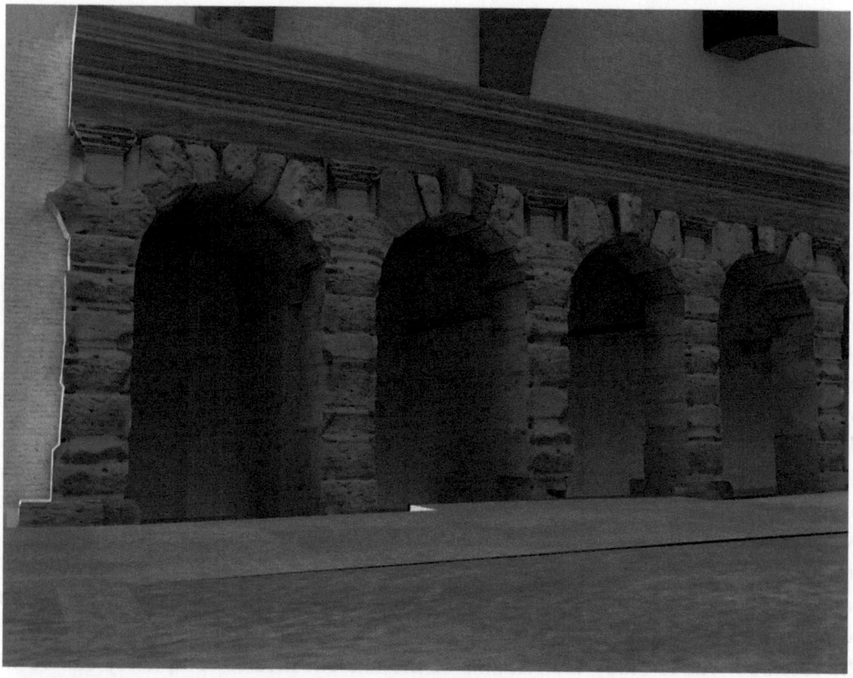

Fig. 19 Temple of Divus Claudio—Rome, The Porticus

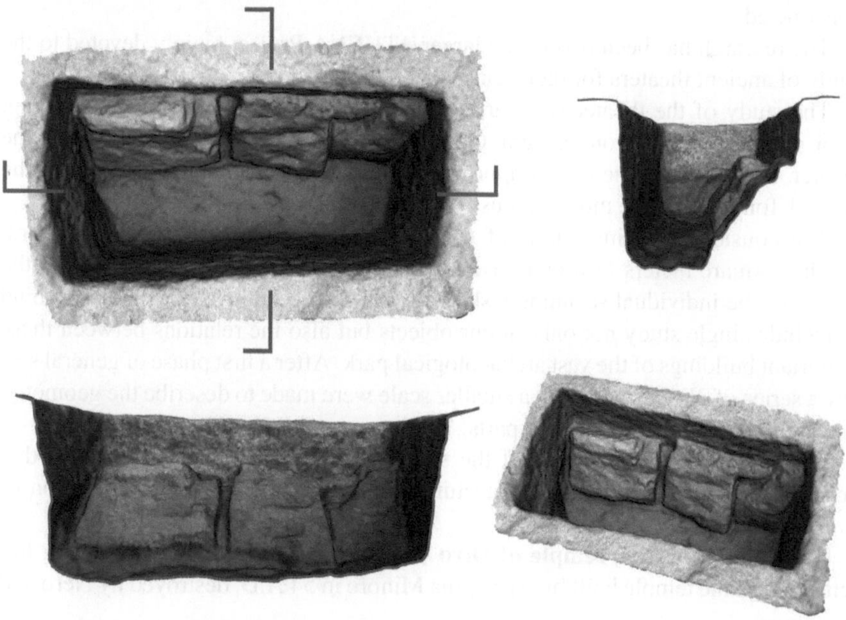

Fig. 20 Crustumerium—Rome, one of the excavated tombs

surveying methods as well as the timing for the operations conducted in situ and for those leading to representation.

Relying on this forecast, eventually integrated by a prototype activity in situ, the following operations have been articulated in two successive, interrelated paths: 1. *Surveying* (data acquiring) and 2. *Survey*, that is the selection, interpretation and representation activities described in previous paragraphs.

Large scale: the Petra site (Figs. 21 and 22) For the Petra archaeological site it was decided to combine different surveying methods and instruments. The underlying idea was that the traditional, proven direct surveying techniques would be flanked at all times by technologically advanced instruments that can more readily scan large surfaces, with the older methods used only as a backup when it was not possible to proceed otherwise. Accordingly, long-range 3D laser scanners, total stations, photo modeling and digital photography were combined and integrated [2, 9, 19]. The data capture stage is thus a fundamental aspect of producing survey deliverables, and consequently of passing from the real object to its 2D/3D representation through a geometrical model and a scaled-down model. The city of Petra, capital of the Nabatean Arabs, located at a distance of 262 km to the south of Amman, is the most important archaeological site in Jordan. It is composed of a series of archaeological remains of structures that go back to the third century AC and today witness the wealth of a civilization that vanished around the seventh century. The purpose of the research was to study the remains of the ancient theater completely carved in the rock by the Nabataeans over 2,000 years ago and which overlooks the terminal path of the "Siq", a canyon around which most of the monuments of the area were constructed.

The research has been part of the larger ATHENA Project mainly devoted to the study of ancient theaters for their reuse [3].[6]

The study of the theater was carried out with no-contact integrated surveying, laser scanner, total station, camera. Quite apart from drawing up the survey of the theater, the study put the most important monuments in the area—the Theater, the "Royal Tombs" and the most famous "Treasury"—in one virtual space.

The considerable dimensions of the intervention covering an area of several hundred square meters lead us to use non-contact sensing technologies and so the results of the individual scanning tasks with a high-precision surveying has to bind to include single study not only in our objects but also the relations between these important buildings of the vast archaeological park. After a first phase of general survey a series of 2D/3D models at a smaller scale were made to describe the geometry, and the proportions of the single parts.

The result of the first phase of the survey was a series of 2D/3D models that describe the geometrical and architectural structure analyzing each proportion of every single part.

Building scale: the Temple of Divo Claudio in Rome (Fig. 23) Nothing has remained of the temple built by Agrippina Minore in 54 A.D, destroyed by Nero and

[6] Ancient Theatres Enhancement for New Actualities funded by the EU in the Euromed Heritage IV Programme.

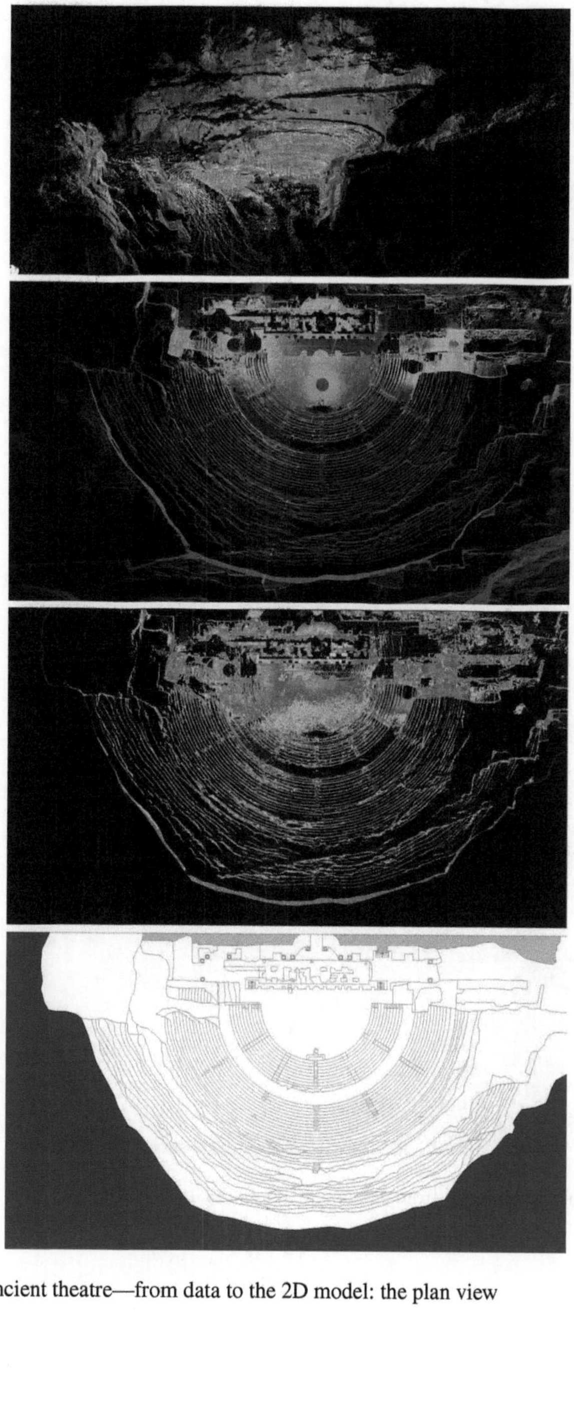

Fig. 21 Petra ancient theatre—from data to the 2D model: the plan view

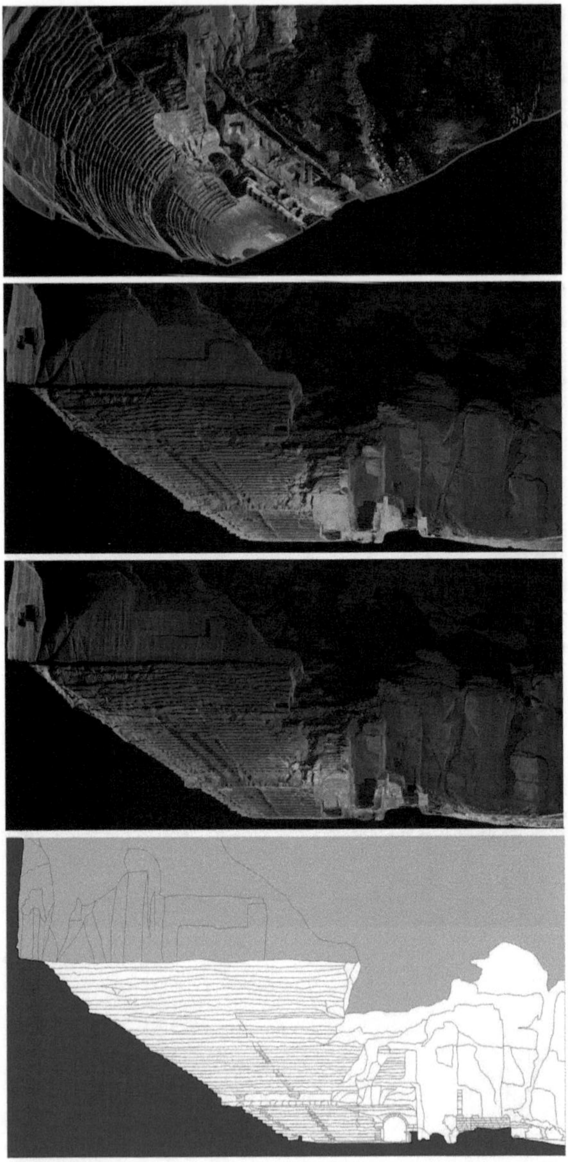

Fig. 22 Petra ancient theatre—from data to the 2D model: cross section

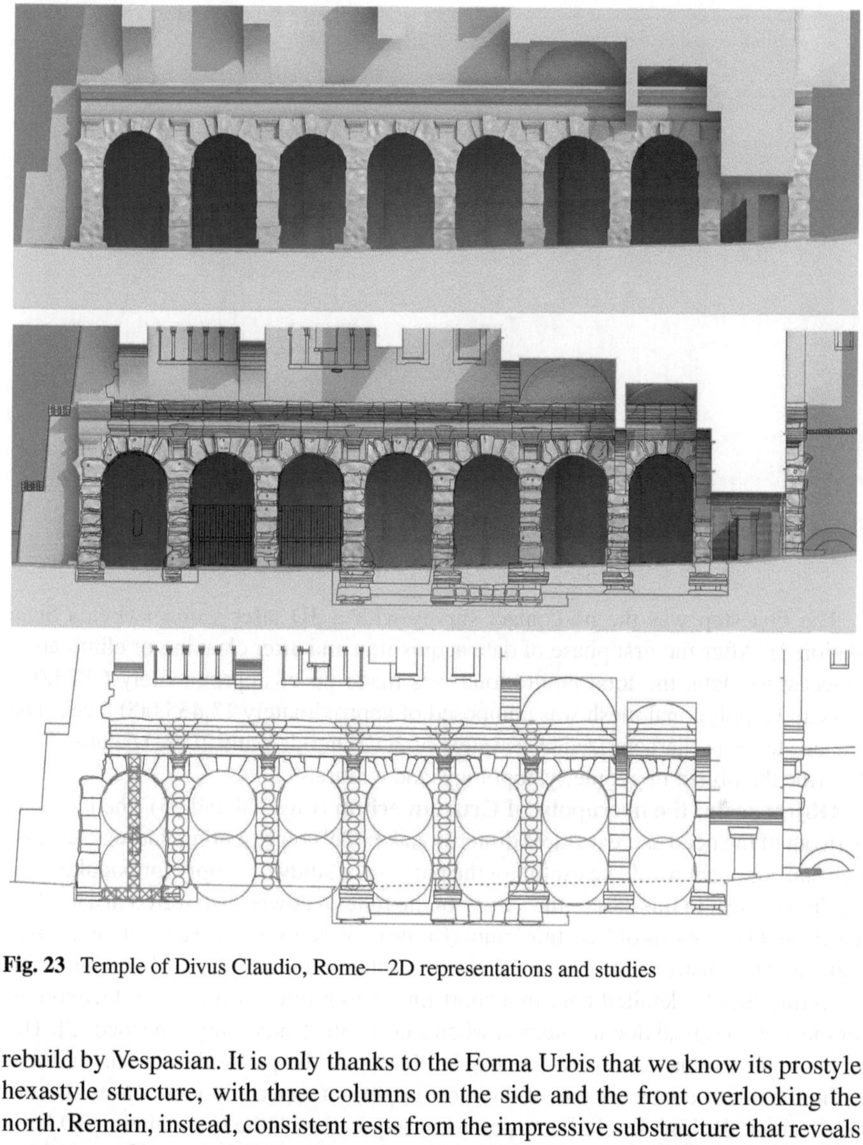

Fig. 23 Temple of Divus Claudio, Rome—2D representations and studies

rebuild by Vespasian. It is only thanks to the Forma Urbis that we know its prostyle hexastyle structure, with three columns on the side and the front overlooking the north. Remain, instead, consistent rests from the impressive substructure that reveals a structure of imposing dimensions of roughly 180 × 200 m, in large part still visible today. The research aimed at identifying procedures and results able to meet the needs and expectations of both research groups (architects and archaeologists). Therefore a system was established capable of managing the information obtained from the survey by different types of knowledge depending on the addressee. Then, analyzing the potential acquired by the detection, it was agreed to proceed with the construction of a facility through a critical survey able to identify the characteristics that define the object.

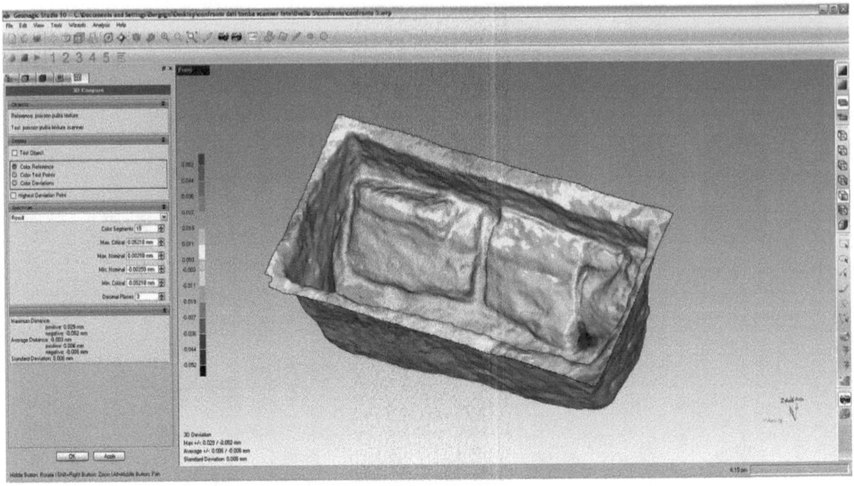

Fig. 24 Crustumerium, Rome—the 3D thematic model

The first step was the no-contact survey with a 3D laser scanner (Leica Scan Station 2). After the first phase of data acquisition and after cleaning or eliminating unnecessary data, the total point cloud was made up of approximately 6,828,000 units and a polygonal mesh was composed of approximately 13,435,000 faces. The second step was characterized by a system of 2D/3Dmodels and 2D/3D details. They describe the object in geometry, topology, and texture.

Object scale: the necropolis of Crustumerium (Figs. 24 and 25) The idea was born out of the need to create three dimensional models representing findings through a virtual copy that would be useful for the purpose of study or simply for popularizing the discoveries. In this case—the survey of the funeral dowry discovered in a tomb at the ancient necropolis of Crustumerium (Rome)—we chose to use a short range laser scanner. This instrument, tried and tested in other experiments, deals mainly with collecting highly detailed data in a short time being thus an important technology for the archeological documentation when a no-contact surveying is needed [2]. The archeological finds are always breakable objects so the possibility to survey them without a direct contact is one of the most important aspects in these cases. Taking into account the high level of data precision acquired with the triangulation 3D laser scanner (Minolta Vivid 9i), $+/-50\,\mu\text{m}$ at the distance of 0.6 m, the result is a virtual 3D reconstruction thanks to which it is possible to discover even the smallest deformations in the surface of the ceramic artifact. It is thus possible to register, for example, tiny fissures, classical stretching of the material, a clear evidence of the technique used in making the artifact, and even to detect the thickness of layer of the decorative pigment.

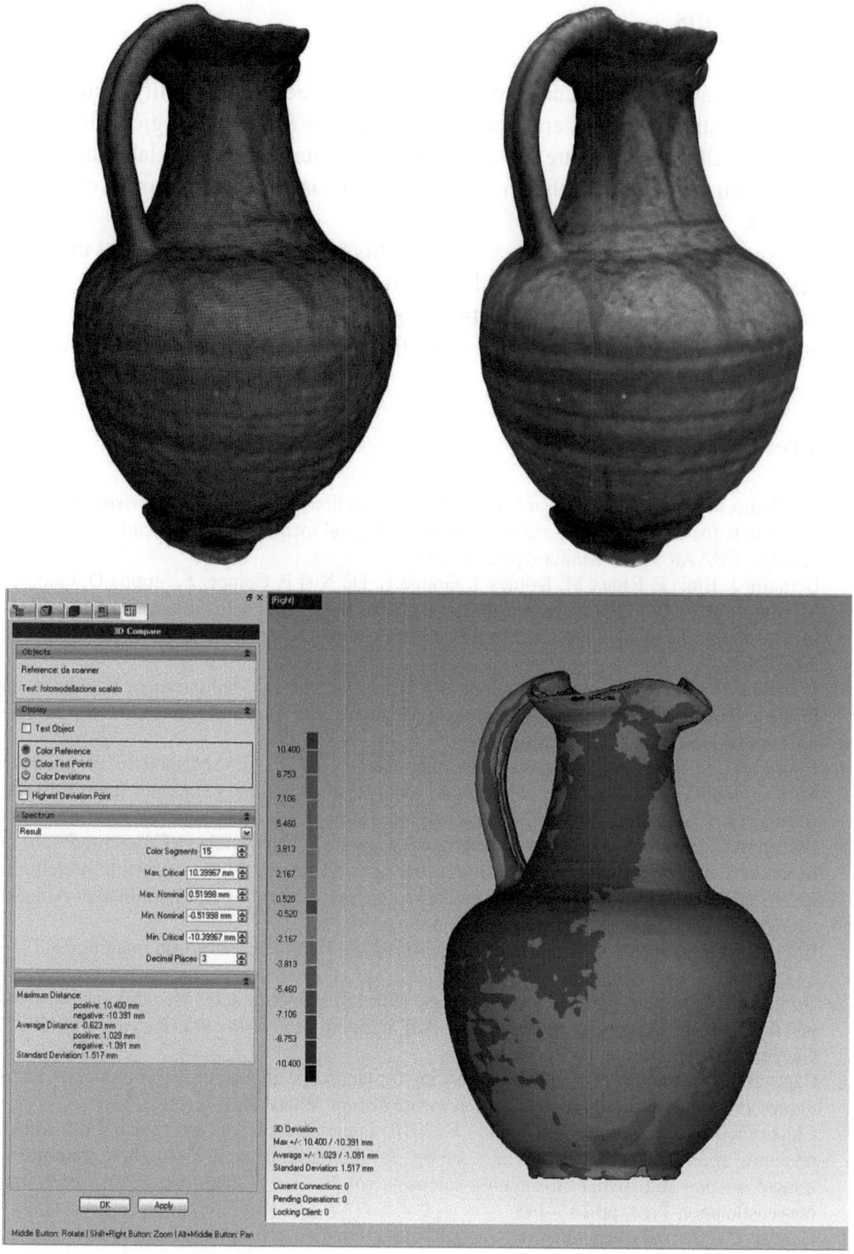

Fig. 25 Crustumerium, Rome—modeling of an artifact

7 Conclusions

Although partial, our experience has clearly enlightened the possibility (and maybe the need) of establishing general operative guidelines for archaeological surveying in order to unify and regulate the procedures of data collection, elaboration and representation that will make the final result scientific in character, i.e. more objective and correct.

The comparison with other experiences in this field, the test of different methodologies on different scale objects will lead to the establishment of flexible *modus operandi* which lends itself to adaptation in specific, concrete cases or to the needs of surveying maintaining, at the same time, the versatile character of the survey.

References

1. Apollonio F, Gaiani M, Baldissini S (2011) Construction, management and visualization of 3D models for cultural heritage GIS systems. In: Digital media and its application in cultural heritage, CSAAR Press, Amman, pp 283–299
2. Beraldin J, Blais F, Rioux M, Domey J, Gonzo L, De Nisi F, Comper F, Stoppa D, Gottardi M, Simoni A (2003) Optimized position sensors for flying-spot active triangulation systems. In: Fourth international conference on 3-D digital imaging and modeling, pp 29–36, 6–10 Oct 2003 Banff,
3. Bianchini C (2012) La Documentazione dei Teatri Antichi del Mediterraneo: le attività del Progetto Athena a Mérida / Documentation of Mediterranean Ancient Theatres: Athena's activities in Mérida. Roma, Gangemi Editore
4. Bianchini C (2012) Rilievo e Metodo Scientifico-Survey and Scientific Method. In: Elogio della Teoria. Identità delle discipline del Disegno e del Rilievo. Atti del Convegno Internazionale (Roma, 13–15 dicembre 2012). Gangemi Editore, Roma, p 391–400
5. Bianchini C, Borgogni F, Ippolito A, Senatore L, Capiato E, Capocefalo C, Cosentino F (2012) From surveying to representation, theoretical background, practical issues, possible guidelines. In: VSMM 2012, 18th international conference on virtual systems and multimedia. Atti del Convegno Internazionale, Milano, pp 507–513
6. Blais F (2004) A review of 20 years of range sensor development. J Electron Imaging 13:231–243
7. Borgogni F, Ippolito A (2011) I modelli 3D nei rilievi di architettura. In: Metodologie integrate per il rilievo, il disegno, la modellazione dell'architettura e della città. Ricerca Prin 2007. Gangemi Editore, Roma, pp 71–78
8. Cantrell B, Michaels W (2010) Digital drawing for landscape architecture: contemporary techniques and tools for digital representation in site design. Wiley, New Jersey, p 320
9. Chiabrando F, Nex F, Piatti D, Rinaudo F (2010) Integration of Tof camera and multi-image matching approach for cultural heritage survey. In: International archives of photogrammetry, remote sensing and spatial information sciences, vol 38, Part 5, commission V symposium. Newcastle upon Tyne, pp 143–148
10. Cundari C (2012). Il rilievo architettonico, Ragioni, Fondamenti, Applicazioni. Aracne, Roma, p 568
11. Dell'Unto N, Wallergård M, Dellepiane M, Lindgren S, Eriksson J, Petersson B, Paardekooper R (2010) An experiment of integrated technologies in digital archaeology: creation of new pipelines to increase the perception of archaeological data. In 38th annual international conference on computer applications and quantitative methods in archeology (CAA 2010) fusion of cultures, pp 1–8, http://vcg.isti.cnr.it/Publications/2010/DWDLEPP10/AnExperimentofIntegratedTechnologiesinDigitalArchaeologyCreation.pdf

12. Docci M, Maestri D, Gaiani M (2011) Scienza del disegno. Città Studi, Torino, p 448
13. Docci M, Bianchini C, Ippolito A (2011) Contributi per una teoria del rilevamento architettonico—papers for a theory of architectural survey.In: Disegnare idee immagini, vol 42. Gangemi Editore, Roma, pp 34–41
14. bib15 El-Hakim S, Gonzo L, Voltolini F, Girardi S, Rizzi A, Remondino F, Whiting E (2007) Detailed 3d modeling of castles. Int J Architect Comput 05(02):199–220. http://www.inf.ethz.ch/personal/whitinge/resources/pubs/IJAC-5-2-El-Hakim.pdf
15. Entwistle J, McCaffrey K, Abrahams P (2009) Three-dimensional (3D) visualisation: the application of terrestrial laser scanning in the investigation of historical Scottish farming townships. J Archaeol Sci 36:860–866
16. Gaiani M, Benedetti B, Apollonio F (2011) Teorie per rappresentare e comunicare i siti archeologici attraverso modelli critici. In: SCIRES-IT SCientific RESearch and Information Technology Ricerca Scientifica e Tecnologie dell'Informazione. CASPUR—CIBER Publishing, vol 1(2), pp 37–70
17. Ippolito A (2007) Dalla nuvola di punti alla superficie. Analisi e problematiche. In: Metodi e tecniche integrate di rilevamento per la costruzione e fruizione di modelli virtuali 3D dell'architettura e della città. Ricerca Cofin 2004, Gangemi Editore, Roma, pp 32–43
18. Molyneaux B (2011) The cultural life of images visual representation in archaeology. Routledge, London, p 296
19. Stanco F, Tanasi D, Gueli A (2012) Computer graphics solutions for dealing with colors in archaeology. In: CGIV 2012, 6th European conference on colour in graphics, imaging, and vision, Amsterdam, pp 97–101
20. Vrubel A, Bellon O, Silva L (2009) A 3D reconstruction pipeline for digital preservation. In: Proceedings of IEEE conference on CVPR, pp 2687–2694. http://www.isprs.org/proceedings/XXXVIII/part5/papers/100.pdf

Architectural Heritage and 3D Models

Mario Centofanti, Stefano Brusaporci and Vittorio Lucchese

Abstract Architecture represents the physical space built by man—in its immanent and tangible presence—and a spatial and temporal event. The architectural 3D digital model is the mediator between intellect and tangible reality, and it takes the form of a digital replica of the observable phenomenal reality. Thereby the model expresses—i.e. contains—the history and it's passage through time; a *visual narration* that is part of the historical process and critical analysis. It's an interpretable *document*, but also a genuine critical-historical text, expressed with the figurative language of the virtual dimension. Presupposition of this methodology for historical analysis, it's a careful architectural surveying, a wise modeling project and an intelligent and critical use of the digital model.

Keywords Architecture · 3D digital models representation

1 Introduction

Information and modelling digital technologies have produced profound changes in architectural surveying and representation, accordingly to the use of 3D models.

If in the past the outcome of an architectonical representation was made by two dimensional drawings, nowadays they are integrated by 3D models.

M. Centofanti · S. Brusaporci (✉) · V. Lucchese
DICEAA, Department of Engineering Faculty, University of L'Aquila, via G. Gronchi 18, 67100 L'Aquila (AQ), Italy
e-mail: stefano.brusaporci@univaq.it

M. Centofanti
e-mail: mario.centofanti@univaq.it

V. Lucchese
e-mail: vittoriolucchese@gmail.com

P. Di Giamberardino et al. (eds.), *Computational Modeling of Objects Presented in Images*, Lecture Notes in Computational Vision and Biomechanics 15,
DOI: 10.1007/978-3-319-04039-4_2,

Architectonical heritage's 3D modelling is conceptually related to knowledge: it's required the values understanding and their appropriate documentation and representation. Digital models are architectural medium, in this way meta-models that describe the buildings, namely a complex system made by spaces, surfaces, materials, constructive technologies and degradation, with modification and stratification processes witnesses of events and cultures that have occurred over time. Therefore this kind of models are the antithesis of that digital non-places offered by video games' platforms, because they have to be representative of architectural individuals, with own characteristics, result of historical defined events, belonging to a precise context.

The chapter is divided into four sections: the second one is about the nature of the model for the historical architecture (Mario Centofanti); the third one illustrates an analysis' method, developed in the Italian experience, based on the use of interpretative models (Stefano Brusaporci); the fourth one is about a specific case study (Vittorio Lucchese).[1]

2 The Role of the 3D Model in the Cognitive/Planning Process of Historical Architecture

The final product of an architectural survey is the representative model.

The meaning and essence of the changes in architectural models, in the transition from traditional surveying to surveying using 3D optical measuring techniques, above all with reference to the reciprocal interactions between subject, phenomenal reality and model, have all been amply explored.

Models can be generated by CAD software using manual modelling, or directly generated by automatic scanning, be static or dynamic, be manipulable and interactive, and demand the creation of suitable standards.

The model, in its role as mediator between the intellect and tangible reality, is the tool people use to organize their mental representations of perceptible, phenomenal reality. In the contemporary period this takes the form of a *digital replica*, with its own autonomy, and a level of verisimilitude and immersive potential that raises doubts over its being an integral substitute for reality within the cognitive process. Yet it is not possible to overcome the *otherness* between the model and the phenomenal manifestation of the real object; in a hermeneutic key, in the sense of an *isomorphic* relationship, intended not as identity but analogy [64, p. 491].

The model, in its role as a medium between the subject and the phenomenon, represents by its very nature a modification of the latter. This mutation is connected to the transit through the human mind and the patterns that significantly involve the subjective perception of the observer, and also to the reduction of the object/phenomenon represented to an entity which is in any case discretized, irrespective of the pro-

[1] The models of modern buildings presented in the paper are made by Stefano Brusaporci and Vittorio Lucchese.

grammed precision and definition. From a perceptive point of view, about the digital reproduction of the architectural reality, we recall the concepts expressed by Walter Benjamin in his classic "*The Work of Art in the Age of Mechanical Reproduction*" (1936):

> the architecture as prototype of a work's collective use through a distracted perception, that is fragmented, jerky; the substitution of the cultural value with the expositive value.

The study of architectural history focuses on the physical space constructed by man, its immanent, tangible presence and its dimension as event, as spatial and temporal happening.

The cognitive act is the experiential act. But it is the lived experience of the event as a sequence of spatial/temporal events, up to the event in the present that sums up all the previous ones. The model thus expresses — in the sense that it contains — the history and the passage of time of the situation explored from its conception, to its creation, to its transformations, up to the current period: historic/synchronic and diachronic sections, reconstructions and/or visualizations of modified situations, or intentions and prefigurations never actually implemented, or simply narrated.

If we refer to Paul Ricoeur's reflections on the narrative dimension of architecture and the temporal dimension of architectural space [58], we can reconsider the model itself as a *visual account* of an architectural narration.

The structured, complex model, as explained thus far, figures in the process of historical/critical analysis as a 'document' therefore itself open to interpretation, but also a genuine *historical/critical text* expressed with the language of figuration in the virtual dimension.[2]

The premise of a restoration project is the necessary relationship with something pre-existing. Surveys and models therefore play a strategic role as a cognitive act—Brandi's notion of recognition—and as a fundamental instrumental support, with regards to the *specular* relationship we expect between a descriptive/interpretative model and a planning model.

From the theoretical/methodological point of view we can draw parallels with the procedure of Reverse Modelling, in which a digital survey of surfaces and the construction of the relative digital model using polygonal or polynomial modelling represent a starting point for designing industrial products [44].

The specific nature of the architectural model however demands that we go beyond what is visible, exploring the intimate make-up of an architectural organism, namely its structural elements. The concept of duality that Brandi [9, p. 10] expressed with regards to works of art:

> matter as the revelation of the image manifests the bipolar rapport between matter as appearance and matter as structure

also applies to historic architecture, where the matter/structure itself forms the architectural space. In this regard mention has been made of the notion of an *anatom-*

---

[2] " [...] a serious graphic apparatus is first and foremost a record and at the same time a genuine historical/critical 'text', not expressed in the usual verbal language, but in the language of figuration." [18, p. 472]. Also see [17, 19, 40].

ical survey, which implies the creation of a descriptive model including structural components and elements [23–25]. The latter must be explored and identified by means of the usual operations of documental analysis and non-destructive diagnosis as a precautionary measure, and then by monitoring while work in is progress.

Models of this kind integrate our interpretation of geometrical and dimensional data and formal, figurative, architectural and spatial values, providing an analysis of the material and structural characteristics. To quote Vitruvius, this kind of model provides the correct premise for restoration projects that should succeed in combining the necessary *firmitas*, or solidity (reducing seismic vulnerability) with *venustas*, beauty (spatial and figurative restoration), and *utilitas*, usefulness—in terms of restoring function or repurposing. In the process of *critical restoration* the model fulfils various tasks when it comes to monitoring work in progress and any modifications to ongoing work; in terms of comparing the transformations wrought by the restoration work to the previous state of the building, and in the ongoing monitoring of the building after the restoration work for the purposes of planned maintenance.

3 From the "Graphical Analysis" to 3D Models for Architectural Analysis: The Italian Experience

In 1989 Mario Docci published a paper titled "*Disegno e rilievo: quale didattica?*" [Drawing and surveying: what didactics?], in the first issue of the journal "*Disegnare Idee Immagini—Drawing Ideas Images*"[3] [31], concerning a methodology for architecture analyzing, tested by the author and his staff in the Course of Design and Surveying held at the Faculty of Architecture of the University of Rome "La Sapienza" from the academic year 1975–1976. The chapter recalls what he has already published in 1983 in the book "*Disegno e analisi architettonica*" [Drawing and architectural analysis] [33].

Aim of the chapter is presenting how drawing, in addition to be suitable for project communication, can be an instrument to study building's characteristics. Referring to the structuralism lesson, drawing is regarded as a meta-language, that is a graphical language able to analyze another language, the architecture's one.[4]

Although in the didactic field, it's developed a research method for critical analysis, believing that going thought the projects of great masters—modern and of the past—with drawing is a useful way to understand the architectural values.

[3] The journal "Disegnare Idee Immagini—Drawing Ideas Images" is edited by the Department of Representation and Surveying (now Department of History Drawing and Restoration of Architecture) of Rome University "Sapienza", published in Rome by Gangemi, indexed by Thomson Institute for Scientific Information (AHCI Arts and Humanities Citation Index) ISSN 1123-9247. Over the years the journal has been a constant reference for those who studies architectural analysis and representation, publishing many of the most relevant Italian assays. Except for the cited paper published in 1989, all the others issues that will be quoted from this journal are in full English text; in references there are the original Italian titles.

[4] In general for a semiology approach to architecture:[8, 34].

In particular Docci quotes the expression "graphical analysis" from the book "*Analisi grafica dei valori architettonici*" [Graphical analysis of architectonical values] of the mid-fifties (then 1960) by Vincenzo Fasolo, professor of History and Styles of Architecture since 1925; he also widely uses the instrument of drawing for reading, analyzing and comparing historic buildings in his essay "*Guida metodica per lo studio della storia dell'architettura*" [Methodological guidebook for studying the history of architecture] [36].

In the graphical analysis Docci identifies a methodology based on rigorous criteria, that allows to study proportions, volumes, forms, configurations and structures, and the relationship between all the elements that contribute to the conformation of the architectural language. In particular Docci focuses on the usefulness of schematizations, seen as a real interpretative models of architectural language [31, pp. 38–39]:

> The graphic medium is used to create models for architecture, or urban space, understanding, to get a sense and analyse it as a scientist artificially reproduces a phenomenon in his laboratory. In this way drawing identifies with the model's concept, or better with a knowledge's graphical model. In this regard it should be noted that a model is really a model when it is composed of set of elements linked together by the same rules which govern the elements constituting the space, described by the model; therefore it couldn't represent the building as it appears, but it establishes an analogy to point out the laws that regulate the organization of the work. Then it's a process of reduction of the complex architectural reality, to exalt the significant characteristics, highlighting them in a schema.

On an operational level we have to do different analysis, but aware that they represent specific thematizations, and there should be a final re-composition of the results. In particular Docci suggests to conduct distributive, formal, spatial and structural analysis, of the relation between the building and its context, associated to synchronically and diachronically studies between it and others of the same architect and of other authors.

By surveying and representation digital technologies' developing, there have been many applications related to historic buildings, especially aimed at its communication, enhancement, enjoyment and management. The debate on the relationship between new technologies and representation of architecture was, and still it is, wide-ranging [63, 65–67].

If at the beginning the studies involved on unavoidable problems of computer graphics—we remember the example of the model of the abbey of Cluny, made by IBM France in 1992—, through the years the technological progress of 3D modeling and rendering, especially real time rendering, has favored the development of virtual reality, in particular of virtual heritage that combines Information and Communication Technologies with the field of architectural heritage; moreover the technologies of augmented reality contribute to implement immersive, dynamic and interactive experiences [45]. Virtual reality allows the interacting simulation and real-time processing of all the information that is contained in the model; this aspect promotes the development and diffusion of virtual museums [59].

At the same time the graphical analysis methodology has found a way of developing in 3D modeling technologies, producing a field of study where the digital model acquires the function of "meta-model", that is an instrument for architecture's critical[5]—and in particular historical-critical—analysis. Compared to traditional graphical analysis, made by two-dimensional drawing such as plants, elevations, sections, perspective and axonometric projections, 3D models allow a continuous multi-dimensional and multi-level interpretations, favoring visualizations and synthetically simulations.

Modelling and semantics problems—not more and not just issues of computer graphics—are related to the architectonic ones, so the digital model's characteristics are inseparably linked to the ones of architecture (for example if it's a ruin of classical age, a renaissance palace, a baroque church, a modern building) and to the ones of the specific and individual building under study. From this point of view the process of model's construction is particularly important, as critical synthesis and integration of architectural survey and analysis of historical documents; of particular importance it is the study of the transformation phases, of the relationships with the context, of the constructive elements. Moreover such models can be used as core aggregator and organizer of documental information, that is as framework for architectural information systems [10].

In the Italian experience numerous researches can be attribute to the area of 3D modelling for architectural analysis. According to a first classification, it's possible to distinguish between studies on historical architectures and studies on modern buildings, for which especially may be available original project; these graphical documents require a careful study, both from an historical point of view than in relation to the building.

A second classification can be made between studies on existing buildings and not more existing ones (or profoundly transformed). In the second case it is required the virtual reconstruction of missing conformations, philologically reconstructed. To this field can be attributed many of the experiences on surveying and virtual reconstruction of archaeological sites; among all we remember the researches coordinated by Francesca Fatta on the archaeological sites in Northern Africa and in Southern Italy: models are built referring to a systematic study of archaeological maps, essays on architectural and archaeological history, drawings made for excavations since the eighteenth century, artefacts in museums [37].

On 3D models for historical critical analysis, it's significant the experience coordinated by Mario Docci regarding the digital reconstruction of the Sangallo's project for the St. Peter's Basilica, based on the drawings made for Pope Paul III in 1537–1538 and on the reverse modeling of the original wooden model in 1:30 scale. Known are the criticisms advanced by Michelangelo about low lighting, excessive decorations and too many orders of columns; on the whole, he said that the project wasn't conforming to classical language. The digital model allows us to verify the values of the Sangallo's project, to study the shape of the dome, to increase proportional analysis and, last but not least, to understand the author's concept [7, 32].

[5] The "historical-critical method" refers to a set of criteria for the historical and philological study of the architectural heritage; the building it's intended as a synthesis of modification and transformation that conduced it to the current configuration, results of architectural cultures and interventions that have taken place over time [15].

Not different experience it's the one proposed by Marco Carpiceci, who presents the 3D digital reconstruction of architectures drawn by Leonardo da Vinci, considered emblematic of his thought. The study was conducted according to a philological and hermeneutic point of view, which aims to reveal Leonardo's ideas [21].

The research unit guided by Marco Gaiani presents an hypothesis of attribution to Palladio of a drawing regarding Villa Contarini a Piazzola sul Brenta (secc. XVI–XVII–XIX). Being available limited drawings, the study develops issues of model's semantization in order to built the whole model of the planned building [2].

In the chapter on the Palazzo Mattei di Giove in Rome (XVI–XVII), Livio Sacchi uses the digital model to study geometrical, proportional and constructive building's rules [61].

Mario Centofanti applies the method of 3D modeling to the study of architectural heritage, using the analysis and views made by the digital model to explore the architectural characteristics of the building of Margaret of Austria in L'Aquila (XVI–XIX centuries) [25].

On the virtual reconstruction of no more existing configurations of historical buildings, we cite the work of Stefano Brusaporci about the churches of St. Justin and St. Paul near L'Aquila (XIII–XVIII–XX centuries), churches that in 1946 have been subjected to restorations. In particular the first one was reconfigured it in a medieval way. Brusaporci virtually re-built the church as it was before according to architectural survey and archival data; the historical photographic documentation of 1946 made it possible—through techniques of digital photogrammetry, used in analogy to what happens in forensics and accident fields—to define the architectural elements now missing ([14]), (Figs. 1 and 2).

Important contributions are related to the modern architecture. The publication of 2001 titled *Architettura Disegno Modello* [Architecture Drawing Model], editors Piero Albisinni and Laura De Carlo, proposes an experience based on the use of 3D models for the graphical analysis of the works of Giovanni Michelucci, Maurizio Sacripanti and Leonardo Savioli. The study, that starts from original drawings, favours the analysis of these authors and of their works in relation to their historical context. 3D models, sectioned and/or exploded, with the analysis of selected components, promote critical representations [1].

Livio Sacchi, aiming to a close examination of the theories underlying compositional choices, presents the virtual reconstruction of some unrealized buildings—the buildings represented in Studi per la Città Nuova by Antonio Sant'Elia (1913–1914) and the Danteum by Giuseppe Terragni (1938)—as well as of a series of architectures built in the modern age, in particular the ones of the EUR district (1935–1936) in Rome [66].

Among the studies on the use of models guided by Riccardo Migliari, we remember those who have, as case studies, the Maison Citrohan of Le Corbusier and the Danteum of Giuseppe Terragni. In particular, with regard to the second one we observe the particular attention placed in setting the project, not realized, in the historical context of the city of Rome [52].

The theme of modern movement studying through digital modelling, in order to investigate and experience buildings no longer existing, it's presented by Francesco

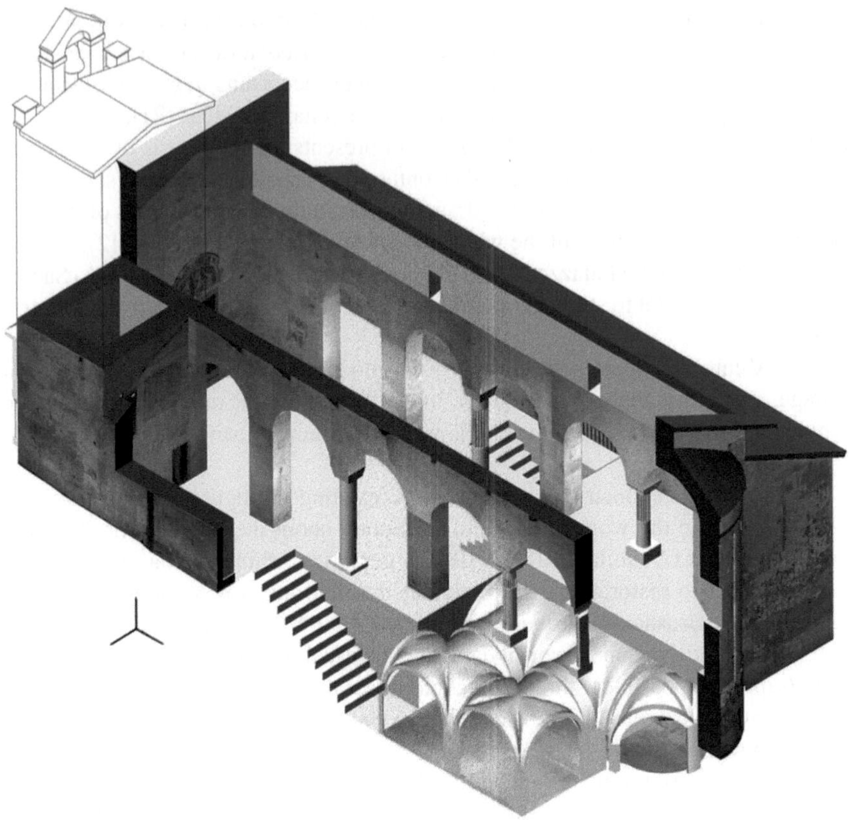

Fig. 1 Digital model of S. Justin's church. It allows to represent building's architectural characteristics

Maggio and Marcella Villa with the digital reconstruction of houses realized for the V Triennale of Milan in 1933, and then demolished [47]. Francesco Maggio also deals with the study of two existing buildings in Agrigento: the Balilla's House by Enrico del Debbio (1929) and the Post Office building by Angiolo Mazzoni (1931–1939) [46].

And similarly Stefano Brusaporci uses 3D models in his essay on modern Italian architecture [14] (Figs. 3, 4, 5, 6 and 7).

Rodolfo Maria Strollo, in a study on the complex of the observatory of Tusculum (1939), not only presents the surveying model, but uses models—derived from original drawings—to compare different planning solutions, in order to analyze for each one the figurative and material values, and at the same time to reconstruct the events that led to the final design configuration [63].

The condition of the digital model to be freely represented, interrogated and browsed, in time and space, according to broader media, semiotic and epistemological schemes, compared to traditional 2D drawings, favours the study and the

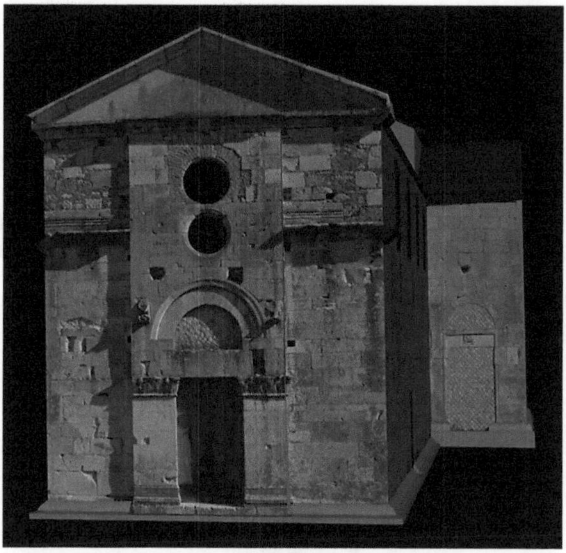

Fig. 2 3D photorealistic model of the church of S. Paul near L'Aquila (XIII–XVIII–XX centuries)

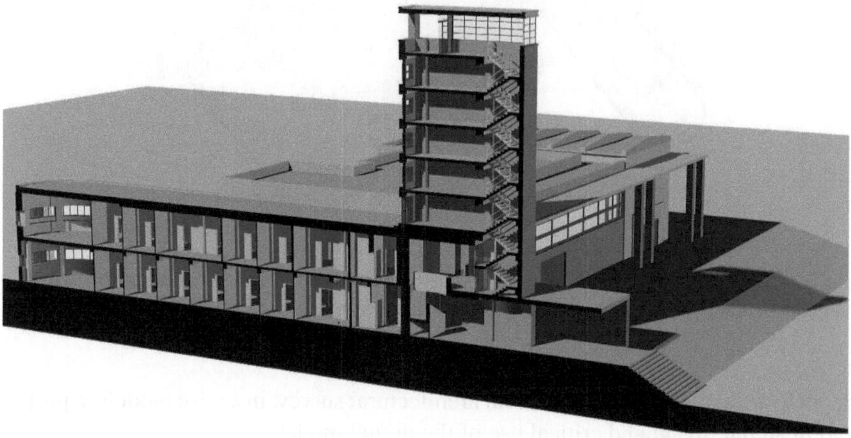

Fig. 3 Casa del Balilla in Ascoli Piceno (1933–1934). Rendering with the perspective section of the tower and office block

communication of architectonical heritage's values and characteristics. With a risk of aestheticization own sake [48]—a "*Dionysian tension*" of "*absolute appear*" in the words of Purini [56, p. 95])—but with new and relevant scientific virtue.

Obviously the case studies cited are not exhaustive; they want to represent the contents of a line of research that can benefit greatly from the development of information technology but which has the presupposition of its methodological application in a

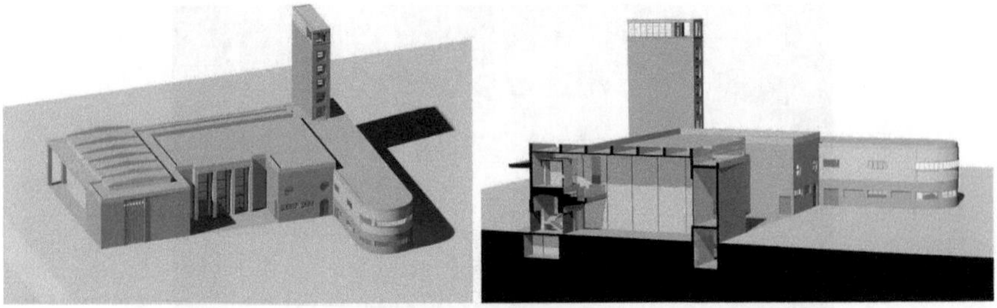

Fig. 4 Casa del Balilla in Ascoli Piceno Isometric rendering and perspective section of the cinema. You can see the office block with a tower, the hall of the gym, cinema

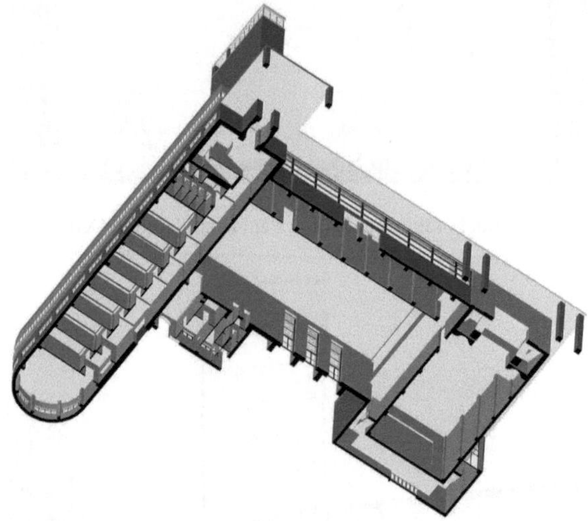

Fig. 5 Casa del Balilla in Ascoli Piceno. Render isometric split from the bottom. Although internally the buildings are connected, each has its own entrance on different elevations

depth historical analysis, in a careful architectural survey, in a wise modeling project and in an intelligent and critical use of the digital model.

4 Case Study: The "Cinema Massimo" in L'Aquila

The "Cinema Massimo" in L'Aquila, commissioned by the *Istituto Nazionale Fascista Assicurazione contro gli Infortuni sul Lavoro*, was planned by the roman architect Luigi Ciarlini between 1940 and 1941 and built between 1943 and 1947 [14]. The project is part of the renovation of the historical cities and belongs to that process of *social buildings* development, promoted by the Fascist government. In this period were built many constructions for directional activities and social services

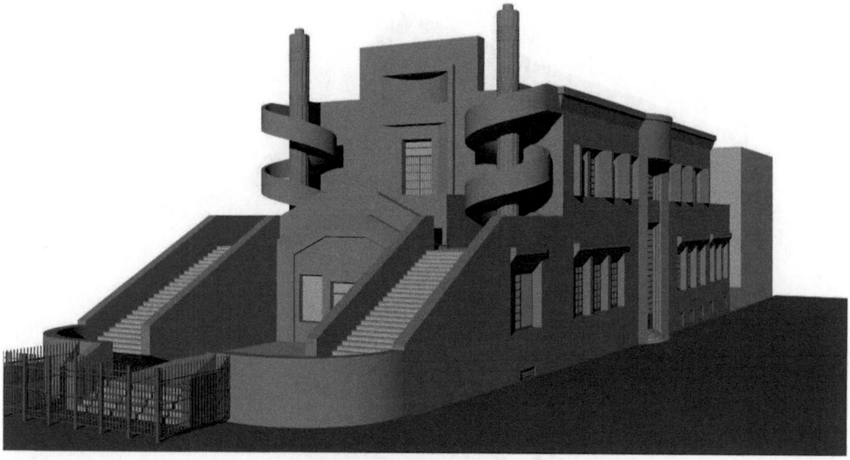

Fig. 6 Opera Nazionale Dopolavoro in Chieti (1933–1934). Rendering of the principal front, characterized by two helical stairs to reach the roof garden

such as schools, hospitals, government agencies offices, *case del Fascio*, buildings for workers' club, etc. There are "new" building typologies and among them a particular importance was given to the cinema for cultural purposes and propaganda. The renovation of L'Aquila historical city had already begun in the second half of the nineteenth century [22], focusing on the widening of Corso Federico II, the main axis of the urban plan, with the purpose, never fully completed, to build continuous porticos along the main street's sides.

The typological-distributive system of the Cinema Massimo follows from the requirements of context insertion, with the integration of the external space of the portico with the building project (Fig. 8). From the porticos, characterized by columns with entasis, you can enter in the foyer which is placed beside to the hall and interior service spaces. On the other side, the hall overlooks directly the outside through safety exits. From a constructive and formal point of view, the building is fully into the architectural and historical context of the '30s and '40s in Italy, when it began the structures building with reinforced concrete, but without the figurative value present in the European avant-garde. In fact, the Italian architecture keeps a close relationship with the formal solutions previous to the introduction of frame-systems with the presence of walls, no-loadbearing function, and of composite structures. Besides for the period are important: the search for a modern monumental style by the using of classical language without decorative elements, the admixture of elements in an eclectic style and the search on finishing materials, conditioned by the needs of autarchy. In fact in the final period of the fascist regime, the Italian state was isolated in the international context.

From a methodological point of view, the building study was deal with the elaboration of the 3D model, starting with the integrated survey (direct and photogrammetric), the analysis of the old documentation related to the project

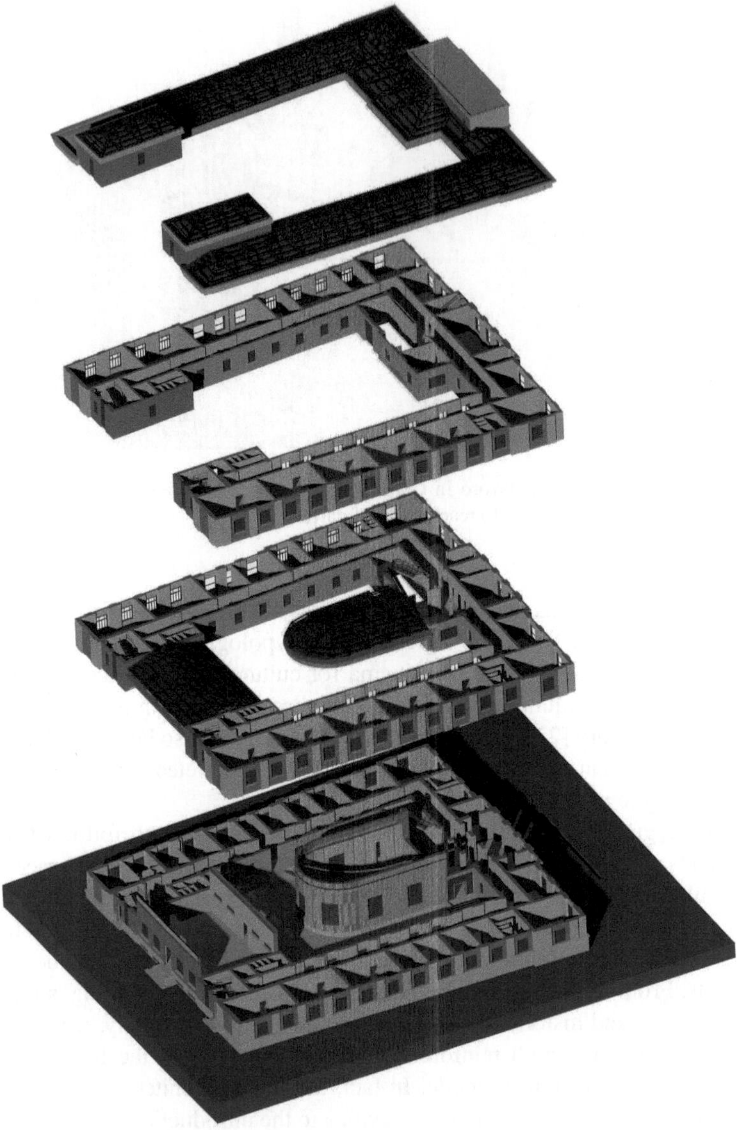

Fig. 7 School in Teramo. Isometric render split from the bottom. In correspondence with the entrance there is the Aula Magna in the courtyard; in front there is the gym that can communicate with the court or directly to the backside

(Fig. 4), a survey made in 1963 and a survey made in 2005 (Rolli G, Rilievo e Restauro dell'edificio Cinema Massimo all'Aquila. Dissertation, Università dell'Aquila, Facoltà di Ingegneria, Corso di Laurea in Ingegneria Edile-Architettura, a.a. 2004–2005, supervisor Prof. Mario Centofanti). In order to study the modern architecture,

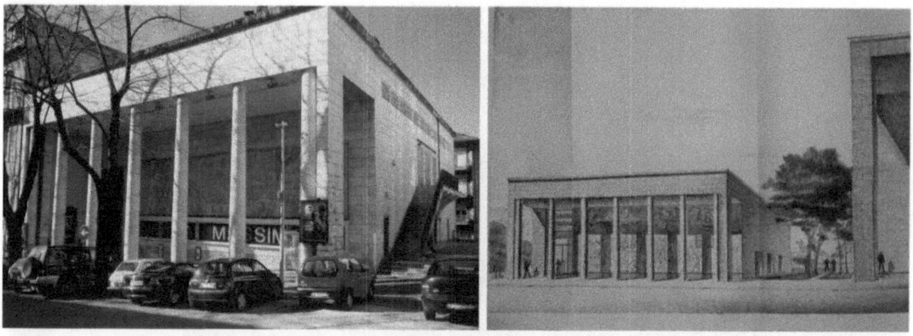

Fig. 8 Cinema Massimo in L'Aquila. The principal front in an actual photo and in a project's perspective drawing

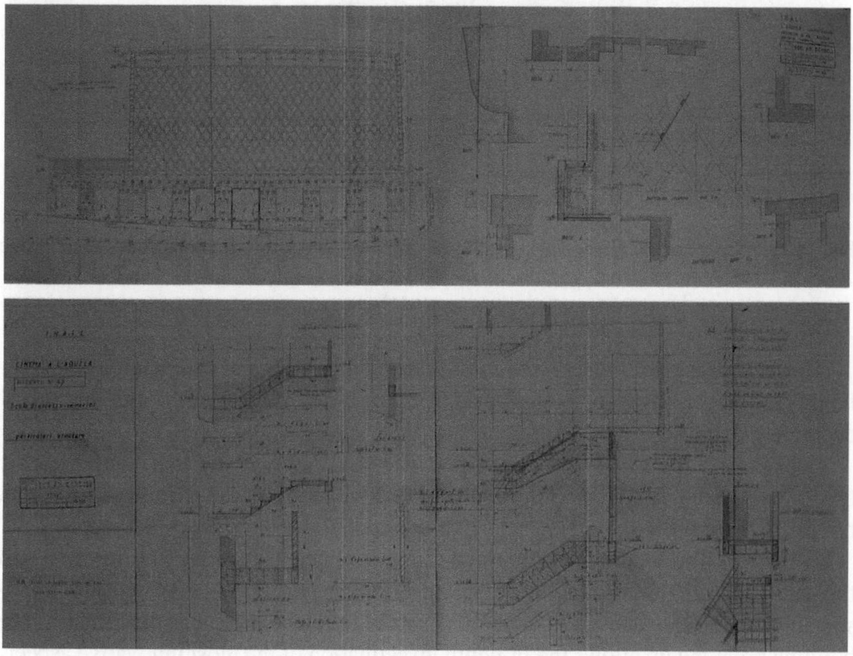

Fig. 9 Original project drawings of Cinema Massimo in L'Aquila: Carpentry and executive façade with constructive details

the analysis of project's drawings is a useful tool, also to understand construction elements not visible and not directly detectable. The available drawings about the Cinema Massimo are placed in the Historical Archive INAIL in Rome, binder "I.N.A.I.L. L'Aquila—Cinematografo"; there are plans, elevations, sections, perspective views, carpentry with details and structural calculations, some construction details until to the scale1:2 (Fig. 9).

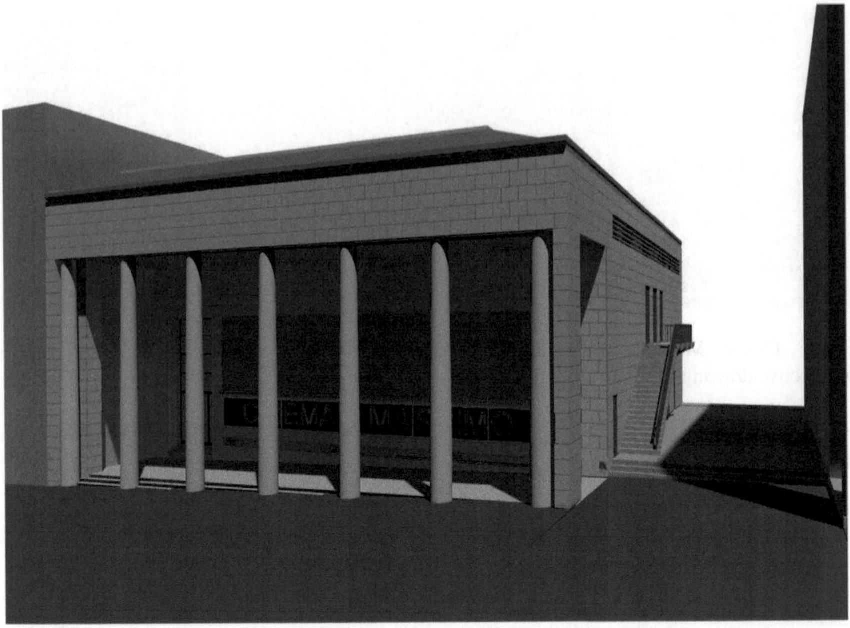

Fig. 10 3D Model of the Cinema Massimo in L'Aquila. Rendering with perspective view of the principal front.

The tridimensional model was realized with modalities and characterizations differentiated in various restitution scales, from the urban context to the architecture or decorative details.

Considering the importance of the restrictions imposed by the context to the typological planning, the model was integrated with volumetric sketches of the next buildings, in order to understand the existent spatial relations (Figs. 10 and 11).

In the building model are combined the spatial and volumetric information and the study and the representation of the constructive system. In particular, the representation ways were chosen to better understand relations between constituents. The building breaking up allows the in-depth investigation of the most innovative aspects of typological and distributive features (Figs. 12 and 13).

E.g., the perspective cross section in Fig. 12 shows the typological element that characterize the distribution system of Cinema Massimo, that is the foyer, placed beside the hall, that provides a distribution on the whole length of the hall itself, but on a single side. This distributive articulation is realized with elevations variability, which ends in helical stairs to enter in the rooms placed in the upper level, behind the hall. Skylights provide to light the foyer through curvilinear false ceiling that follows the elevations variation. Figure 13 shows the hall, that is organized in two levels, with stalls area and upper gallery, both with lateral access, covered by a false ceiling. The stage has a little space behind the screen that allows to use the hall as an auditorium or conference hall.

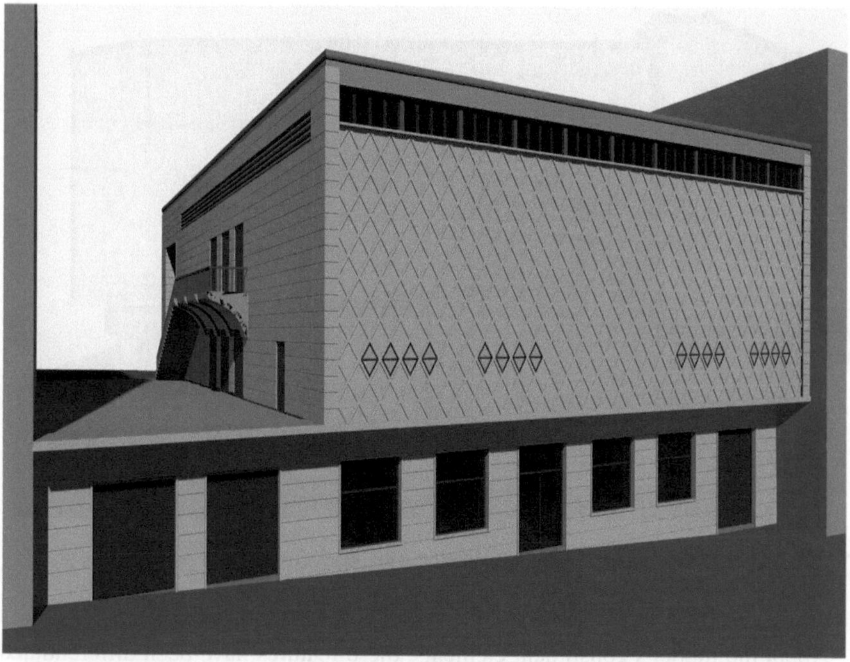

Fig. 11 Cinema Massimo in L'Aquila. Rendering with perspective view of the back front

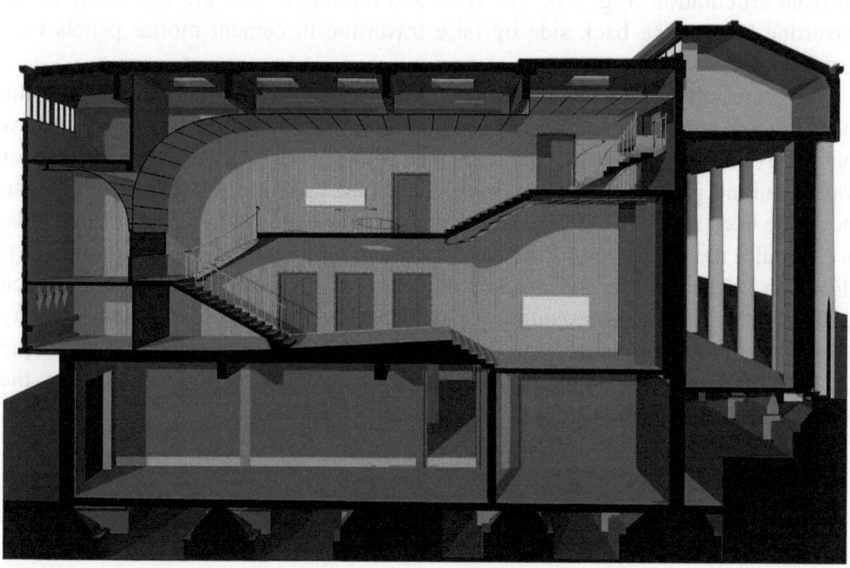

Fig. 12 Cinema Massimo in L'Aquila. Rendering with perspective section of the foyer

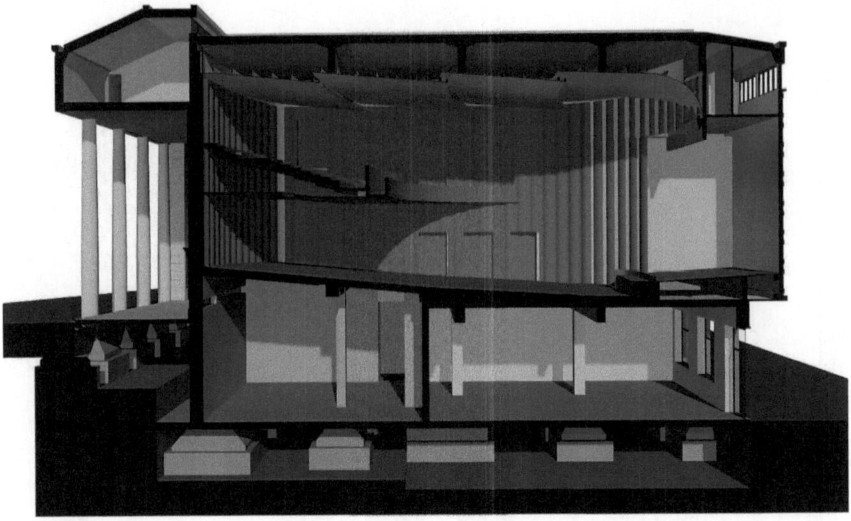

Fig. 13 Cinema Massimo in L'Aquila. Rendering with perspective section of the hall

About the model's constituent elements, these features have been differentiated according to the foundations, the reinforced concrete loadbearing frame, the floors recognizing the brick and concrete elements, the partition walls, the skylights, the false ceilings of the foyer and the hall, the fixtures, the floors, the plaster, the inner lining of the hall walls and others finishing elements, with particular highlighting on front articulation (Fig. 14). The front and the lateral side are characterized by travertine blocks, the back side by false travertine in cement mortar panels with lozenges.

The representation through components allows a suitable comprehension of the most original technological and finishing solutions, also linked to the use of new materials of the period, such as linoleum in the gallery floor, wavy plaster in the foyer walls, Murano glasses etc. These decorative elements characterize the building, so they have been in-depth studied, reducing the scale, using suitable survey methods. In particular the restitution of the bas-relief with a representation of L'Aquila city, placed on the front under the arcades, above the "Cinema Massimo" sign, has been realized with digital photogrammetry techniques, building textured meshes, starting with a point cloud and inserted in the general building model. The same technique has been experimented on the backside front of the building, characterized by the particular solution of the lozenges made of false travertine.

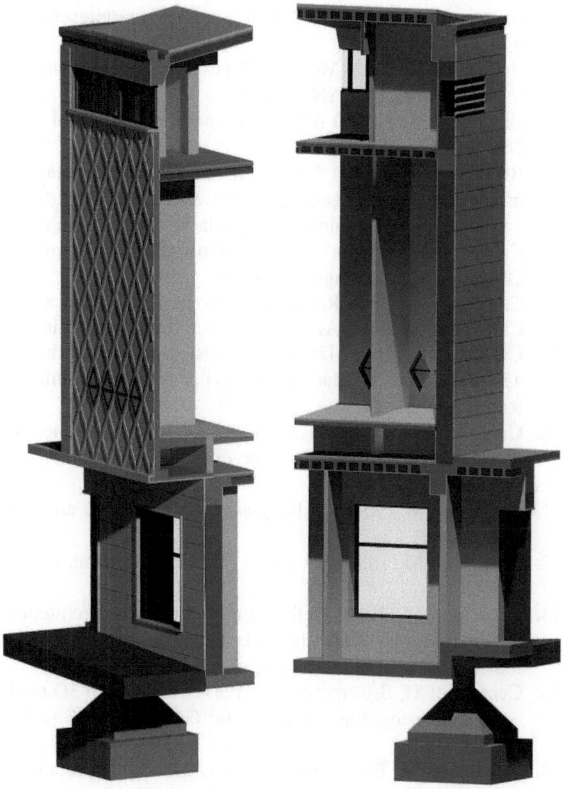

Fig. 14 Cinema Massimo in L'Aquila. Isometric render with detail's representation of the constructive system

References

1. De Albisinni P, Carlo L (eds) (2001) Architettura disegno modello. Gangemi, Roma
2. Apollonio FI et al (2011) Villa Contarini a Piazzola sul Brenta: studi per un'ipotesi di attribuzione palladiana servendosi di modelli tridimensionali. Disegnare Idee Immagini 42:2–55
3. Baculo A (ed) (2000) Architettura e informatica. Electa Napoli, Napoli
4. Benjamin W (1955) Das Kunstwerk im Zeitalter seiner techniscen Reproduzierbarkeit. Suhrkamp, Frankfurt am Main
5. Bettetini G (1991) La simulazione visiva. Bompiani, Milano
6. Bianchini C (2007) Dal reale al virtuale (e ritorno): il modello ligneo di Antonio da Sangallo per il nuovo San Pietro in Vaticano. Disegnare Idee Immagini 34:36–49
7. Bianchini C (2011) Modelli discreti e modelli continui nel rilievo e rappresentazione informatizzata dell'architettura. Disegnare Idee Immagini 22:51–60
8. Brandi C (1967) Struttura e architettura. Einaudi, Torino
9. Brandi C (1977) [1963]) Teoria del restauro. Einaudi, Torino
10. Brusaporci S (ed) (2010a) Sistemi informativi integrati per la tutela la conservazione e la valorizzazione del patrimonio architettonico e urbano. Gangemi, Roma
11. Brusaporci S (2010b) Sperimentazione di modelli tridimensionali nello studio dell'architettura storica. In: Brusaporci S (ed) Sistemi Informativi Integrati per la tutela la conservazione e la valorizzazione del patrimonio architettonico e urbano. Roma, Gangemi, pp 58–64

12. Brusaporci S (2011a) Modelli digitali per la rappresentazione dell'architettura. DisegnareCon 8:107–115
13. Brusaporci S (2012) Modelli 3D per il progetto di restauro. In: Papa ML (ed) Il disegno delle trasformazioni. CLEAN, Napoli
14. Brusaporci S (2010b) Architetture per il sociale negli anni Trenta e Quaranta del Novecento. Gangemi, Roma
15. Brusaporci A (1983) Metodi di ricerca storico-critica sull' architettura. Aggiornamenti e prospettive. In: Proceedings of the XXI Congresso di Storia dell' Architettura, Roma, 12–14 October 1983. Centro Studi per la Storia dell' Architettura, Roma, pp 23–42
16. Cannella M (2011) La Cappella Palatina di Palermo: misura, interpretazione, rappresentazione. Disegnare Idee Immagini 43:56–69
17. Carbonara G (1990) Restauro dei monumenti. Guida agli elaborati grafici, Liguori
18. Carbonara G (1997) Avvicinamento al restauro, Teoria, Storia. Monumenti, Liguori
19. Carbonara G, Fiorani D (2000) Analisi, descrizione e interpretazione storico-critica nel disegno a fini di restauro.In: Martone M (ed) La normazione nella rappresentazione dell'edilizia. Kappa, Roma, pp 39–49
20. Carnevali L, Cundari C (2012) Modello materiale e modello digitale a supporto della didattica della rappresentazione. Graphic expression applied to building, vol 2. Editorial Marfil S.A, Alicante, pp 481–487
21. Carpiceci M (2010) Filologia/ermeneutica dell'architettura leopardiana. Disegnare Idee Immagini 41:18–29
22. Centofanti M (1984) L'Aquila 1753–1983. Il restauro della città. Edizioni Libreria Colacchi, L'Aquila.
23. Centofanti M (2010) Della natura del modello architettonico. In: Brusaporci S (ed) Sistemi informativi integrati per la tutela la conservazione e la valorizzazione del patrimonio architettonico e urbano. Roma, Gangemi, pp 43–54
24. Centofanti M, Brusaporci S (2012a) Architectural 3D modeling in historical buildings knowledge and restoration processes. In: Gambardella C (ed) Less More. La Scuola di Pitagora, Napoli
25. Centofanti M, Brusaporci S et al (2012b) Interpretative 3D digital models in architectural surveying of historical buildings. In: Di Giamberardino P (ed) Computational modelling of objects represented in images. CRC Press, London
26. Chiavoni E, Fanone A (2006) Moretti ritrovato: il caso dell'ex GIL di Trastevere. Disegnare idee immagini 33:46–55
27. Clini P (2008) Architetture al CAD Metodi e tecniche per la rappresentazione. Pitagora, Bologna
28. Colombo F (1990) Ombre sintetiche. Liguori, Napoli
29. Cundari C (2006) Il Disegno. Ragioni Fondamenti Applicazioni. Kappa, Roma
30. De Luca L et al (2011) A semantic-based platform for the digital analysis of architectural heritage. Comput Graph 35:227–241
31. Docci M (1989) Disegno e rilievo: quale didattica? Disegnare Idee Immagini 37–54
32. Docci M (2007) La Basilica Vaticana non costruita. L'opera di Antonio da Sangallo. Disegnare Idee Immagini 34:24–35
33. Docci M et al (1983) Disegno e analisi architettonica. Università degli Studi di Roma "La Sapienza" Dipartimento di rappresentazione e Rilievo, Roma.
34. Eco U (1968) La struttura assente. Bompiani, Milano
35. Fasolo V (1960) Analisi grafica dei valori architettonici. Facoltà di Architettura, Università di Roma, Roma, Lezioni del prof. Vincenzo Fasolo. Istituto di Storia dell'Architettura
36. Fasolo V (1954) Guida metodica per lo studio della storia dell'architettura. Edizioni dell'Ateneo, Roma
37. Fatta F (2011) La rappresentazione dell'Africa romana. In Giovannini M, Prampolini F (eds) Spazi e culture del Mediterraneo, vol 3. Centro Stampa d'Ateneo, Reggio Calabria, pp 221–240
38. Fatta F et al (2012) A net of small museum for policies of planning, safeguard and government of mediterranean archeological landscape. In: Gambardella C (ed) Less more architecture. Napoli, La Scuola di Pitagora, pp 1261–1268

39. Filippa M et al (eds) (2011) Metodologie integrate per il rilievo, il disegno, la modellazione dell'architettura e della città. Gangemi, Roma
40. Fiorani D (2004) Restauro architettonico e strumento informatico. Guida agli elaborati grafici, Liguori
41. Gaiani M (ed) (2006) La rappresentazione riconfigurata. POLI.design, Milano
42. Gambardella C (ed) (2012) Less more architecture design landscape. Le vie dei Mercanti _X Forum Internazionale di Studi, La Scuola di Pitagora, Napoli
43. Giovannini M, Prampolini F (eds) (2011) Spazi e culture del Mediterraneo. Luoghi mediterranei. Centro Stampa d'Ateneo, Reggio Calabria
44. Guidi G et al (2010) Acquisizione 3D e modellazione poligonale. McGraw-Hill, Milano
45. Ippoliti E (2011) Media digitali per il godimento dei beni culturali. DisegnareCon 8:2–13
46. Maggio F (2008) Enrico Del Debbio e Angiolo Mazzoni ad Agrigento. Disegnare Idee Immagini 37:58–71
47. Maggio F, Villa M (2008) Architettura demolita. Edizioni Caracol, Palermo
48. Maldonado T (1992) Reale e virtuale. Feltrinelli, Milano
49. Maldonado T (1997) Critica della ragione informatica. Feltrinelli, Milano
50. Marotta A (2010) Metodologie di analisi per l'architettura: il rilievo come conoscenza complessa in forma di database. In: Brusaporci S (ed) Sistemi informativi integrati per la tutela la conservazione e la valorizzazione del patrimonio architettonico e urbano. Gangemi, Roma, pp 70–73
51. Migliari R (2003) Geometria dei modelli—rappresentazione grafica e informatica per l'architettura e per il design. Kappa, Roma
52. Migliari R (ed) (2008) Prospettiva dinamica interattiva. Kappa, Roma
53. Mingucci R (2010) Modellazione digitale Informativa per l'analisi e la rappresentazione del Paesaggio Urbano. In: Brusaporci S (ed) Sistemi informativi integrati per la tutela la conservazione e la valorizzazione del patrimonio architettonico e urbano. Gangemi, Roma, pp 144–155
54. Negroponte N (1995) Being digital. Alfred A, Knopf, New York
55. Novello G, Bocconcino M (2011) CAD, BIM, GIS and other tricks of the computer science in the education of the Building Engineer. In: IMProVe 2011- international conference on innovative methods in product design. Libreria Cortina, Padova
56. Purini F (2003) Digital divide. In: Sacchi L, Unali M (eds) Architettura e cultura digitale. Skira, Milano, pp 87–96
57. Ribichini L (2007) I Modelli. Storie di diverse vicende e realizzazioni. Disegnare Idee Immagini 34:50–61
58. Ricoeur P (2008) Architettura come narrazione. In: Rocca E (ed) Estetica e architettura. Il Mulino, Bologna
59. Ronchi AM (2009) eCulture: cultural content in the digital age. Springer, Berlin
60. Sacchi L (2003) Rappresentazione fra realtà e utopia. Disegnare Idee Immagini 27:42–53
61. Sacchi L (2005) Il rilevamento di palazzo Mattei di Giove a Roma. Disegnare Idee Immagini 31:68–81
62. Sacchi L, Unali M (eds) (2003) Architettura e cultura digitale. Skira, Milano
63. Strollo RM (2008) L'Osservatorio Astronomico del Tuscolo - rilevamento e progetti. Aracne, Roma
64. Toth I (1997 [1967]) Aristotele e i fondamenti assiomatici della geometria. Prolegomeni alla comprensione dei frammenti non euclidei del "Corpus Aristotelicum" [Das Parallelenproblem im Corpus Aristotelicum], Milano.
65. Unali M (ed) (2006) Lo spazio digitale dell'architettura italiana. Kappa, Roma
66. Unali M (ed) (2008) Abitare virtuale significa rappresentare. Kappa, Roma
67. Unali M (2009) Qual è il modello di rappresentazione complesso nella rivoluzione informatica? Disegnare Idee Immagini 38:30–39
68. Valenti R (2003) Architettura e simulazione. La rappresentazione dell'idea dal modello fisico al modello virtuale, Biblioteca del Cenide, Reggio Calabria
69. Zerlenga O (2008) Rappresentazione geometrica e gestione informatica dei modelli. La scuola di Pitagora, Napoli

Flow Patterns in Aortic Circulation Associated to the Mustard Procedure

G. D'Avenio, S.Donatiello, A.Secinaro, A.Palombo, B.Marino, A. Amodeo and M. Grigioni

Abstract The transposition of the great arteries (aorta and main pulmonary artery) is a pathological condition which is faced with negative outcome in the very first years of life, if left untreated. A surgical procedure for restoring a more physiological situation is the Mustard procedure, which allows total correction of transposition of the great vessels, by means of surgical redirection of caval blood to appropriate atria. In the Mustard procedure, pulmonary and systemic circulation are driven by the left and right ventricle, respectively. With respect to the physiological case, after the Mustard operation the ascending part of the aorta, immediately downstream of the ventricle, has a lower curvature. The present study is meant to characterize, by means of patient-specific modelling and computational simulation, the aortic hemodynamics in patients operated on with a Mustard procedure, in order to highlight whether the

G. D'Avenio (✉) · M. Grigioni
Department of Technology and Health, Istituto Superiore di Sanità, Rome, Italy
e-mail: davenio@iss.it

M. Grigioni
e-mail: grigioni@iss.it

S. Donatiello · A. Secinaro · A. Amodeo
Pediatric Hospital "Bambino Gesù", Rome, Italy
e-mail: salvatored111@libero.it

A. Secinaro
e-mail: aurelio.secinaro@opbg.net

A. Amodeo
e-mail: antonioamodeo@yahoo.it

A. Palombo
Department of Clinical and Molecular Medicine, 'Sapienza' University of Rome, Rome, Italy
e-mail: alessandro.palombo@uniroma1.it

B. Marino
Department of Pediatrics,'Sapienza' University of Rome, Rome, Italy
e-mail: bruno.marino@uniroma1.it

P. Di Giamberardino et al. (eds.), *Computational Modeling of Objects Presented in Images*, Lecture Notes in Computational Vision and Biomechanics 15,
DOI: 10.1007/978-3-319-04039-4_3,

native connection of the aorta to the right ventricle can cause particular concerns, with respect to the physiological case.

Keywords Cardiovascular surgery · Aortic circulation · Fluid dynamics

1 Introduction

A not negligible series of cardiac pathologies of the newborn implies the transposition of the great arteries (aorta and main pulmonary artery). Since the functional difference between right and left ventricle, the right ventricle, which in such a case is destined to sustain the systemic circulation, will be overloaded. This type of circulation is thus faced with negative outcome in the very first years of life, if left untreated.

A surgical procedure for restoring a more physiological situation is the Mustard procedure, which allows total correction of transposition of the great vessels, by means of surgical redirection of caval blood flow to the left atrium and then to the left ventricle, which pumps the deoxygenated blood to the lungs (it must be recalled that in a normal heart the deoxygenated blood is pumped instead by the right ventricle into the lungs). In the Mustard procedure, pulmonary and systemic circulation are driven by the left and right ventricle, respectively. With respect to the physiological case (Fig. 1), after the Mustard operation the ascending part of the aorta, immediately downstream of the ventricle, has a lower curvature.

The present study is meant to characterize the aortic hemodynamics in patients operated on with a Mustard procedure, in order to highlight whether the native connection of the aorta to the right ventricle can cause particular concerns, with respect to the physiological case.

2 Materials and Methods

MRI images of a patient operated on with Mustard procedure at the Bambino Gesù Pediatric Hospital, Rome, were processed with Mimics software (Materialise, Belgium), allowing the construction of a 3D model of the aorta, from the aortic root downstream to the abdominal aorta, including the supra-aortic arteries. The model was built by means of suitable (upper and lower) thresholds for intensity of the image.

The 3D model was subsequently imported into 3-matic software (Materialise, Belgium), in order to prune the parts not belonging to the aortic circulation. 3-matic offers design modification, design simplification, 3D texturing, remeshing, forward engineering, at the level of STereoLithography (STL) representation. STL is a file format developed by a stereo-lithography CAD software (3D Systems), but also supported by many other software packages. STL files describe only the surface geometry of a three dimensional object without any representation of color, texture or other common CAD model attributes. Since an STL file describes a raw unstructured

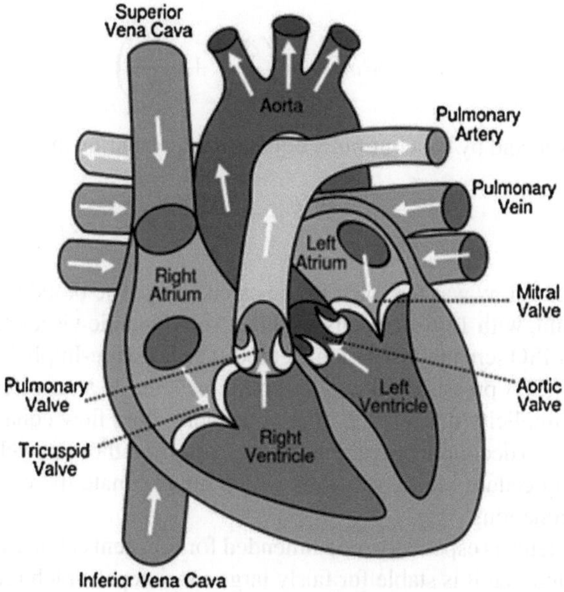

Fig. 1 Circulation in normal subjects: the *aorta* is connected to the *left ventricle*, and is subjected to a large curvature in the ascending part. Patients who are eligible for the Mustard procedure have instead the aorta congenitally connected to the *right ventricle* (figure source: http://upload.wikimedia.org/wikipedia/commons/thumb/e/e5/Diagram_of_the_human_heart_%28cropped%29.svg/600px-Diagram_of_the_human_heart_%28cropped%29.svg.png)

triangulated surface, by means of the unit normal and vertices of the triangles, it gives a rather low-level model representation, which requires powerful software tools to be effectively further processed.

In particular, the possibility to design or repair missing or badly rendered components after thresholding of MRI images was very useful to build a realistic 3D model of the aortic district.

A volume mesh of about 2.75 millions tetrahedral was then created and imported in Ansys Fluent 12.1, a flexible general-purpose computational fluid dynamics software package used to model flow, turbulence, heat transfer, and other physical phenomena [1, 6].

Suitable boundary conditions were set at the input and outputs of the model. The flow (at the inlet section) and pressure (at the outflow sections, i.e., the cerebral arteries and the descending aorta) values were imposed according to the typical values in the subjects at the age of the candidate for the Mustard procedure.

The flow motion was described by the principle of momentum conservation, expressed by the Navier-Stokes equations:

$$\frac{\partial U_i}{\partial t} + U_j \frac{\partial U_i}{\partial x_j} = \frac{1}{\rho} \frac{\partial \sigma_{ij}}{\partial x_j} \qquad (i, j = 1, 2, 3) \tag{1}$$

where

$$\sigma_{ij} = -P\delta_{ij} + \mu\left(\frac{\partial U_i}{\partial x_j} + \frac{\partial U_j}{\partial x_i}\right) \tag{2}$$

is the stress tensor, and by the continuity equation, representing the principle of mass conservation:

$$\frac{\partial U_i}{\partial x_i} = 0 \tag{3}$$

Steady, laminar flow was assumed in the calculation. The blood was modeled as a Newtonian fluid, with 1.06 g/cc density and 3.5 cP dynamic viscosity.

We used the PISO scheme as solution method. The Pressure-Implicit with Splitting of Operators (PISO) pressure-velocity coupling scheme is a non-iterative method for solving the implicity discretised, time-dependent, fluid flow equations [4]. This technique allows to decouple operations on pressure from those on velocity. At each time-step, the procedure yields solutions which approximate the exact solution of the difference equations.

The PISO scheme is especially recommended for transient calculations, but it was also demonstrated that it is stable for fairly large time steps, which renders it useful for steady-state calculations as well [3]. Its usefulness is even more appreciable in case of steady-state simulations with distorted meshes. Actually, the unstructured tetrahedral mesh provided by the 3D reconstruction of the aortic model from MRI images was somewhat distorted, hence the PISO scheme allowed an improvement over faster but less accurate algorithms (e.g., SIMPLE).

As for pressure interpolation, the PREssure STaggering Option (PRESTO!) Scheme was used, as recommended for flows in strongly curved domains. The PRESTO! scheme uses the discrete continuity balance for a "staggered" control volume about the face to compute the "staggered" pressure (face pressure).

A custom software was written in the Matlab environment, in order to process the velocity and pressure data yielded by the CFD analysis for each section, and saved by the user in an ASCII file. The software enables to do a suitable transformation of the common coordinate system, in order to decompose the velocity vectors in two components, parallel and perpendicular to the given section. This feature enabled, in particular, an easy calculation of secondary flows.

Similarly to previous studies [7], we chose to evaluate the results in two sections, immediately downstream of the left subclavean artery (LSA) and in a section positioned in the descending aorta, at 14 cm below the center of the latter. These two sections will be denoted henceforth as Sects. 1 and 2, respectively.

Figure 2 shows the outline of the mesh for CFD simulation, with the two sections referred to above.

Moreover, we evaluated the results also on a sagittal plane. The latter was defined here as the plane passing through the centers of mass of Sects. 1 and 2, and parallel to the vertical direction.

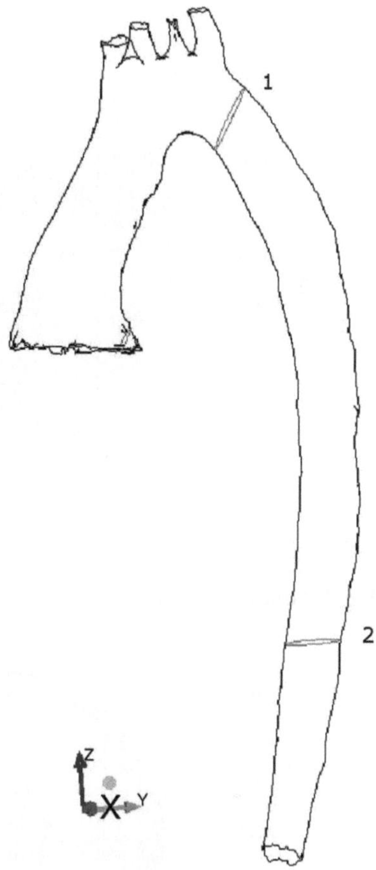

Fig. 2 Outline of the mesh used in the CFD simulations. The borders of Sects. 1 and 2 are depicted

3 Results

Figure 3 shows the static pressure distribution in Sect. 1, downstream of the LSA. The inner part of the bend is towards the bottom part of the figure. The section is viewed form the upstream side, and the patient's right-hand side is towards observer's left. The pressure values are higher towards the convex part of the aortic arch, the pressure difference in the section is 0.66 mmHg.

Figure 4 shows the axial velocity with respect to the plane of Sect. 1, downstream of LSA. A region of peak velocity can be seen, at the top of the graph, i.e., immediately downstream of the LSA inlet.

Referring again to Sect. 1, Fig. 5 shows the in-plane velocity vectors, as seen from the upstream side.

Figure. 6 shows the static pressure distribution in Sect. 2, close to the exit of the fluid domain. The section is viewed form the upstream side. The antero-posterior direction is along y, whereas patient's right hand side is towards observer's left.

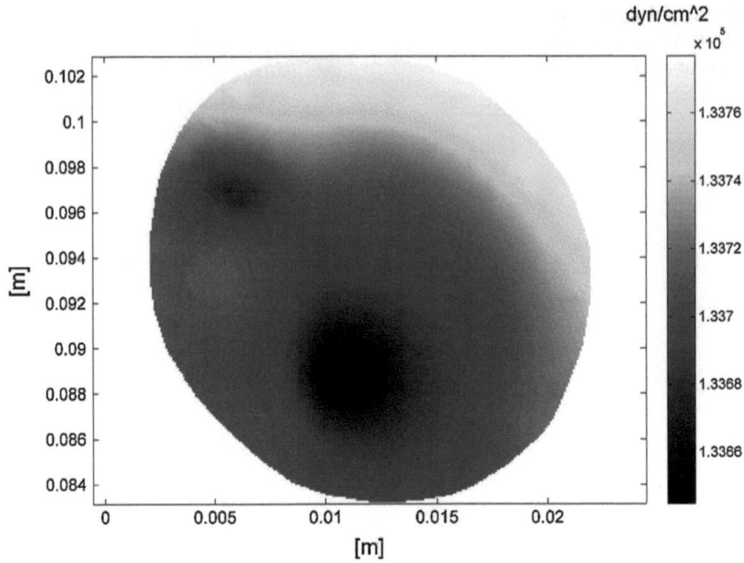

Fig. 3 Static pressure [dyn/cm^2] in Sect. 1, downstream of LSA

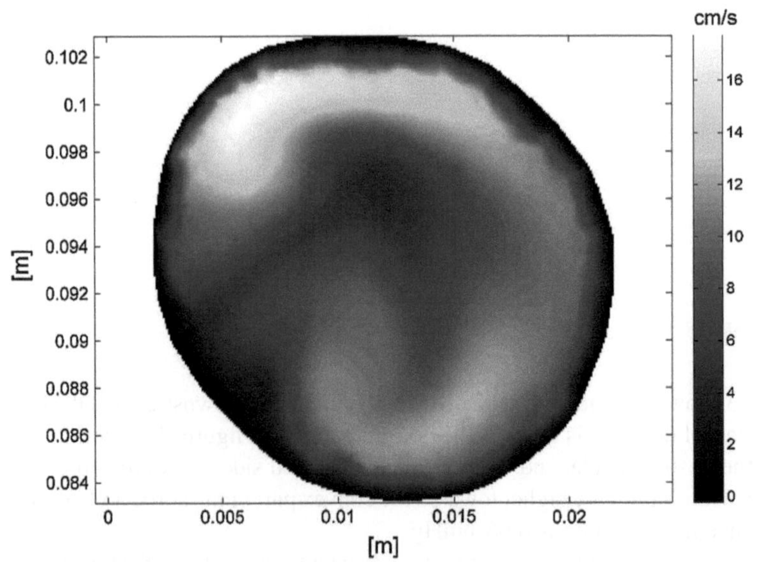

Fig. 4 Axial velocity [cm/s] (positive towards the descending aorta) in Sect. 1, downstream of LSA

It can be observed how the region of higher pressure has rotated clockwise with respect to the pressure distribution downstream of the LSA (Fig. 3). This correlates well with the overall clockwise rotation of the vector field in Fig. 5, downstream of the LSA.

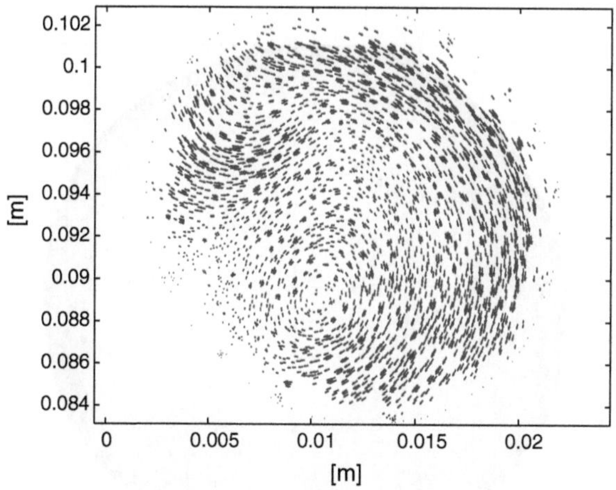

Fig. 5 In-plane velocity in Sect. 1, downstream of LSA

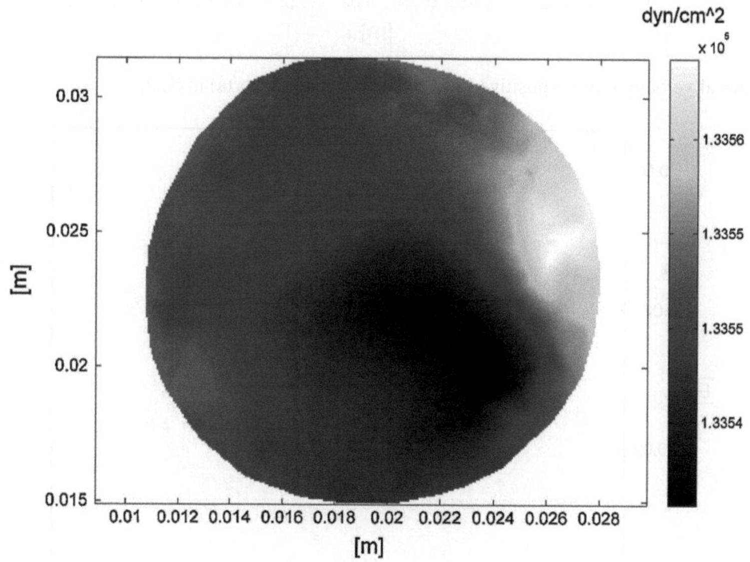

Fig. 6 Static pressure [dyn/cm^2] in Sect. 2

Figure. 7 reports the axial velocity at Sect. 2, as seen from above. The flow field here is less complex than at Sect. 1, due to the distance travelled by the blood, which smoothes out the asymmetry of the velocity distribution.

Figure 8 reports the in-plane velocity vectors for Sect. 2. These secondary flows are still complex at this relatively high downstream distance, even though there is no clear recirculation zone as in Fig. 5.

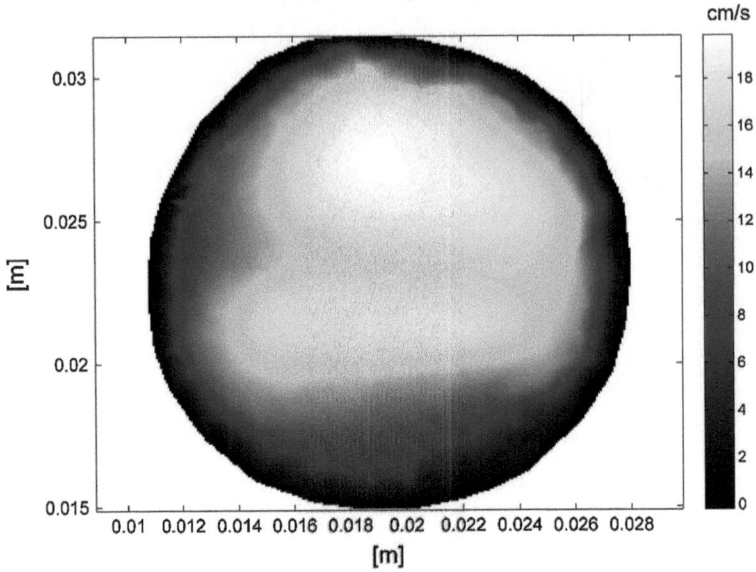

Fig. 7 Axial velocity [cm/s] (positive towards the descending aorta) in Sect. 2

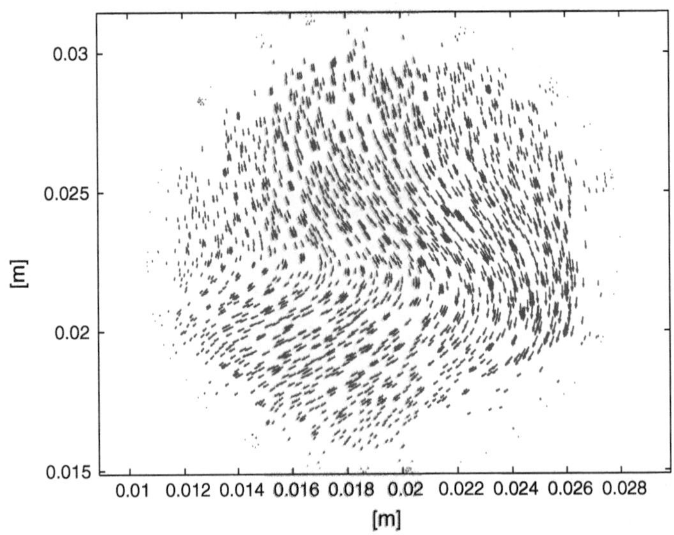

Fig. 8 In-plane velocity in Sect. 2

Another view of the in-plane flow is given by the vorticity component aligned with the normal to the section: Figs. 9 and 10 show this quantity, with the in-plane vector field superimposed on it, for Sects. 1 and 2, respectively.

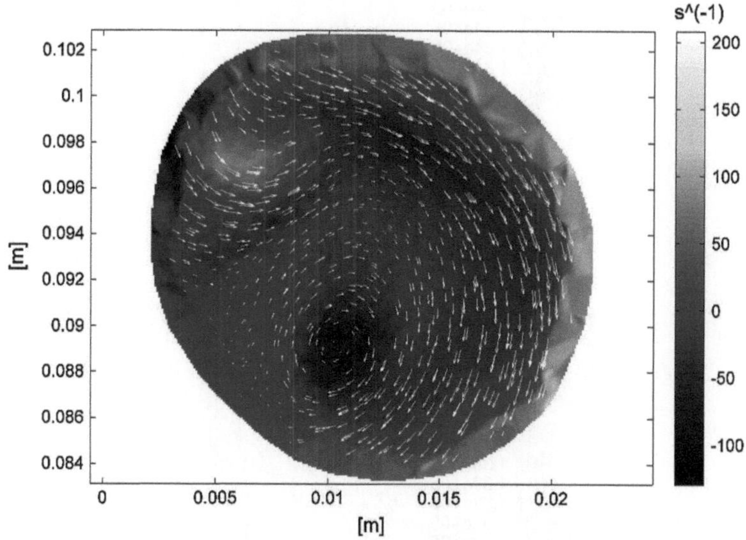

Fig. 9 The out-of-plane vorticity is superimposed on the decimated vector field (1 every 4 vectors are displayed, for sake of clarity), Sect. 1

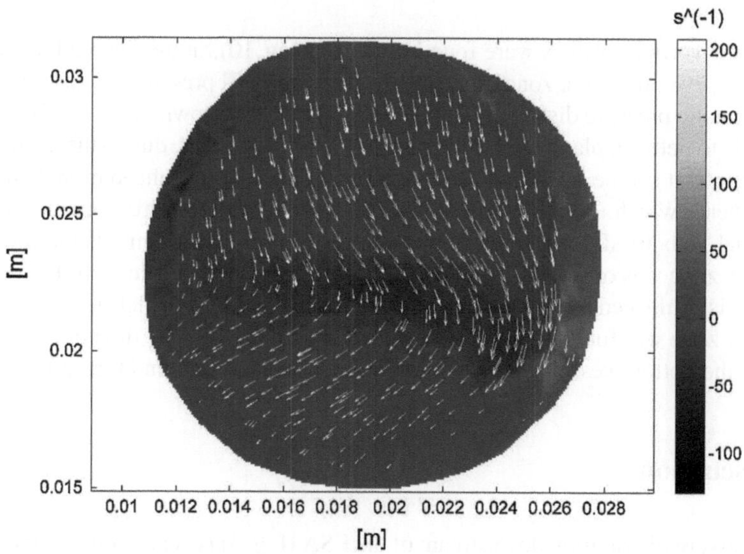

Fig. 10 The out-of-plane vorticity is superimposed on the decimated vector field (1 every 4 vectors are displayed, for sake of clarity), Sect. 2

The vorticity component has a clear negative peak at the bottom of Sect. 1 (at the opposite side of the LSA attachment to the aorta), correlated with the velocity recirculation.

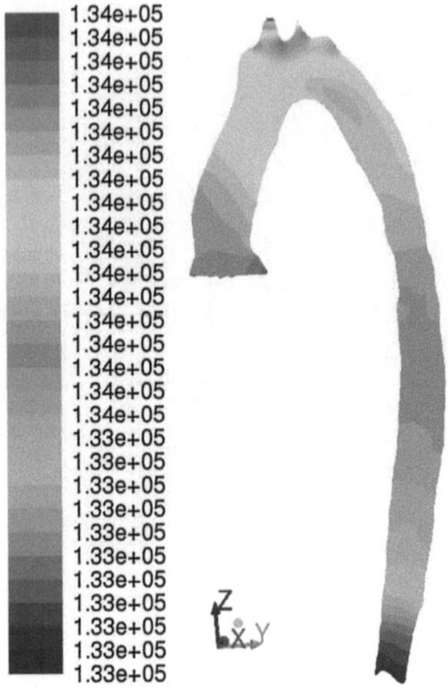

Fig. 11 Static pressure [dyn/cm^2] in the sagittal plane

Lower vorticity values were found in Sect. 2 (Fig. 10), in the descending part of the aorta, even though a zone of negative values was still present.

The static pressure distribution in the sagittal plane is shown in Fig. 11. It was not possible to define a plane intersecting all supra-aortic arteries, due to the anatomical constraints. It can be seen that there are pressure minima just ahead of and after the aortic bend, which is a condition promoting flow separation. This notwithstanding, the axial velocity did not show flow reversal, even though a remarkable low flow velocity zone was observed close to the concave side of the aortic arch (Fig. 12).

This is confirmed by the in-plane velocity field (Fig. 13), in which a strong upward velocity zone was found until the aortic bend, where the velocity direction could not follow the bottom vessel wall, and a low velocity zone was found thereafter.

4 Discussion

The pressure distribution downstream of the LSA (Fig. 3) is very similar to the result in [7]. Generally, the results hereby presented share the characteristic patterns of physiological aortic flow, even though a zone of separated flow was not observed, contrary to, e.g., [5] and [7]. These studies, however, reported results relative to flow in the unstable regime (late systole), when flow separation and, possibly, disturbances can be expected. In the present study a stationary condition was instead considered, which should be referred more realistically to peak systole, at minimal inertial effects (in fact, at peak systole the derivative of flow rate is zero).

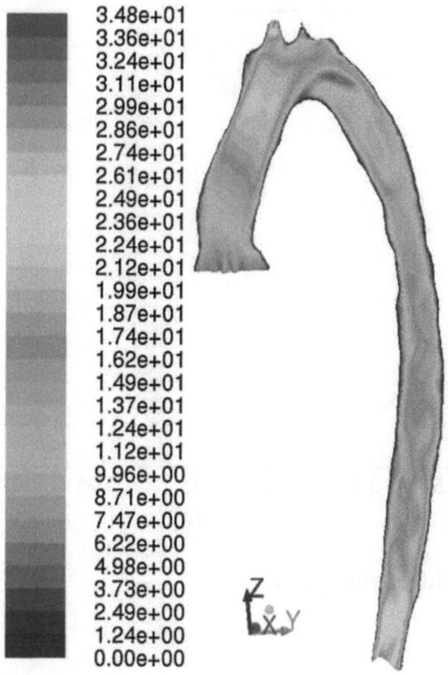

Fig. 12 Velocity magnitude [cm/s] in the sagittal plane

As already recalled in [7], retrograde flow appears in zones of initially slower antegrade velocities, under the retarding pressure gradient in late systole, therefore the low velocity zone at the bend of the arch in Fig. 12 can be associated to the already investigated flow reversal zone in the physiological aorta [5].

It must be underlined that many of the characteristic signatures of aortic flow can be appreciated. For instance, secondary flow is clearly seen in Sect. 1 (Fig. 5). The rotation is mainly right-handed, as already observed by [5] for the ascending and upper aortic arch in late systole.

This clockwise rotation can also explain the rotation of the location of peak axial velocity, from Sects. 1 to 2, which can be seen in Figs. 4 and 7, respectively.

Recent investigations with time-resolved three-dimensional (3D) phase-contrast magnetic resonance imaging [2] enabled to compare different anatomic structures in the ascending aorta with regard to the associated secondary flows. In particular, the incidence of (mainly right-handed) secondary flows was found to be more pronounced in subjects with dilated ascending aorta, compared with subjects presenting a normal aorta. A similar difference was also found in patients with a dilated ascending aorta, comparing patients with a bicuspid valve to those with a tricuspid valve. These findings suggest that the features of aortic flows may be indicative of pathological states, and possibly useful for predicting the evolution of the patient's conditions in the long term. More generally, the identification of aortic flow structures, in principle, can be a tool for the classification of the patient's state, allowing the evaluation of the effectiveness of, e.g., surgical reconstructions. It can be foreseen that future investigations will enable to improve the prediction of the clinical outcome in such critical procedures as the Mustard operation.

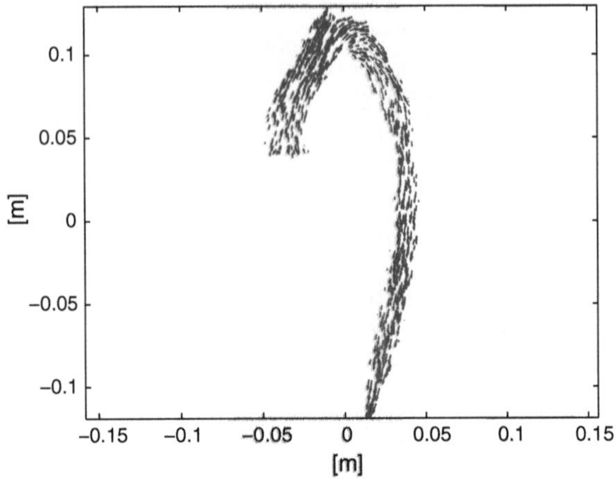

Fig. 13 In-plane velocity field (*sagittal plane*)

5 Conclusions

The results of the study indicate that the aortic flow after the Mustard procedure, even though driven by the right ventricle, retains the properties of the physiological aortic flow. In particular, the lower curvature of the ascending part of the aorta, immediately downstream of the ventricle, in comparison to the physiological case (i.e., ascending aorta connected to the left ventricle), was not found to be associated to significant differences with respect to the previously characterized aortic flow patterns in the physiological case, confirming the effectiveness of the operation on the hemodynamical point of view.

References

1. Carroll GT, McGloughlin TM, Burke PE, Egan M, Wallis F, Walsh MT (2011) Wall shear stresses remain elevated in mature arteriovenous fistulas: a case study. J Biomech Eng 133(2):021003
2. Hope MD, Hope TA, Meadows AK, Ordovas KG, Urbania TH, Alley MT, Higgins CB (2010) Bicuspid aortic valve: four-dimensional MR evaluation of ascending aortic systolic flow patterns. Radiology 255(1):53–61
3. Issa RI (1986) Solution of the implicitly discretised fluid flow equations by operator-splitting. J Comput Phys 62(1):40–65
4. Issa RI, Gosman AD, Watkins AP (1986) The computation of compressible and incompressible recirculating flows by a non-iterative implicit scheme. J Comput Phys 62(1):66–82
5. Kilner PJ, Yang GZ, Mohiaddin RH, Firmin DN, Longmore DB (1993) Helical and retrograde secondary flow patterns in the aortic arch studied by three-directional magnetic resonance velocity mapping. Circulation 88(5 Pt 1):2235–2247

6. Redaelli A, Bothorel H, Votta E, Soncini M, Morbiducci U, Del Gaudio C, Balducci A, Grigioni M (2004) 3-D simulation of the St. Jude Medical bileaflet valve opening process: fluid-structure interaction study and experimental validation. J Heart Valve Dis 13(5):804–813
7. Wood NB, Weston SJ, Kilner PJ, Gosman AD, Firmin DN (2001) Combined MR imaging and CFD simulation of flow in the human descending aorta. J Magn Reson Imaging 13(5):699–713

Fuzzy Image Segmentation: An Automatic Unsupervised Method

Silvana G Dellepiane and Sonia Nardotto

Abstract A new method is here proposed for the unsupervised, automatic, global region segmentation of digital images, hereinafter referred to as the "Automatic Fuzzy Segmentation" (AFS). Starting from the fuzzy intensity-connectedness definition (χ -connectedness) and the related growing mechanism, it allows a strict and very simple integration between the analysis of topological connectedness and grey level similarities of the pixels belonging to the same region. By overcoming the previous drawback due to the need of some seed points selection, an iterative processing is here developed, able to adapt to the image content. The automatic selection of seed points is driven by intermediate connectedness results which alternates the analysis of inter-region similarities with inter-region separation measurements. The robustness of the method with respect to the three required parameters is discussed. Example cases related to real application domains are here presented and discussed.

Keywords Segmentation · Fuzzy processing · Connectedness · MS lesion detection

1 Introduction

For many years, image segmentation, or rather the process of identifying regions of interest starting from a digital image or volume, has been a major problem in image processing and a subject of extensive research work. Segmentation purpose is to partition an image into regions with homogeneous properties that faithfully correspond to the objects or parts of the objects of interest [5]. Among the methods and solutions suggested in the literature, the ones exploiting fuzzy logic have proved

S. G. Dellepiane (✉) · S. Nardotto
Università degli Studi di Genova, DITEN via Opera Pia 11a – I16145, Genova, Italy
e-mail: silvana.dellepiane@unige.it

S. Nardotto
e-mail: sonia.nardotto@edu.unige.it

P. Di Giamberardino et al. (eds.), *Computational Modeling of Objects Presented in Images*, Lecture Notes in Computational Vision and Biomechanics 15,
DOI: 10.1007/978-3-319-04039-4_4,

to be very promising. In fact, fuzziness is an inherent feature of real images, which are created through imaging devices and are naturally affected by defects, such as resolution limitations, blurring, noise, etc. Another hindrance to image analysis is the heterogeneity of the materials of the objects under examination, as occurs in the Biomedical and Remote Sensing fields, where it is necessary to observe the internal organs of living beings or to observe the Earth's surface. Even when acquired from a single class, the imaging signal may be characterized by various levels of intensity. Fuzzy logic has been widely used in image segmentation, mainly to cluster the signal based on punctual features. Although the spatial and topological properties of images are important, only a few methods are able to exploit such an additional dimension [18]. In this context, fuzzy connectedness [8] may help to solve these problems identifying precisely the elements composing an image and belonging to the same region of interest, despite the existing uncertainties and variations in the original signal intensity levels. The aim of the proposed work is to extend the multi seed segmentation (MSMC) method proposed in Angiati et al. [1] for a fully automatic processing, thus achieving the so-called "Automatic Fuzzy Segmentation (AFS)" method. The core of the method is the fuzzy intensity-connectedness approach [8], here applied starting from a number of seed points which are automatically selected with the goal of the global image segmentation. This new method implements an iterative procedure which starts from a random selection of a few seed points, and stops with the complete segmentation of the image. Each iterative step alternates addition of new significant seeds and deletion of useless ones. This is a random process based on fuzzy operators, it is unsupervised and is only driven by the original data and intermediate results. It makes use of only three parameters and robustness can be easily proved, as reported in the evaluation session. The extensive experimental session has also proved good performances, when compared with other methods. The outline of the chapter is as follows. In Sect. 2, we shall briefly review the main segmentation approaches that are related to our method. Then the formulation of the proposed automatic segmentation method is presented. In Results section the applications of AFS will be reported and compared with already published methods. The conclusions section ends the chapter.

2 Proposed Method

Even though the spatial and topological properties of images are of major importance, they are only partially exploited by literature methods. A few approaches have been developed able to exploit the topological information in a fuzzy-logic framework [8, 17]. They are based on a close examination of the connectedness between pairs of image pixels and the relevant paths, in addition to the actual signal intensity. In Saha and Udupa [14] the so-called "relative fuzzy connectedness" method has been proposed where various objects in the image "are let to compete among themselves in having pixels as their members". In the experiments there proposed, some seeds are utilized to specify a class of objects and some others correspond to different co-objects in the background. In the present work, starting from the fuzzy intensity-connectedness concept and the related computational method, Dellepiane et al. [8], new image processing steps are defined and introduced to realize an automatic unsupervised fuzzy image segmentation.

The proposed *Automatic Fuzzy Segmentation (AFS)* method represents an innovative extension of the system proposed in Angiati et al. [1] where a multi-region fuzzy seed-based segmentation has been described, devoted to the global segmentation of a given image.

Notation

Let an n-dimensional Euclidean space $\mathbb{R}^n$ be subdivided into hypercubes called spels (an abbreviation for "space elements"). When n = 2, spels are called pixels and they are represented by $p = p(x, y)$. When n = 3 spels are called voxels and they are represented by $p = p(x, y, z)$. Let L be an n-dimensional lattice of size D^n, made of the v_i 's, with $i = 1, \ldots, D^n$. An original digital image (or volume) is the field

$$\boldsymbol{Z} = \{(v_i, \xi(v_i))\, / v_i \in L\} \tag{1}$$

whose values range from 0 to the maximum grey-level, defined on the n-D lattice L. A fuzzy field M is a fuzzy subset defined in the following [13]:

$$\boldsymbol{M} = \{(v_i, \mu(v_i))\, / v_i \in L\} \qquad \mu \in [0, 1] \tag{2}$$

In fact, every digital picture/volume can be represented by an equivalent fuzzy field since, as stated in [6], there always exists a rational value r such that, for each spel v_i, we can write:

$$\mu(v_i) = r \cdot \xi(v_i) \tag{3}$$

As it is well known, the purpose of image segmentation is the partition of an image $\boldsymbol{M}$ into a set of regions, $\{R_k\}$ where each R_k is a connected component and it holds that:

$$\bigcup_k R_k = \boldsymbol{M}$$

$$R_k \cap R_h = \Phi \; for\; k \neq h \tag{4}$$

The automatic segmentation method here proposed is based on five steps that are iterated until the stop condition is verified. They are introduced in the following and will be described in detail in the next sections.

I. Fuzzy χ-connectedness Map Computation: A fuzzy χ-connectedness map is independently computed for each selected seed. Unlike the method described in [1] where seeds are manually located by the user, in this method the seed points are automatically placed during the processing, in an adaptive way with respect to the actual image content.

II. Redundant Seeds Reduction: This step detects and obviates the situation where more than one seed is representing the same region.

III. Total Connectedness Map Computation: The seeds-related membership maps are merged into a single "Total-connectedness map" that is used to drive the next processing steps.

IV. Residual Detection and Seed Generation: It automatically finds new seeds when the previously selected ones are not sufficient to achieve a complete segmentation result.

V. Stopping Criterion and Labeling : appropriate stopping criterion and the labeling step are defined in subsection V.

The first iteration starts from a set of seed points randomly selected.

2.1 Fuzzy χ-connectedness Map Computation

Before talking about χ-connectedness we introduce the classical Fuzzy Connectedness concept. Given the generic fuzzy field ***M*** described in Eq. (2), we define the path $P(p,q)$ as a connected sequence of spels $< p_1, p_2, \ldots, p_Q >$ from a spel $p_1 = p$ to a spel $p_Q = q$, where Q is the length of the path that joins the point p to the point q. We can express the conventional fuzzy degree of connectedness from p to q as in [12], that is:

$$c_\mu (p,q) = conn (\mu, p, q) = \max_{P(p,q)}[\min_{z \in P(p,q)} \mu_z] \tag{5}$$

where the max is applied to all paths $P(p,q)$ from p to q (thus referring to the optimum path connecting p with q), and the minimum is applied to all points z along the optimum path.

This definition implies the following properties [3]:

- c_μ is symmetrical, i.e.,

$$\forall\ (p,q) \in L^2, \qquad c_\mu (p,q) = c_\mu(q,p);$$

- c_μ is transitive, i.e.,

$$\forall\ (p,q) \in L^2, \qquad c_\mu (p,q) \geq \max_{P_{(q,p)}} \left[\min(c_\mu (p,x), c_\mu(x,q))\right]$$

- c_μ is weakly reflexive [10], i.e.,

$$\forall\ (p,q) \in L^2, \qquad c_\mu (p,p) \geq c_\mu (p,q)$$

From the above definition, it follows that a fuzzy connected component associated with a generic point q is a fuzzy subset that can be expressed as:

$$\forall\, p \in L,\ \Gamma_{\mu}^{q}(p) = \max_{P_{(q,p)}}\left[min_{z \in P_{(q,p)}} \mu(z)\right] = c_{\mu}(q, p) \tag{6}$$

For each spel p, its degree of connectedness to q in $\boldsymbol{M}$ is obtained as its membership in $\Gamma_{\mu}^{q}(p)$. In other words, a fuzzy connected component (in terms of grey-level homogeneity and topologic connectedness) can be identified for each image point. This approach is very similar to the segmentation process for some object, provided that a point q belonging to the object is selected. However, the objects of interest in a real image neither are always characterized by light or dark areas (tops or bottoms), nor they correspond to image plateaux, nor they are necessarily surrounded by high contrast background areas. The above definition of degree of connectedness does not take into account these considerations. Therefore, it is necessary to make the connectedness value independent of the reference grey-level. Moreover, it is worth noting that the classical c_{μ} is not equivalent for both a signal and its complement, as differences are considered in an absolute way, not in a relative one. c_{μ} follows the behaviour of the field $\boldsymbol{M}$ for decreasing μ values, whereas it is independent of increasing μ values. In the context of digital images this fact is a limitation, but it can be faced by using the definition of χ-connectivity, introduced in Dellepiane and Fontana [7]. In order to exploit the definition of connectedness for the purpose of image segmentation, we consider a modified field (with respect to a generic reference spel a, in the following referred to as a seed point) expressed as:

$$\chi^{a}(p) = 1 - |\,\mu(p) - \mu(a)\,| \tag{7}$$

The χ − connectedness associated with the seed spel a can therefore be determined by applying Eq. (5) to the field

$$\boldsymbol{X}^{a} = \left\{\left(v_i, \chi^{a}(v_i)\right) / v_i \in L\right\}$$

It takes the name of intensity connectedness or χ-connectedness and turns to be:

$$c_{\chi^{a}}(p) = conn\left(\chi^{a}, a, p\right) = max_{P(a,p)}[min_{z \in P(a,p)} \chi^{a}(z)] \tag{8}$$

It can easily be shown that this is equivalent to computing:

$$c_{\chi^{a}}(p) = 1 - \min_{P(a,p)}[\max_{z \in P(a,p)} |\mu(z) - \mu(a)|] \tag{9}$$

For a generic spel at any intensity level equal to $\mu(a)$, the formula corresponds to the shiftment the signal $\mu(p)$ to $\mu(p) + 1 - \mu(a)$ and, simultaneously, to the reverse of $\mu(p)$ with respect to $\mu(a)$ for each point with $\mu(p) > \mu(a)$.

Let $p(a, v_i)$ be a connected sequence of spels from a to the generic v_i given by $< a,\ v_1,\ v_2, \ldots,\ v_{i-1},\ v_i >$. It can be deduced that for two spels belonging to the best path from the seed (i.e., the path that satisfies the max operator), the degree of connectedness reduces to

$$c_{\chi^a}(v_i) = \min_{z \in P(a,v_i)} \chi^a(z) = \min\left[\min_{z \in P(a,v_{i-1})}\left(\chi^a(z)\right), \chi^a(v_i)\right] \quad (10)$$

that is,

$$c_{\chi^a}(v_i) = \min\left[c_{\chi^a}(v_{i-1}), \chi^a(v_i)\right] \quad (11)$$

In other words, the intensity-connectedness of a spel v_i is equal to its value in χ^a or, if its χ-connectedness has not the minimum value in that path, to the intensity connectedness of the previous spel along the best path from a to v_i.

The core of the image segmentation method refers to the particular growing process that was firstly described in [7, 8].

2.2 Redundant Seeds Reduction

At the beginning, the seed points are randomly placed, then it is required to determine the eventual cases where more than one seed is associated to the same region, before calculating the total map. It is thus necessary to define and search these situations, in order to collapse more seeds into one. To this aim, we define the so-called "redundant seeds". To find the redundant seeds, a distance between the connectivity map generated from seed a and the one generated from seed b is computed:

$$d(v_i) = \left|c_{\chi^a}(v_i) - c_{\chi^b}(v_i)\right| \quad (12)$$

associated to the distance energy value:

$$\alpha = \sum_i d(v_i) \quad (13)$$

A decreasing sigmoidal fuzzy membership function "low_s", with flex point in s, is also defined:

$$low_s :\rightarrow [0, 1] \begin{cases} \lim_{\alpha \to 0} low_s = 1 \\ \lim_{\alpha \to 1} low_s = 0 \end{cases} \quad (14)$$

In such a way, two seeds a and b are considered to be redundant if the energy of the distance field is low, given that the original grey level of the two seeds are similar enough. Thanks to the second constraint, only (T-1) comparisons are required at each iteration, starting from a list where seeds are ordered on the basis of their original grey level, being T the actual number of seed points.

2.3 Total Connectedness Map

Let v_{at}, $t = 1 \ldots T$ be T random seed-points, each corresponds to a different class or region. The Multi-Seed Multi-Class (MSMC) method allows to separately identify a region associated to a seed. For each seed point v_{at}, the corresponding intensity-connectedness field $C_t = \{(v_i\ ,\ c_{\chi^a}(v_i))\quad v_i \in L\}$ is generated. To this end, for each intensity-connectedness map a parallel processing is executed, by running the growing mechanism starting from each seed v_{at}, independently to each other. In this way, each intensity-connectedness field C_t separately contains information about the region/object corresponding to the related seed point. The computation of all the membership values assigned to a spel is equivalent to the generation of a hyper-matrix similar to the c-fuzzy-partition matrix defined in Bezdek [2]. A single final-intensity-connectedness-map field, $\hat{C}$, integrating information derived from all the seeds, is generated by applying the fuzzy union:

$$\hat{C} = \bigcup_{t=1}^{T} C_{\chi t} \tag{15}$$

where

$$c(v_i) = \bigcup_{t=1}^{T} c_{\chi t}(v_i) = \max_t\{c_{\chi t}(v_i)\} \tag{16}$$

2.4 Residual Detection and Seed Generation

2.4.1 Residuals' Map Calculation

When a significant region is not located by any of the selected seeds, a new seed point must be appropriately looked for. Once it is found it is added to the already existing seeds list and the related χ-connectedness map is generated. To the end of such a new seed selection, the intermediate total connectedness map is used. In fact, when a region has not been properly identified, some "residuals" appear in the map and can be automatically located. We here define "residuals" as those spels that have low values in the total-connectedness map, thus indicating that they are not appropriately represented by any of the selected seeds. The residual map, P, is then derived by assigning to each spel site the value:

$$\rho(v_i) = low_\rho\{c(v_i)\} \tag{17}$$

Since the location of new seed points is based on the residual map, a post-processing step devoted to its regularization is applied as explained in Sect 2.4.2.

2.4.2 Residual Map Regularization and Seed Generation

Due to the complexity of the images at hand, the presence of noise, and the low contrast between regions, many spurious spels are usually detected in the residual map. For such reasons, and in order to avoid the selection of seeds related to too small regions, a regularization step is proposed before the new seed selection task. To this end, the erosion operator of Mathematical Morphology (also called Minkowski difference) is applied to the residual map. A 3×3 structuring element (SE) is used and is applied to the whole residual map. Erosion of the residual field P is defined in Shapiro and Stockman [16]. The so obtained P_E map has homogeneous bright areas from where we can extract the new seed points. These areas passing from P to P_E, are reduced in size, decreasing the number of spels corresponding to the potential seeds and improving the probability of placing a seed far from the region border. The new seeds are randomly placed inside the brightest areas of the eroded residual map P_E and the iterative process is repeated starting from the first step. The stopping condition is based on the disappearance of any residual.

2.5 *Stopping Criterion and Labeling*

2.5.1 Stop Condition

The stop condition φ is essential because it determines when it is no longer necessary to find new seed points. Since the new seed points are searched directly on the eroded residuals' map P_E, just on this field P_E the stop condition is evaluated. Each time a residual is calculated and a new seed is determined (actually we may look for more seeds at a time), a new temporary connectivity map $C_{\chi^{v_a}}$ is calculated. Consequently, each time a new residuals' map P_E is calculated with its connectivity map $C_{\chi^{v_a}}$. For each temporary residuals' map P_E, the occurrence of bright spels on the whole image are calculated (φ_j) as the average map integral value. This is a percentage measure that will have a decreasing trend until it reaches a minimum value. The stop condition is then defined as the minimum percentage number, φ, of final residuals accepted in the stop condition. When the stopping criterion is verified, no more seeds are added or deleted and an intermediate label map is generated from the final total-connectedness map. It associates each image pixel to the most-connected seed (as defined in Eq. (16)):

$$\lambda(v_i) = \arg\{\max_t\{c_{\chi^t}(v_i)\}\} \tag{18}$$

As in the classical fuzzy Pattern Recognition, a map is created by a Maximum-Membership criterion that achieves a hard partitioning starting from the fuzzy results. In this way, it is possible to keep track of the origin of different regions into the final maps (Fig. 1). Due to the presence and integration of the results derived from more than one seed, the detected regions are no more assured to be connected components,

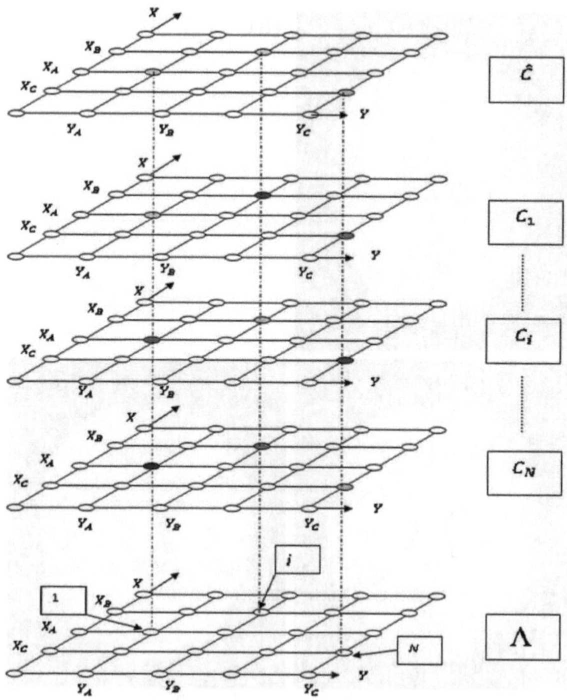

Fig. 1 Fuzzy Union of N intensity connectedness fields and generation of a label map (example on a 2D lattice)

as it was described in Dellepiane and Fontana [7] and more than one connected component can be found for each of the processed seeds. In all the processing steps only a few parameters have to be selected: the value s of the function low_s in Eq. (14), the value ρ of the function low_ρ in Eq. (17), and the number, φ, of final residuals accepted in the stop condition. In Sect. 3 the robustness of the AFS method with respect to these parameters is discussed, together with a preliminary comparison with other methods.

3 Results

3.1 AFS of Brain Healthy Tissues

To evaluate the AFS method performances, MRI brain volumes have been considered, addressing the segmentation of intracranial brain tissues, i.e., Cerebrospinal Fluid (CSF), White Matter (WM) and Gray Matter (GM). In order to make the test results comparable with other works in the literature, the Brainweb dataset [4], which

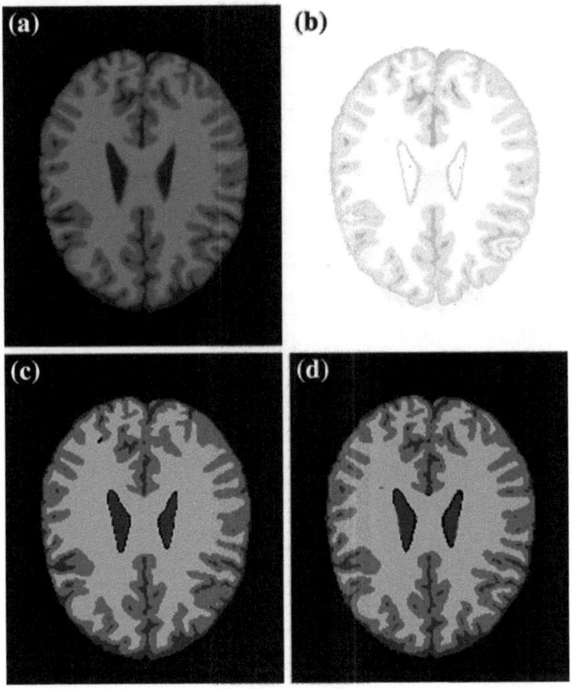

Fig. 2 Simulated T1-weighted MR image, 100th slice: 0 % noise **a** Original T1 image. **b** Final total-connectedness maps; **c** Label map; **d** Phantom

provides simulated MRI volumes for normal brain, has been used. In order to evaluate the robustness with respect to various parameters configuration (s, ρ, φ), some tests with different setting are proposed. As regards the Brainweb dataset, the segmentation performances achieved on T1, T2 and PD volumes with different noise levels (from 0 to 3 %) have been evaluated. Intensity non Uniformity—RF—is always set to 0 % since specific algorithms are available to face this problem that is not the focus of the present work. In each case the image slice is made of 181 × 217 pixels, pixel size being 1 mm^2. Figure 2a shows, as an example, the 100th brain T1-weighted slice, without noise that will be used as the example case in the following. Intermediate steps of the proposed algorithm, corresponding to singular intensity-connectedness maps C_t of the first four seed points are depicted in Fig. 3. After the reduction of eventual redundant seeds, the temporary total-connectedness-map C is obtained that is the basis for the residuals analysis.

In Fig. 4 successive residual maps are presented as achieved by running the process some iterations after the four random seeds described in Fig. 3. Five subsequent residual maps P are shown in the left image portion, the corresponding eroded residual maps P_E are in the right part. In each eroded residual map P_E the new seed point are looked for, until the stop condition is verified. In this example the φ_j's percentage measures are 1.45, 1.38, 0.89, 0.46, and 0.15 %, respectively. Since the stop condition

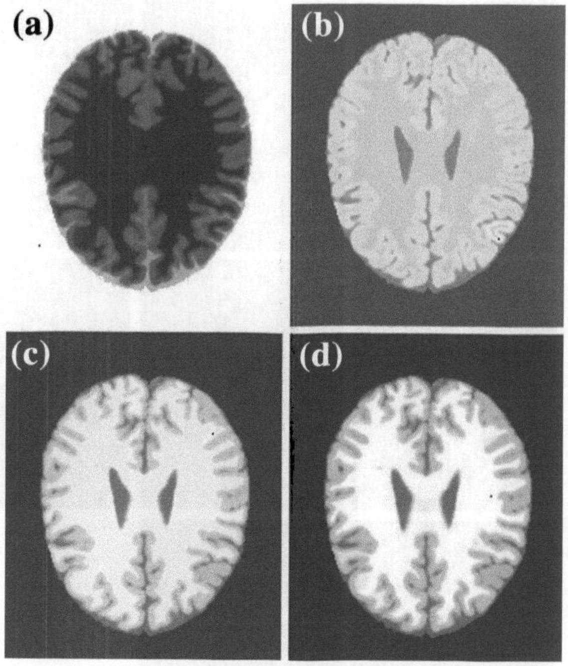

Fig. 3 Singular intensity-connectedness maps C_t of first seed points. **a** First seed point map. **b** Second seed point map. **c** Third seed point map. **d** Fourth seed point map

φ was set to $= 0.3\,\%$, the process came to an end with the residual map shown in Fig. 4j.

For each iteration a new seed point is put randomly in the space, but only the bright spels of the eroded residual map P_E may actually become seed points. In Fig. 5 the new seed points derived from the given residuals are shown, together with the corresponding singular-intensity-connectedness maps. At the end of the shown session the final total seed points are eight and their coordinates are shown in Table 1. Starting from these seed points the final-intensity-connectedness-map $\hat{C}$ is calculated and its related label map Λ is derived as presented in Fig. 2c. Figure 6 shows the binary map of the labelled components for each seed point as derived from the label computation proposed in Eq. (18).

3.2 *Evaluation of Brain Healthy Tissues Segmentation*

The global segmentation turns to be quite accurate, and a small over segmentation is achieved since the same class of interest can be associated to more than one label. As it is well known, Dellepiane [5], when running a segmentation method, over segmentation and under segmentation errors need to be limited, and not contemporary present at the same time. In the present context, where a segmentation result is

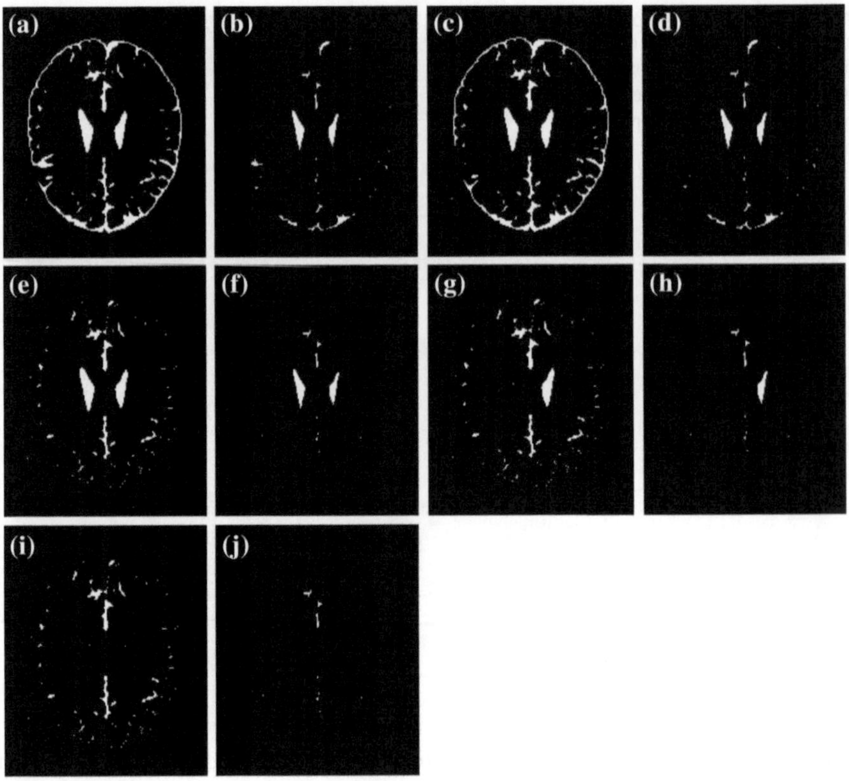

Fig. 4 Residuals'map P (*left*) and eroded residuals' map P_E (*rights*) with **a**, **b** $\varphi_j = 1.45\,\%$, **c**, **d** $\varphi_j = 1.38\,\%$, **e**, **f** $\varphi_j = 0.89\,\%$, **g**, **h** $\varphi_j = 0.46\,\%$, **i**, **j** $\varphi_j = 0.15\,\%$

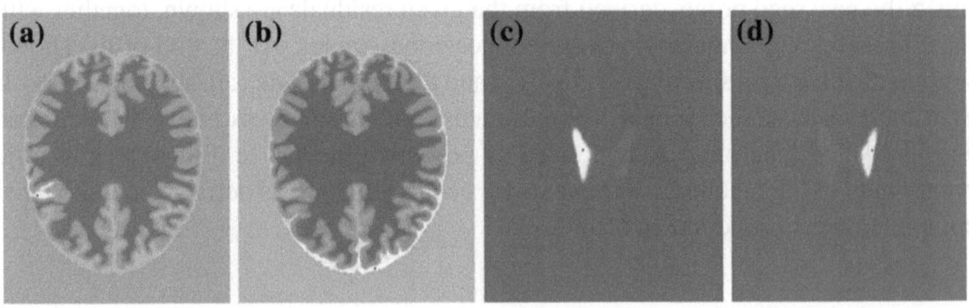

Fig. 5 Singular intensity-connectedness maps after new seed points selection. **a** Fifth seed point map. **b** Sixth seed point map. **c** Seventh seed point map. **d** Eighth seed point map

preliminar to a classification step, over segmentation errors are much better accepted than under segmentation errors. In fact, the former type is corrected by merging regions in the classification step at a symbolic level. The latter requires a backtracking to correct the error at the numerical level. By looking at Fig. 6, one can notice

Table 1 Final seed points' coordinates

x	y
21	166
137	160
135	65
133	104
33	136
104	191
75	103
108	104

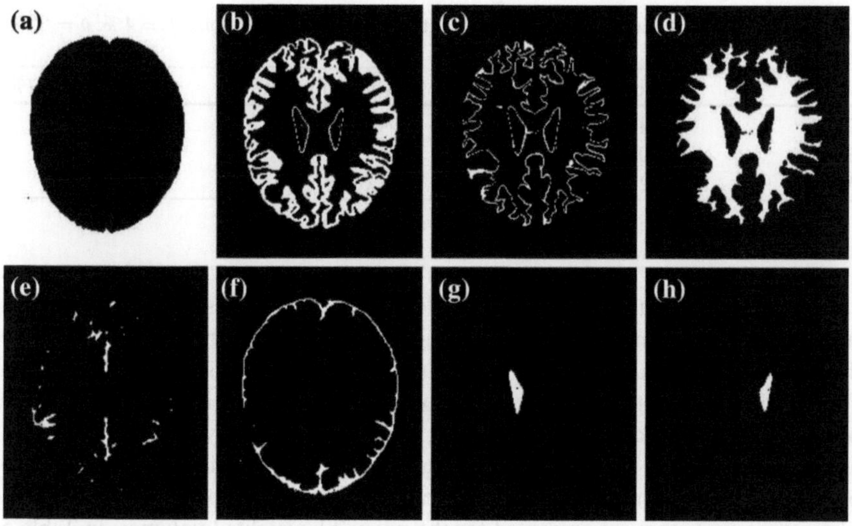

Fig. 6 Binary label map of **a** first seed point, **b** second seed point, **c** third seed point, **d** fourth seed point, **e** fifth seed point, **f** sixth seed point, **g** seventh seed point, **h** eighth seed point

that spels corresponding to a seed's label are not necessarily connected, as it was expected by Eq. (15). If required, a classical connected components labelling step can be applied to the labelling map. For a visual comparison between the segmentation result and the reference result proposed by the web site, Fig. 2c, d shows the final method result (left) and the true segmentation provided by the Brainweb phantom (right). For a better visualization and for a comparison test, each connected component is assigned a label corresponding to the most similar class of the phantom. By leaving unchanged the parameters' configuration, different tests have been executed, to evaluate the repeatability of the method and the reliability of the results in the various random trial repetitions. For a robustness analysis, this same procedure is repeated by changing the parameter setting. Two features are considered: the final connected components' number (CC) and the final seed points' number (SP). As one

Table 2 Connected components' number (CC) and seed points' number(SP) for T1-weighted MRI, 0 % noise

$s = 4\,\%, \rho = 85\,\%, \varphi = 0.3\,\%$		$s = 3\,\%, \rho = 90\,\%, \varphi = 0.3\,\%$	
CC	SP	CC	SP
86	9	127	11
119	9	105	10
11	8	86	7
97	8	94	11
96	7	97	11
107	9	95	8

Table 3 Example accuracy results for T1-weighted MRI volume, 0 % noise, $s = 4\,\%$, $\rho = 85\,\%$, $\varphi = 0.3\,\%$

	Specificity (%)	Sensitivity (%)	Accuracy (%)
CSF	99.47	94.39	98.90
GM	95.08	99.06	97.15
WM	98.25	91.69	96.05

can appreciate from the examples in Table 2, these two values are within a range. In the reference phantom connected components are 79. To numerically evaluate the performances of the proposed segmentation, different measurements have been computed, referring to the phantom. In particular, the following parameters have been extracted for each class: Specificity, Sensitivity, Accuracy [9], as presented in Table 3 for the given example. The average accuracy values of the results obtained by the six independent trial tests described above has been considered in Table 4. The same parameters are presented for the noisy T1-weighted volumes, in Table 5 (1 % noise) and Table 6 (3 % noise), showing very high values. A slight decrease as the noise increases is observed. The same parameters are presented for the noisy T2-weighted volumes, in Table 7 and for the noisy PD- weighted volumes, in Table 8 (noise level 1 % in both cases). A slight values' decrease is noticed for these two types of acquisition, due to the generally less contrasted and less clean original volumes. In fact, as it is well known, the T2-weighted and the PD volumes are more affected by noise than T1- weighted volumes and also the contrast between the regions is lower. For a better discussion clarity, Fig. 7 shows the ROC scatter plot applied to six different parameter configurations in the processing of the T1-weighted image, 3 % noise. The three different colors represent the three classes: CSF (blue), GM (red), WM (green) and each configuration is represented by a symbol.

The configuration represented by the small solid diamonds ($s = 3\,\%, \rho = 90\,\%, \varphi = 0.3\,\%$) corresponds to the largest spread between classes, which then turn out to be unbalanced. In fact, performances are better for CSF than WM. As deals with CSF and GM the best class changes if we consider the sensitivity or the specificity. The configurations represented by the circle ($s = 6\,\%, \rho = 90\,\%, \varphi = 0.3\,\%$)

Table 4 Average Accuracy results for T1-weighted MRI volume, 0 % noise, s = 3 %, $\rho = 90\,\%$, $\varphi = 0.3\,\%$

	Specificity (%)	Sensitivity (%)	Accuracy (%)
CSF	99.35	94.25	98.76
GM	97.81	98.67	98.32
WM	98.00	95.26	97.09

Table 5 Accuracy results for T1-weighted MRI volume, 1 % noise, s = 4 %, $\rho = 90\,\%$, $\varphi = 0.3\,\%$

	Specificity (%)	Sensitivity (%)	Accuracy (%)
CSF	98.99	95.51	98.61
GM	98.83	98.69	98.92
WM	98.40	95.60	97.53

Table 6 Accuracy results for T1-weighted MRI volume, 3 % noise, s = 6 %, $\rho = 95\,\%$, $\varphi = 0.3\,\%$

	Specificity (%)	Sensitivity (%)	Accuracy (%)
CSF	98.88	94.57	98.44
GM	97.28	98.34	97.84
WM	97.77	93.51	96.28

Table 7 Accuracy results for T2-weighted MRI volume, 1 % noise, s = 3 %, $\rho = 95\,\%$, $\varphi = 0.3\,\%$

	Specificity (%)	Sensitivity (%)	Accuracy (%)
CSF	99.12	94.71	98.64
GM	97.92	97.32	97.62
WM	96.94	94.93	96.28

and by the triangle ($s = 6\,\%$, $\rho = 90\,\%$, $\varphi = 0.3\,\%$) characterize the three classes with a better balance.

3.3 Comparison with Other Methods

In Tables 9 and 10, a comparison with other methods is shown for Brainweb T1-weighted volumes. For the AFS method the average of the values obtained by the six tests described above has been considered. The MSMC method refers to the fuzzy segmentation described in paper Angiati et al. [1], where seeds have been manually placed. The Fuzzy Vectorial method, reported in Zhuge et al. [20] makes

Table 8 Accuracy results for PD-weighted MRI volume, 1 % noise, s = 4 %, ρ = 95 %, φ = 0.3 %

	Specificity (%)	Sensitivity (%)	Accuracy (%)
CSF	98.14	81.06	96.09
GM	98.96	97.94	98.50
WM	95.02	94.06	94.75

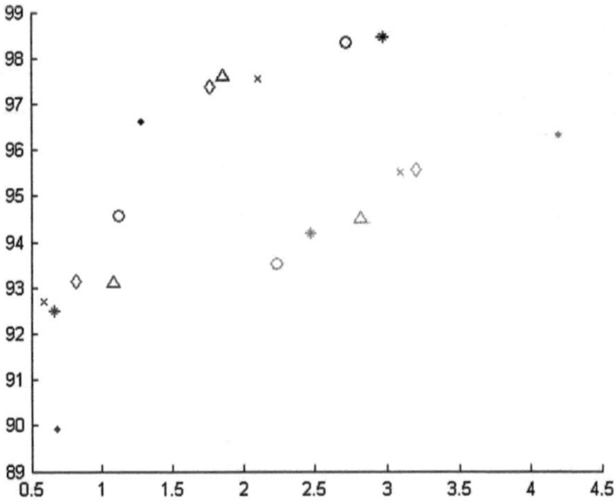

Fig. 7 ROC scatter plot of CSF (*blue*), GM (*red*), WM (*green*) for six different parameters' setting: s = 3 %, ρ = 90 %, φ = 0.3 %, s = 4 %, ρ = 95 %, φ = 0.3 %, s = 5 %, ρ = 90 %, φ = 0.3 %, s = 6 %, ρ = 90 %, φ = 0.3 %, s = 7 %, ρ = 90 %, φ = 0.3 % s = 8 %, ρ = 90 %, φ = 0.3 % for T1-weighted MRI volume, 3 % noise

use of the multiparametric volumes, by exploiting T1-weigthed, T2-weigthed and PD images at the same time. As one can notice all the AFS results are favourably comparable with the results of the other methods. Taking into account that the MSMC method does not work on volumes and the Fuzzy Vectorial works on T1-weighted and T2-weighted and PD data fusion, we should expect some improvements by AFS extension to 3D and multiparametric input. In Fig. 8 the ROC scatter plot related to the three methods are shown: AFS(red), MSMC(green) and Fuzzy Vectorial (blue). The graph refers to a T1-weighted image with 1 % noise, with s = 3 %, ρ = 95 %, φ = 0.3 %, and it presents all three classes CSF (circle), GM (triangle), WM (diamond). AFS performs always better than Fuzzy Vectorial method, both in terms of specificity and sensitivity. It was considered important also to report the ROC scatter plot for the six tests in the same parameters' setting (s = 8 %, ρ = 90 %, φ = 0.3 %) for a T1-weighted image with 3 % noise (Fig. 9). Each class is represented by a color: CFS by red, GM by blue, and WM by green. All three classes present a distribution much concentrated in a range 0–0.045 in terms of specificity and in a range 0.85–1 in terms of sensitivity . This is certainly a positive factor because it validates the

Table 9 Specificity and sensitivity parameters obtained by AFS method (s = 3 %, ρ = 95 %, $\varphi = 0.3\,\%$), MSMC algorithm, and fuzzy vectorial method for volumes with 1 % noise

	AFS-T1		MSMC-T1		Fuzzy vectorial	
	Spec. (%)	Sens. (%)	Spec. (%)	Sens. (%)	Spec. (%)	Sens. (%)
CSF	98.99	95.51	99.68	96.50	93.90	94.10
GM	98.83	98.69	98.13	92.76	94.80	94.80
WM	98.40	95.60	95.27	99.84	96.80	96.40

Table 10 Specificity and Sensitivity parameters obtained by AFS method (s = 8 %, ρ = 95 %, $\varphi = 0.3\,\%$), MSMC algorithm, and Fuzzy Vectorial method for volumes with 3 % noise

	AFS-T1		MSMC-T1		Fuzzy Vectorial	
	Spec. (%)	Sens. (%)	Spec. (%)	Sens. (%)	Spec. (%)	Sens. (%)
CSF	98.92	93.10	99.68	96.50	94.60	94.20
GM	98.14	97.61	98.13	92.76	92.30	95.80
WM	97.18	94.51	95.27	99.84	97.00	93.40

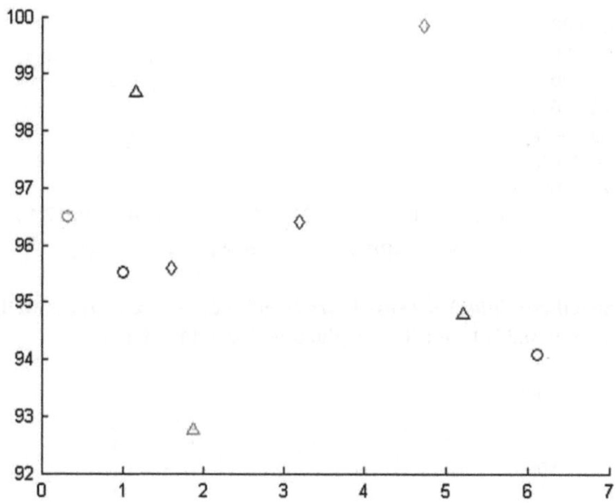

Fig. 8 ROC scatter plot of AFS (*red*), MSMC (*green*) and Fuzzy Vectorial (*blue*) for the three different classes: CSF (*circle*), GM (*triangle*), WM (*diamond*) T1-weighted image with 1 % noise. (s = 3 %, ρ = 95 %, $\varphi = 0.3\,\%$)

hypothesis of robustness and excellent performance of the method. Figures 10 and 11 lead to the same conclusions. Figure 10 shows the trend of Specificity (blue), sensitivity (red) and accuracy (green) indiscriminately for all three classes relative to the same configuration ($s = 8\,\%$, $\rho = 90\,\%$, $\varphi = 0.3\,\%$). As we can see the trend of the single value deviates little from a mean value, except for a negative peak (85 %) of sensitivity.

The same is true for the graph shown in Fig. 11, in which the trend of connected components' number and seed points' number is represented for the same configu-

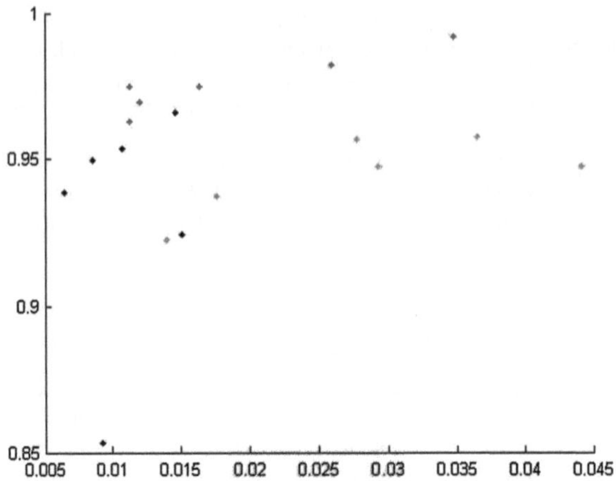

Fig. 9 ROC scatter plot ($s = 8\,\%$, $\rho = 90\,\%$, $\varphi = 0.3\,\%$) for a T1-weighted image with 3 % noise for CSF (*red*), GM (*blue*) and WM (*green*)

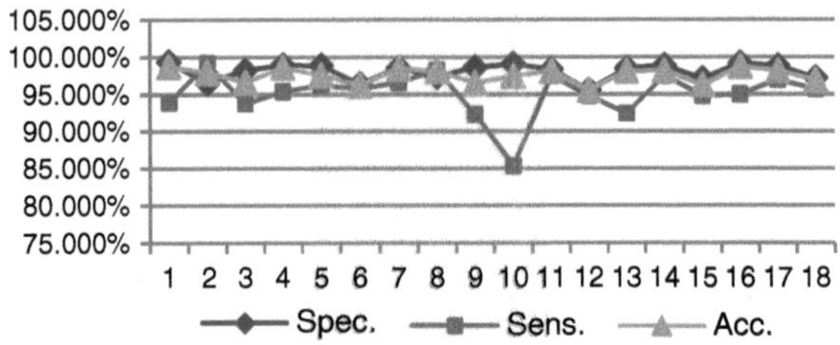

Fig. 10 Trend of Specificity (*blue*), sensitivity (*red*) and accuracy (*green*) for all three classes with ($s = 8\,\%$, $\rho = 90\,\%$, $\varphi = 0.3\,\%$) for a T1-weighted image with 3 % noise

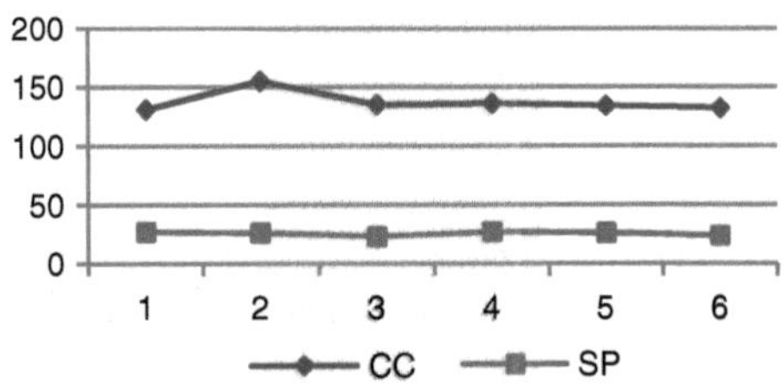

Fig. 11 Trend of connected components' number and seed points' number with $s = 8\,\%$, $\rho = 90\,\%$, $\varphi = 0.3\,\%$ for a T1-weighted image with, 3 % noise

ration ($s = 8\,\%$, $\rho = 90\,\%$, $\varphi = 0.3\,\%$). Also in this graph we can see that both variables oscillate slightly around their mean values ($CC_m = 137,2$ and $SP_m = 25,5$). This confirms again the robustness of the method.

As a final statistical analysis we show the Cohen's Kappa values for the six tests of this configuration ($s = 8\,\%$, $\rho = 90\,\%$, $\varphi = 0.3\,\%$) in Fig. 12. The value k is in

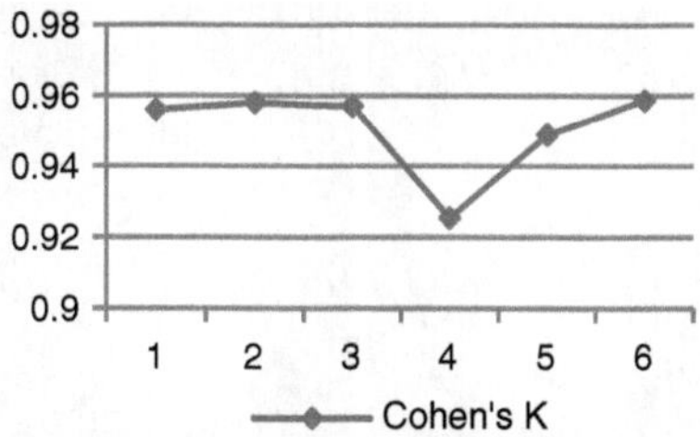

Fig. 12 Trend of Cohen's Kappa of each test with $s = 8\,\%$, $\rho = 90\,\%$, $\varphi = 0.3\,\%$ for a T1-weighted image with 3 % noise

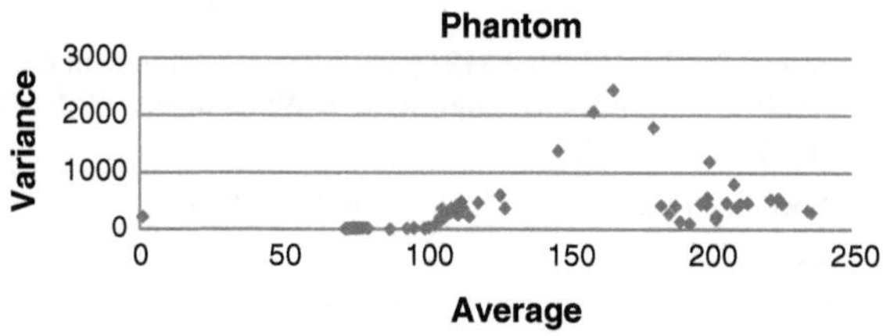

Fig. 13 Scatter plot of phantom's connected components gray levels for a T1-weighted image with 0 % noise

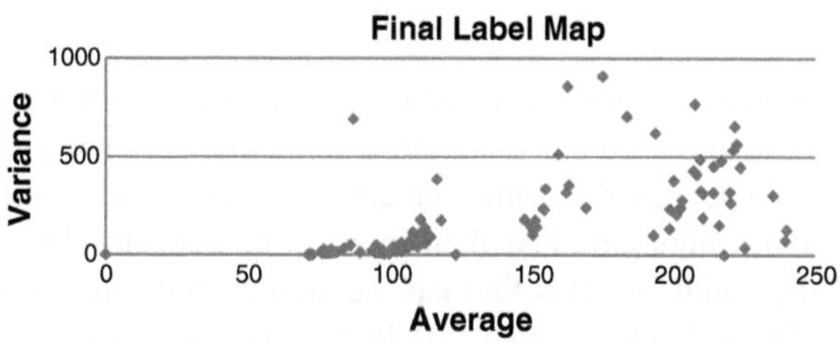

Fig. 14 Scatter plot of final label map 's connected components for a T1-weighted image with 0 % noise

the range (0,1) and k = 1 corresponds to the best case. Each test has a k value included in the range 0.92–0.96 and that means the AFS has good image processing performances (mean value: k = 0.95735). Finally we have done a new evaluation in terms of grey levels, related to each connected component. Figure 13 shows the scatter plot of phantom's connected components (CC = 79) with the grey level average on horizontal axis and the variance on vertical axis. Data are related to the T1-weighted image with 0 % noise and as one can notice, there is not a clear separation between the classes. In fact there are not very distinct clusters and a thresholding segmentation would not be enough to distinguish each region. However, despite this initial condition, the results shown above indicate a good AFS method performances.

Figure 14 shows the same scatter plot related to the connected components of the final label map Λ. As in the phantom's scatter plot the connected components with higher grey levels values are more scattered. It is also possible to notice a

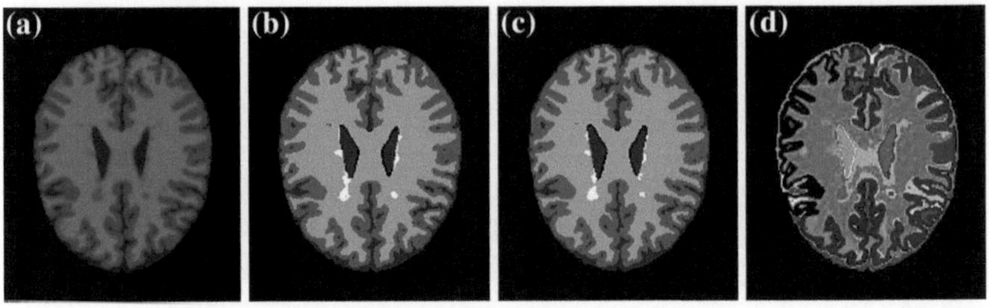

Fig. 15 Simulated T1-weighted MR pathological image, 100th slice: 0 % noise **a** Original image; **b** Label map; **c** Phantom (P), **d** Final label map Λ of the example

Table 11 Accuracy results for T1-weighted MRI pathological volume with 0 % noise , $s = 4\,\%$, $\rho = 95\,\%$, $\varphi = 0.1\,\%$ (CSF = Cerebrospinal fluid , WM = White matter, GM = Gray matter, MS= Multiple sclerosis lesions)

	Specificity (%)	Sensitivity (%)	Accuracy (%)
CSF	98.91	96.95	98.75
GM	96.50	99.23	97.91
WM	99.34	92.70	97.03
MS	88.46	83.83	88.44

greater separation between the classes when considering the average grey level as the discriminating feature. We can distinguish three intensity ranges: 60–120, 140–170 and 200–255. In general the connected components, found by the segmentation procedure, are more numerous and then more homogeneous than the connected components of the phantom. This fact can be appreciated looking at the variance values which are limited in the range 0–1000. This situation is a direct consequence of the segmentation procedure, whose aim is to partition the image into homogeneous regions.

3.4 AFS of Tissues with Multiple Sclerosis Lesions

In the proposed approach it was decided to discard the PD segmentation result because, as shown in the previous Section, it appears to be more affected by noise than T1-and T2-weighted images, thus increasing the confusion degree in the data fusion step. In addition, the information related to MS lesions brought by PD segmentation is very often redundant and coherent with information present in the T2 segmented volumes.

An example result of the just described process of the 100th slice, 0 % noise (Brainweb case) is shown in Fig. 15. The Fig. 15a shows the original image, Fig. 15b the Label map and Fig. 15c the Phantom (P). Figure 15d shows the related final label map Λ represented by a lookup table so that each connected component

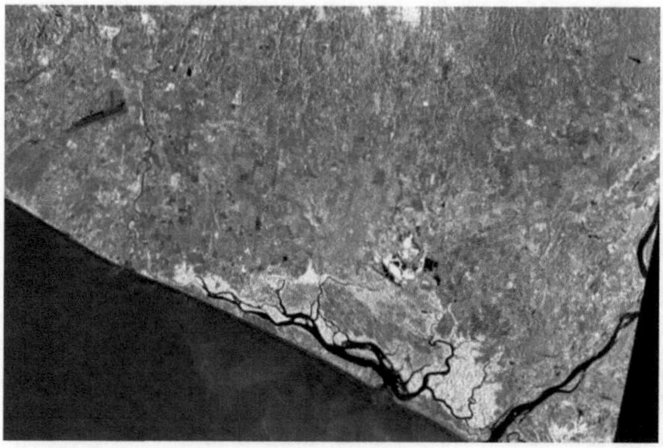

Fig. 16 A satellite SAR image

has a random colour. In Table 11 the obtained results are summarized in terms of sensitivity, specificity, accuracy, connected components' number and seed points' number with increasing noise. A very good specificity and accuracy are achieved for MS class, while sensitivity appears a little smaller. Anyway, it could be shown that very often the segmentation error does not rely on the lesion identification but sometimes an under-segmentation of the single object occurs. So that the error is not in the detection of the lesion but in its dimensionality estimation, that may be less critical if the application goal is limited to guide the medical staff toward a quick identification of the position of the lesions, leaving to a further and deeper step the analysis of original volumes to understand the lesion state. At last to make a full assessment we have to considered computational time. For the simplest case, i.e., a non-pathological T1-weighted image with 0 % noise the CPU time is 48 s. For the worst case, i.e., a pathological T1-weighted with 3 % noise, the CPU time at the prototypal level can be equal to 5 min, taking into account that no effort was spent in reducing processing time. These values can change depending on parameters' settings, but always with variations of a few seconds. Thanks to the specific parallelism intrinsic to the proposed method, the global computation time can be significantly reduced with appropriate SW and HW solutions.

3.5 Other Applications

To prove the general applicability of the AFS method, in this section, we present some tests on real MR volumes and in other application fields than biomedical imaging. Some tests have been performed on a satellite Synthetic Aperture Radar (SAR) image (Fig. 16) that has been acquired in the framework of the "OPERA – Civil protection from floods" project, which was funded by the Italian Space Agency (ASI) [15]. The AFS method has also been applied to a real T1-weighted MR brain image in coronal

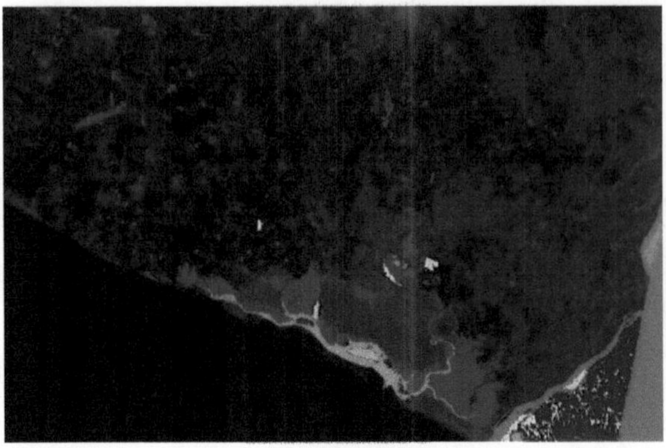

Fig. 17 Label map of satellite image

Fig. 18 IBSR image

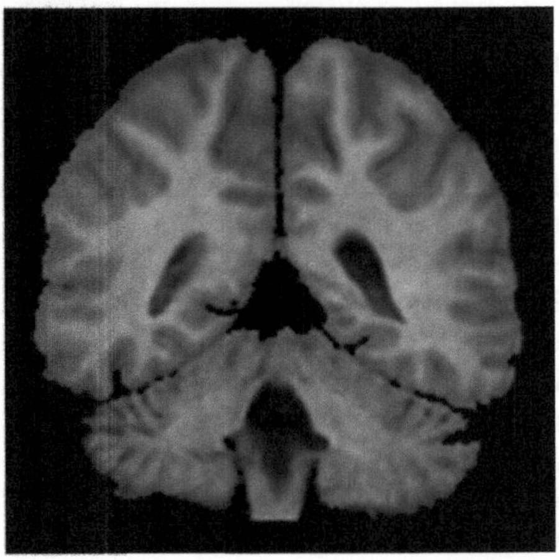

view provided by the Internet Brain Segmentation Repository (IBSR) [19] (Fig. 18). A random parameters' configuration has been tried only to offer the reader a visual result, without any specific evaluation in term of sensitivity, specificity or accuracy. We used the following parameters' setting: $s = 4\,\%$, $\rho = 85\,\%$, $\varphi = 0.3\,\%$. In Fig. 17 the label map Λ is shown related to the satellite image of Fig. 16; in Fig. 19 the label map related to Fig. 18 is shown with random colors. As one can see the AFS method achieves a good segmentation also with other type of images and so it could be used in other application fields.

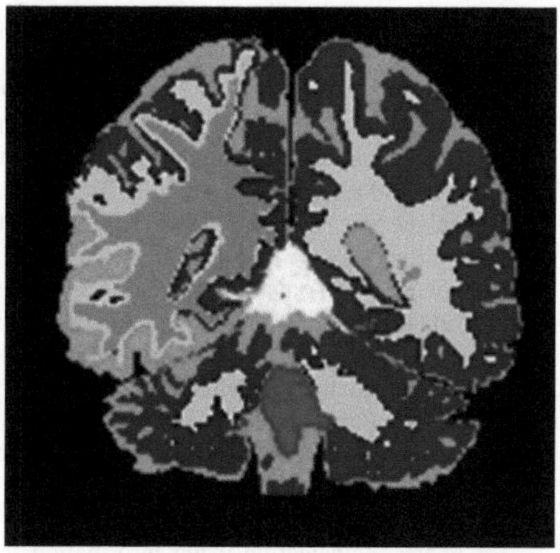

Fig. 19 Label map of IBSR image

4 Conclusions

In the current work, an automatic unsupervised fuzzy method for image segmentation has been proposed, the aim is the total segmentation of a digital image without user intervention. Performance evaluation of the method has been presented. The major advantage is that the present method does not require any a-priori information neither a training phase. As shown above, good results have been achieved, often comparable or superior to those presented in the literature but with the advantage that the present AFS method does not make use of any parameter estimation through a supervised phase. Since the AFS method is also independent on the image content and on the image resolution, it works well for any kind of images. The robustness of the method with respect to the three required parameters has been deeply investigated and has been here briefly discussed, showing very promising behaviours. As a final advantage, the proposed method is very simple and transparent to the user. Its extension to the multiparametric exploitation of more source channels is straightforward and should be related to better performance [11] quality.

References

1. Angiati E, Minetti I, Dellepiane SG (2010) Multi-seed segmentation of tomographic volumes based on fuzzy connectedness. In: De-Shuang H (ed) Advanced intelligent computing theories and applications with aspects of artificial intelligence. Springer, Heidelberg, p 360–367
2. Bezdek JC (1981) Pattern recognition with fuzzy objective function algorithms. Kluwer Academic Publishers, Norwell
3. Bloch I (1993) Fuzzy connectivity and mathematical morphology. Pattern recogn Lett 14(6):483–488
4. Cocosco CA, Kollokian V, Kwan RK-S, Pike GB, Evans AC (1997) Brainweb: online interface to a 3D MRI simulated brain database. NeuroImage 5(4):425

5. Dellepiane SG (1991) Image segmentation: errors, sensitivity, and uncertainty. In: Proceedings of the annual international conference of the IEEE. Engineering in Medicine and Biology Society, vol 13, pp 253–254. 31 Oct–3 Nov 1991. doi:10.1109/IEMBS.1991.683923
6. Dellepiane SG, Carbone V, Nardotto S (2012) An automatic unsupervised fuzzy method for image segmentation. In: Computational modeling of objects presented in images: fundamentals, methods and applications, p 307–312
7. Dellepiane SG, Fontana F (1995) Extraction of intensity connectedness for image processing. Pattern Recogn Lett 16(3):313–324
8. Dellepiane SG, Fontana F, Vernazza GL (1996) Nonlinear image labeling for multivalued segmentation. IEEE Trans Image Process 5(3):429–446
9. Gour CK, Laurence D, Mahbubur RS (2001) Review of fuzzy image segmentation techniques. In: Design and management of multimedia information systems: opportunities and challenges. Idea Group Publishing, Hershey
10. Kaufmann A (1977) Introduction à la théorie des sous-ensembles flous à l'usage des ingénieurs (fuzzy sets theory). Masson
11. Kim J, Fisher JW III, Yezzi A, Çetin M, Willsky AS (2005) A nonparametric statistical method for image segmentation using information theory and curve evolution. IEEE Trans Image Process 14(10):1486–1502
12. Rosenfeld A (1983) On connectivity properties of grayscale pictures. Pattern Recogn 16(1):47–50
13. Rosenfeld A (1984) The fuzzy geometry of image subsets. Pattern Recogn Lett 2(5):311–317
14. Saha PK, Udupa JK (2001) Relative fuzzy connectedness among multiple objects: theory, algorithms, and applications in image segmentation. Comput Vis Image Underst 82(1):42–56
15. Serpico SB, Dellepiane S, Moser G, Angiati E, Boni G, Rudari R, Candela L (2012) Extracting information from remote sensing data for applications to flood monitoring and damage evaluation. In: Advances in radar and remote sensing (TyWRRS), 2012 Tyrrhenian Workshop on IEEE, p 275–282
16. Shapiro L, Stockman G (2001) Computer vision (Chap. 12). New Jersey, Prentice Hall
17. Udupa JK, Samarasekera S (1996) Fuzzy connectedness and object definition: theory, algorithms, and applications in image segmentation. Graph Models Image Process 58(3):246–261
18. Vaccaro R, Smits PC, Dellepiane SG (2000) Exploiting spatial correlation features for SAR image analysis. IEEE Trans Geosci Remote Sens 38(3):1212–1223. doi:10.1109/36.843013
19. Worth A (1996) The Internet brain segmentation repository (IBSR). http://www.cma.mgh.Harvard.edu/ibsr
20. Zhuge Y, Udupa JK, Saha PK (2006) Vectorial scale-based fuzzy-connected image segmentation. Comput Vis Image Underst 101(3):177–193

The e-Slide in the e-Laboratory of Cytology: Where are We?

Daniele Giansanti, Mauro Grigioni, Marco Pochini, Sandra Morelli, Giuseppe D'Avenio, Alberto Boschetto, Luana Bottini and Maria Rosaria Giovagnoli

Abstract The work approaches the new technological scenario relevant to the introduction of the e-slide in the e-Laboratory of cytology. A detailed analysis of the state of introduction of the technology based on the e-slides has been conducted. The analysis focused on the ICT technologies available for both the remote diagnosis and the cooperative diagnosis in the Hospital based using the e-slide. In particular the work critically investigated the scenarios of introduction of the e-slides with particular attention to the client/server technologies, the tablet solutions, the 3D Virtual reality solutions. From a global point of view the chapter showed that the today's technologies using the e-slide have a great potentiality in the digital-cytology.

Keywords Digital pathology · Digital slide · Digital-cytology

1 Introduction

The virtual microscopy is an alternative solution between the static and dynamic tele-pathology. Telemedicine applied to pathology is considered a valid aid to pathologists [9]; in fact it is supposed to allow the remote exchanging of information about a tissue or a cellular group on a slide; in particular:

D. Giansanti (✉) · M. Grigioni · S. Morelli · G. D'Avenio
Dipartimento di Tecnologie e Salute, Istituto Superiore di Sanità, Roma, Italy
e-mail: daniele.giansanti@iss.it

M. Pochini · M. R. Giovagnoli
Dipartimento di Medicina Clinica e Molecolare, Facoltà di Medicina e Psicologia, Università Sapienza, Roma, Italy

A. Boschetto · L. Bottini
Dipartimento di Ingegneria Meccanica e Aereospaziale, Università Sapienza, Roma, Italy

P. Di Giamberardino et al. (eds.), *Computational Modeling of Objects Presented in Images*, Lecture Notes in Computational Vision and Biomechanics 15,
DOI: 10.1007/978-3-319-04039-4_5,

(1) The tele-diagnosis;
(2) The audit of complex cases, by means of shared virtual desktop;
(3) The minimization of resources (more hospitals could share the professionals).

There are two basic methods of Tele-Pathology (T-P). Static T-P consists in the capture and digitalization of images selected by a pathologist or pathologist assistant, which are then transmitted through electronic means remotely. Dynamic T-P consists in the direct communication between two different centres by using microscopes equipped with a tele-robotic system oriented to explore the slide, remotely operated by the tele-pathologist who makes the diagnosis. As an alternative solution between the two methods, widely increasing today is the diffusion of virtual microscopy (VM) [1]. The latter does not refer to the tele-control of microscopes, whilst the glass is scanned as a whole, producing a "e-slide", and a pathologist can navigate remotely (via internet) inside this e-slide or virtual slide in a manner similar to a real microscope.

Until recently the management of the information on the glasses in tele-pathology applications was principally based on the design and construction of a few identical and expensive platforms with microscope units and software tools for both the display and the tele-control (zooming, moving cutting of pieces of images) [3, 6]. In the first applications of these methodologies the latency of information during the transmission caused displacement errors in the positioning of the microscope's mechanics on the glass. For these reasons the need of investigation based on the so called virtual microscopy with virtual navigation on scanned images without using tele-control provided new solutions. Severe problems were also noticed for example in the remote information exchange. The lacking of both a wide-band channel and an ad-hoc visualization strategy strongly delayed the image transmission. It has to be considered that a single file representing a e-slide for cytology applications could reach several tens of gigabytes, more than in the case of applications of tele-echography [3]. Thus the design of an appropriate Visualization Strategy is a basic core aspect. Clearly it is not feasible and reasonable to fully manage a single file of several GB in the World Area Network!

Today the Scenario is completely changed thanks to the introduction of the VM. The principal changes in the world of the Information Technologies affecting Tele Pathology were the following:

- Availability of wide band channels.
- Diffusion of new Visualization strategies.
- Availability of new power image scanners.
- Availability of free visualization software.

The first point was driven by the diffusion of the Information Communication technologies (ICT) for Internet/Intranet/Extranet connections. The second point was driven by the pressing request of very large image exchange by internet. New methodologies today allow the archiving of an image arranged in layers assigned to different magnification factors [6] and answers to the so called internet need "I give you something to see before you become angry!!", as for example in Google Earth and allow

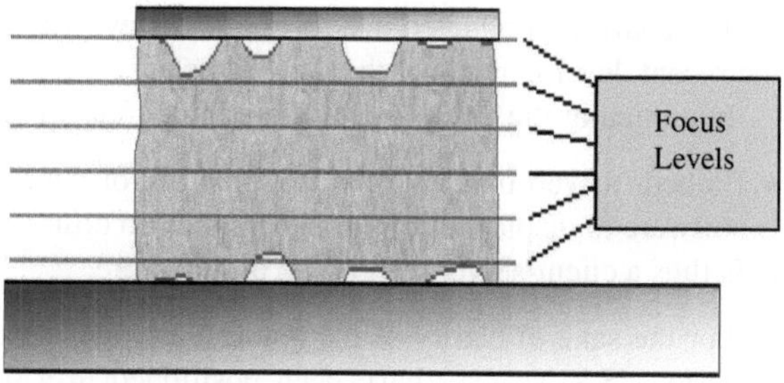

Fig. 1 Example from scanning process in the case of the Z-stack

a remote information exchange using a reasonable wide-band-channel. The third point was driven by the exceptional changes in photonics applied to medicine. Many producers, leaders in photonics, are using their skill to design scanners for virtual microscopy. The fourth point was driven by the diffusion of free web-viewers and by new commercial strategies of the producers of tele-pathology systems. In order to face deeply the introduction of the use of digital cytology we have to make the following basic considerations.

The Tele-pathology mainly relates to the world of histology; the histologist navigates the slide without the need to use the focus function. The e-slide in histology does not require the emulation of the focus function; in histology it is sufficient a flattened vision, in other words the histologist does not need to "smash" in the sample.

When coming to the Digital Cytology (D-CYT) which relates to the world of cytologist, basic problems arise. At first, the cytologist uses a way to navigate completely different from the histologist: she or he in fact widely uses the focus function. Then, we should consider that the cytologist on the contrary to the histologist, uses a lateral area of the eye while navigating (the same used by the primitives to avoid animals attacks); as a consequence of this second aspect a third aspect arises, i.e the stereo-vision is much more important for the cytologist. The focus can be emulated by software, by means of specific functions using also interpolation algorithms not opened to the user. This implies that, at a defined zoom, several focal planes are captured (till 100) for a given sample (depending on the thickness of the sample and the chosen level of magnification). This leads to the generation of very large e-slides during the digitization, and the focus function at a defined zoom should be emulated by generating different images ready for interpolation; in the VM this functionality is called by manufacturers "Z-stack" (Fig. 1). This implies the generation of e-slides tens time larger than in the case of pathology. Furthermore the cytologist's needs are different from the ones of the pathologist when he or she interacts with the VM.

2 Flow of the Work

An analysis has been conducted on the chance to introduce the D-CYT technology in the Hospital and more in general in the dispersed territory.

The analysis conducted in a form of a review was arranged with consideration of the recent developments of the technologies.

In particular the analysis considered that today a system for the D-CYT:

- Embeds a Web-based server as repository of the e-slides and clients with a light software to display, often furnished with no costs.
- Is thus a client-server web-based architecture.

For the sake of clarity of the reader 3 e-slides scanned by means of the Aperio (Aperio, USA) scanner have been positioned in a sever at the URL http://www.diditalslide.it.

Two applications furnished by Aperio allow the reaching of the e-slides by means of the Virtual Navigation and have been used in the study.

The first one is Image-scope which compatible to the Windows OS platforms.

The second one is Spectrum Web Viewer, which is automatically loaded in the browser as soon as the e-slide is reached by the mouse pointer.

Both the two applications can be used in the PC platform, while only the second one seems to be suitable for the use in the Tablets.

The first one has more functionalities; in particular it allows the extraction from the e-slide of separate small images, called snapshots relevant to details useful for example for the diagnosis, useful to exchange because their occupancy is thousands times lower than the e-slide.

The second one, being browser based allows the remote exchange of Url-Links relevant to details useful for the diagnosis [6]. These Url can be exchanged without the need of memory space (being only simple chars) over the WAN.They have been proved to be a useful methodology for telemedicine tele-consulting: one remotely receives the Url and as soon as He or She points on it reaches the details of the e-slide. Figure 2 shows the, to date, standardized accessing to the e-slide using a PC platform. In particular it enlightens:

- The login screen to the web-server (A)
- The interface based on image-scope (B)
- The interface based on Spectrum Web-Viewer (C)

3 ICT and the e-Slides

The study focused on the available ICT technologies allowing client-server web-based architecture for the integration of the use of eslides over the network.

In particular the study investigated the tablet technology, the integration with the 3D technologies and the standardization stage with particular care to the integration with DICOM standard.

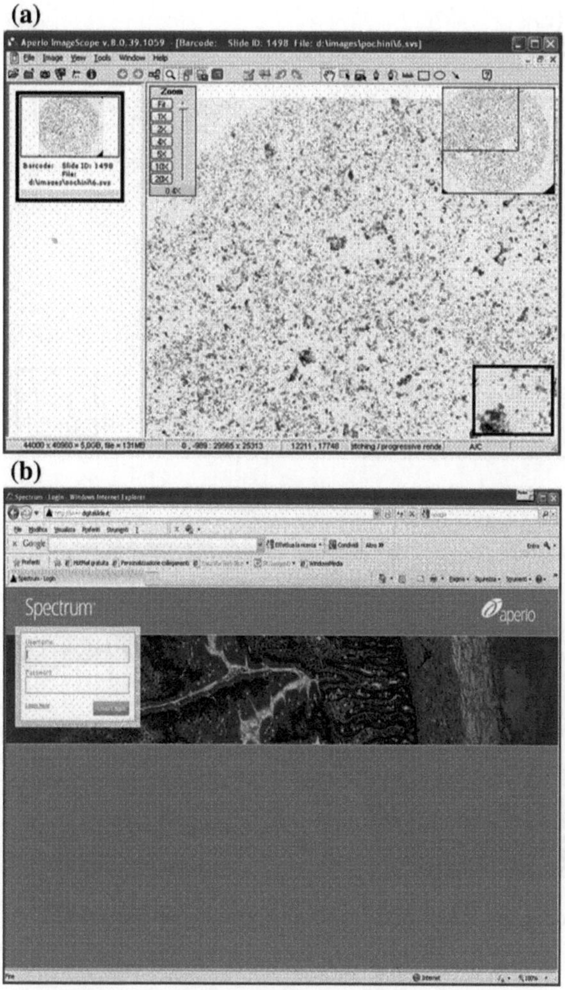

Fig. 2 Accessing to e-slides. **a** The server at the URL www.digitalslide.it. **b** Navigating by means of Image-Scope. **c** Navigating by means of spectrum web viewer

3.1 The Tablet Technologies and the e-Slides

Among the available promising technologies to share image information using the e-slide, the following have been investigated, focusing on D-CYT:

- Smart-phones (wearable-tablet).
- A4-tablet (portable-tablet) such as the Apple Ipad.
- Large touch table (not-portable table) such as the Epson xDesk.

(c)

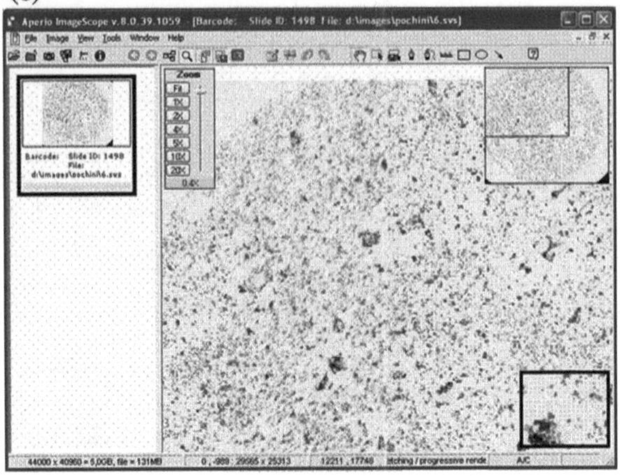

Fig. 2 continued

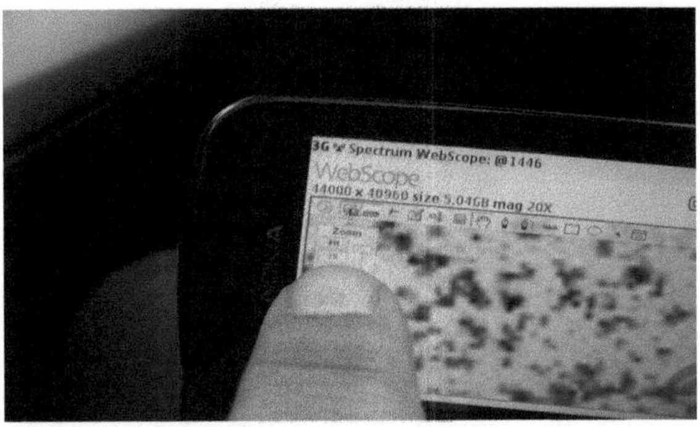

Fig. 3 Example of an application of digital-cytology on a wearable tablet

Starting from the previously described set-up we have accessed to the e-slides remotely positioned in the WEB server at the URL www.digitalslide.it using the three different tablet technologies.

The first two systems, that are widely used for many different purposes, allow to reach everyone in the world, therefore representing a chance for the remote consulting in D-CYT. Regarding the last technology, we focused on the Epson XDesk. Figures 3 and 4 show the access to an e-slide using the Spectrum Web Viewer form Aperio using wearable and portable technologies.

The Epson XDesk (www.epson.it) represents a powerful ICT solution for cooperative analysis and discussion of cases of virtual cytology. In detail, the Epson XDesk is an interactive table; some call it a coffee table because you can put anything on the surface of the table, it works by projections, with the very latest technology on that. This desk is also compatible with Bluetooth communication protocol and as soon as

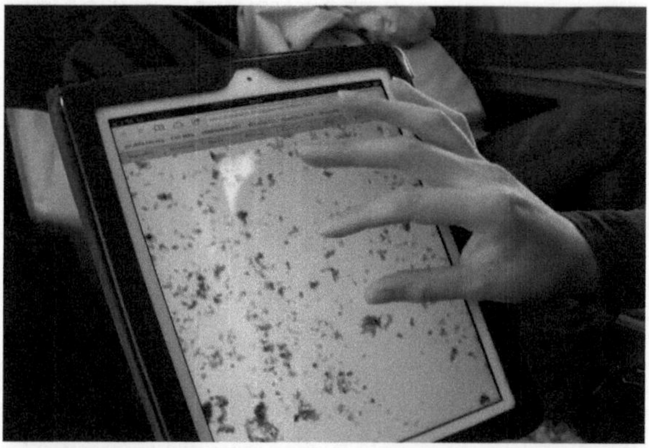

Fig. 4 Example of an application of digital-cytology on a portable tablet

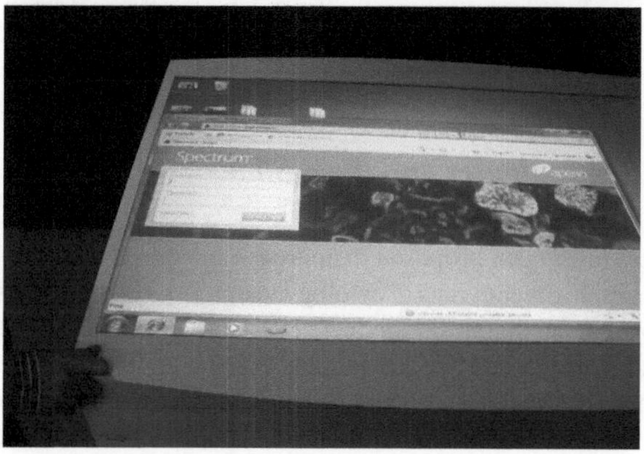

Fig. 5 Remote access and navigation using the xDesk

you put your phone or camera on the surface of the table, the XDesk will be able to see all your files and pictures on the desk. By natural interface pictures on the table can be managed freely and resized, zoomed in and out by finger movements as the iPod touch does, only on a fair larger scale. The Epson XDesk has a 52 inch screen and a 1024×768 touch screen display. It represents the appropriate high technology solution for cooperative discussions, clinical audit, and ultimately the future direction of cooperative virtual microscopy environment. Furthermore it could represent a tool suitable to recover the inheritance of cytology solutions for large screening abandoned because the technology was not so ready for the application, such as PapNet (Neuromedical Systems, Suffern, NY) for computer assisted cervical/vaginal cytology diagnosis [7]. Figures 5 and 6 show a scenario of cooperative decision with XDesk.

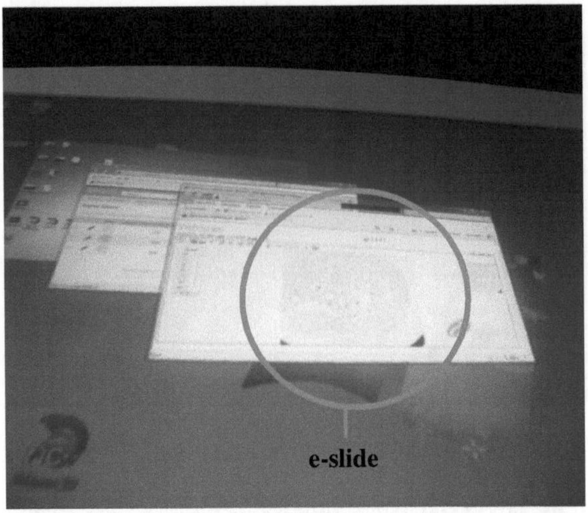

Fig. 6 Detail of an e-slide on the xDesk

3.2 The 3D Technologies and the e-Slides

Different studies have been proposed to approach the introduction of the potentialities of 3D/holographic techniques in cytology vision [8]. However these studies have only dealt with the local diagnosis conducted in stand-alone equipments and have not been conducted over the WAN/LAN in telemedicine applications apart for cardiovascular purpose (the specific targeted research project Collaborative Holographic Environments for Networked Tasks, COHERENT) [2]. The use of these techniques in consideration to the importance of the stereovision of the cytologist, could be of help both to emulate the stereovision thanks to the use of 3D/holographic techniques and to minimize the data transfer among remote nodes as a partial solution for the area occupancy caused by the Z-stack.

3.3 Integration to DICOM of the e-Slides

Two Work Groups (WG)s of the NEMA are facing the integration of the D-CYT into DICOM. The WG26 operates in synergy with the NEMA WG6 [7, 8], the group responsible for the adequacy to the standard, reviewer of the activity of the WG26. The initial objectives of the WG26 were to extend minimal capabilities to describe specimens in DICOM and to create a mechanism to allow exchange and use of whole slide microscopic images within DICOM. The long term goals were to face the integration of also other imaging modalities, such as multi-spectral images, electron microscopy, flow cytometry (another field of D-CYT). The recent approval of the DICOM supplement 145 (Supplement 145: Whole Slide Microscopic Image IOD and SOP Classes) in the 2010/08/24, by the DICOM WG 26 allows today to store the digital pathology images also from D-CYT in a form that is compatible with the same DICOM archive systems used by hospitals and opens new chances for D-CYT. The D-CYT in fact uses very large files in D-CYT (>2GB), the Whole Slide Images (WSI)s produced by digitizing microscope slides at diagnostic resolution. In addition these WSIs have a different type of access regarding the other digital images stored in the PACS systems, due to the fact that the pathologist needs to rapidly pan and zoom images. The WSI representation allows to also consider the Z-stack problem of the D-CYT. The 145 supplement addresses also the considerations available in a previous supplement, the 122 supplement (Supplement 122: Specimen Module and Revised Pathology SOP Classes), about the digital microscopic images. The 145 supplement furnishes now the definitions of the WSI as DICOM Information Object Definitions and describes the WSI image characteristics. Vendors of D-CYT products will make in the next years efforts to adequate their products to the new standards and probably will suggest revisions on the basis of their analysis.

4 Future Perspective of the e-Slides

Today thanks to the development of the information technology, the diffusion of new visualization strategies and the availability of low cost or free visualization proprietary tools, the scenario of the tele-pathology has radically changed: the Virtual Microscopy offers new promising opportunities oriented to the application of D-CYT. This study has investigated the technologies to promote the diffusion of the e-slide via the web-based-client-server technologies. Three important directions have been considered important for the diffusion of the e-slide. The first direction is the use of the tablets. As these technologies are particularly useful for the multimedia image management, using for example the finger based functions, they could be of aid for navigating the e-slide, speeding operation. Three examples of connections to the e-slides, respectively using a wearable/portable and not-potable tablet have been elucidated in the work. Wearable and portable tablets are showing interesting perspectives for remotely tele-consult the e-slide [4, 5]. The not-portable tablets; as for example the Epson Xdesk is showing promising perspectives for the so-called cooperative diagnosis in the e-Laboratory of cytology; in particular it could substitute the traditional methodology based on the multiple-heads-scope. The second direction is the 3D technology, which could be particularly useful for navigating the e-slides in D-CYT were there is the need of emulating both the focus functions and the stereo-vision. Furthermore it could reduce the amount of data to exchange [4].The third direction is the integration to DICOM. It is basic for the integration of the e-slides in the routine Hospital applications as in the case of the digital-radiology [7]. It should be considered, as final global consideration, that specific methodologies of HTA should be introduced to investigate the performances and acceptance of the technology [3, 6]. At the moment we are investigating the design of a HTA tool specific for the D-CYT and the tablets.

References

1. Çatalyürek Ü, Beynon MD, Chang C, Kurc T, Sussman A, Saltz J (2003) The virtual microscope. IEEE Trans Inf Technol Biomed 7(4):14–22
2. D'Avenio G, Balogh T, Grigioni M (2007) Holographic display as innovative training tool. In: ESAO 2007, XXXIV annual congress european society for artificial organs, Krems, Austria, 5–8 Sept 2007
3. Giansanti D, Morelli S, Macellari V (2007) Telemedicine technology assessment part I: setup and validation of a quality control system. Telemed J E Health 13(2):118–129
4. Giansanti D, Castrichella L, Giovagnoli MR (2008) Telepathology training in a master of cytology degree course. J Telemed Telecare 14(7):338–341
5. Giansanti D, Castrichella L, Giovagnoli MR (2008) Telepathology requires specific training for the technician in the biomedical laboratory. Telemed J E Health 14(8):801–807
6. Giansanti D, Castrichella L, Giovagnoli MR (2008) The design of a health technology assessment system in telepathology. Telemed J E Health 14(6):570–575
7. Giansanti D, Grigioni M, D'Avenio G, Morelli S, Maccioni G, Bondi A, Giovagnoli MR (2010) Virtual microscopy and digital cytology: state of the art. Ann Ist Super Sanita 46(2):115–122
8. Giansanti D, Cerroni F, Amodeo R, Filoni M, Giovagnoli MR (2010) A pilot study for the integration of cytometry reports in digital cytology telemedicine applications. Ann Ist Super Sanita 46(2):138–143
9. Weisz-Carrington P, Blount M, Kipreos B, Mohanty L, Lippman R, Todd WM, Trent B (1999) Telepathology between richmond and beckley veterans affairs hospitals: report on the first 1000 cases. Telem J 5(4):367–373

Fatigue Loading of a Ferritic Ductile Cast Iron: Damaging Characterization

Vittorio Di Cocco, Daniela Iacoviello, Francesco Iacoviello and Alessandra Rossi

Abstract Ductile cast irons offer and interesting combination of overall mechanical properties and technological peculiarities, allowing to obtain a high castability (peculiar of cast irons) with good tensile strength and toughness values (peculiar of steels). This result is due to their chemical composition that allows to obtain graphite elements in nodular shape directly from the melt. Ductile cast iron mechanical properties are strongly influenced both by the matrix microstructure and by the graphite nodules. The role of these elements cannot be merely ascribed to a simple matrix-graphite "debonding" damaging mechanism, but, according to previously published results, this role is more complex. In this work, customized image processing procedures were optimized to analyze the evolution of the damaging micromechanisms in a fatigue loaded ferritic ductile cast iron, focusing the graphite elements.

Keywords Ferritic ductile cast iron · Image analysis · Damage characterization

1 Introduction

Since 1948, from the first announce by Henton Morrogh during the AFS Convention, ductile cast irons (DCIs) have offered very interesting mechanical properties only by means of the chemical composition control: neither high temperature nor long

V. Di Cocco · F. Iacoviello · A. Rossi
Dipartimento di Ingegneria Civile e Meccanica, Università di Cassino e del Lazio Meridionale, Cassino, Italy

D. Iacoviello (✉)
Dipartimento di Ingegneria Informatica Automatica e Gestionale Antonio Ruberti, Sapienza Università di Roma, Rome, Italy
e-mail: iacoviello@dis.uniroma1.it

P. Di Giamberardino et al. (eds.), *Computational Modeling of Objects Presented in Images*, Lecture Notes in Computational Vision and Biomechanics 15,
DOI: 10.1007/978-3-319-04039-4_6, © Springer International Publishing Switzerland 2014

duration heat treatments were no more necessary to obtain the desired shape of graphite elements (nodules), with a consequent strong cost reduction. DCIs combine the good castability of gray irons and the toughness of steels and in the last decades, different chemical compositions and heat treatments have been optimized in order to control the matrix microstructure and obtain different combinations of mechanical properties [11, 12]. DCIs are widely used for transportation of raw and tap water, sewage, slurries and process chemicals (in the form of ductile iron pipes), in safety related components for automotive applications (gears, bushings, suspension, brakes, steering, crankshafts) and in more critical applications as containers for storage and transportation of nuclear wastes.

The most common DCIs grades are characterized by ferritic, pearlitic and ferritic-pearlitic matrix and are usually used in the as-cast conditions:

- Ferritic DCIs are characterized by good ductility and a tensile strength that is equivalent to that of a low carbon steel: these grades can be produced either "as-cast" or by means of annealing heat treatments.
- Pearlitic DCIs show higher strength values, good wear resistance and moderate ductility, and their machinability is higher than steels of analogous mechanical properties.
- Ferritic-pearlitic DCIs are the most common grades and are usually produced in the "as cast" conditions: their properties are intermediate between ferritic and pearlitic ones, with good machinability and low production cost.

DCIs can be also alloyed and/or heat treated, obtaining a wide variety of additional grades (Fig. 1) characterized by really interesting mechanical properties:

- Martensitic DCIs show very high strength and wear resistance, but with low toughness and ductility values.
- Bainitic DCIs are characterized by a high hardness.
- Austenitic DCIs show good corrosion resistance, good strength and dimensional stability at high temperature.
- Austempered DCIs (ADI), the most recent grades in the DCI family, are produced by heat-treating cast ductile iron to which small amounts of nickel, molybdenum, or copper have been added to improve hardenability. Austempered DCIs are characterized by increased toughness values, high tensile strength (up to 1750 MPa) and good wear resistance.

DCIs good ductility is mainly due to the peculiar graphite elements morphology and a good graphite nodules nucleation, morphology and distribution is always recommended for all the applications. In order to characterize and improve the DCIs mechanical behavior, an intense research activity has been developed to analyze the effect of the microstructural characteristics on the mechanical properties, considering both the matrix and the graphite nodules. The contribution of graphite nodules

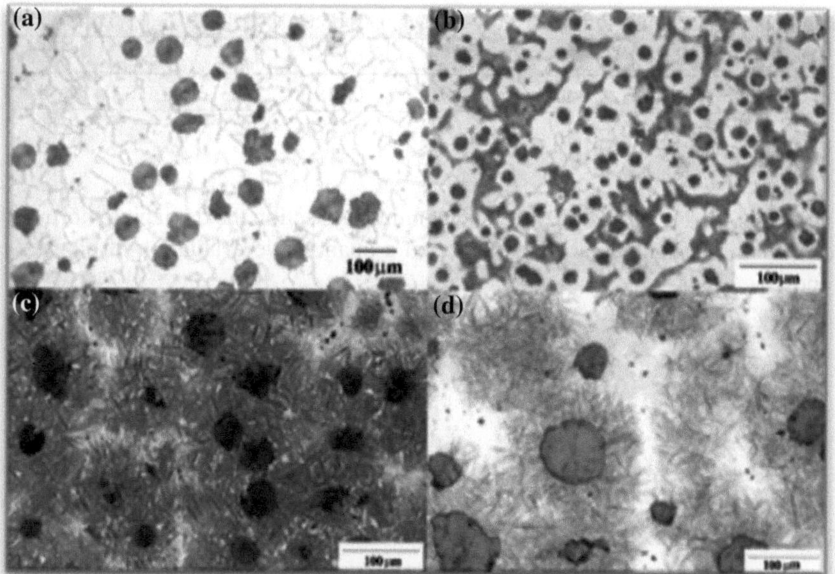

Fig. 1 **a** Ferritic DCI; **b** ferritic-pearlitic DCI; **c** and **d** two different ADI

to the developing of the internal damage during a static or cyclic loading of a DCI is not univocally determined, [1–5, 9, 10, 14–19]. Some authors consider the graphite nodules as "rigid spheres" not bonded to the matrix and acting like voids under tension. Other authors consider graphite nodules as "crack-arresters", due to their peculiar shape that minimizes the stress intensification at the crack tip. Other authors, in fatigue crack propagation conditions, consider graphite nodules as "crack closure effect raisers", due to the role they play at the lower values of the applied stress intensity factor (K_{min}).

Image analysis may help in the identification and characterization of damage. The aim is to obtain an objective evaluation of damage without the supervision of an operator. The main difficulty is related with the quality of the data that may be corrupted for the presence of dust or scratches or non uniform illumination. By considering the image before the damage took place, it would be possible to decide a suitable preprocessing procedure to reduce the effects of degradation. In particular for the analyzed data a second order statistic filter and an adaptive histogram equalization were the main image analysis operations adopted, as will be shown in the next section. The chapter is organized as follows: in the first part of the Material and Methods Section the damaging micromechanisms acting on the investigated alloy are described, whereas in the second part the image analysis procedure adopted is

Table 1 Investigated fully ferritic DCI chemical composition (GJS 350-22)

C	Si	Mn	S	P	Cu	Cr	Mg	Sn
3.62	2.72	0.19	0.011	0.021	0.019	0.031	0.047	0.011

outlined. In the Numerical Results and Comments Section the damaging morphologies in graphite nodules are identified and a quantitative evaluation of damage is proposed.

2 Materials and Methods

In this section, the investigated alloy and the damaging micromechanisms are described, along with the image analysis procedure adopted and the damage evaluation criteria considered.

2.1 Materials

Investigated DCI chemical composition is shown in Table 1. It is characterized by a fully ferritic microstructure and by a very high graphite elements nodularity (higher than 85 %, with a volume fraction of graphite elements of about 9–10 %; 132 nodules/mm^2).

Fatigue tests were performed considering microtensile specimens (25 × 2 × 1 mm). Specimens were ground and polished and fatigue loaded intermittently with a tensile holder and observed in situ using a Scanning Electron Microscope (SEM), considering 20 graphite elements. During fatigue tests, specimens deformation and applied load were measured by means of a Linear Variable Differential Transformer (LVDT) and two miniature load cells (10 kN each), respectively. Figures 2a, b show the tensile holder and the tensile test machine, respectively.

Fatigue tests were repeated three times and performed under load control conditions ($\sigma_{max} = 320$ MPa; $\sigma_{min} = 120$ MPa), with a loading frequency of 0.03 Hz. In order to perform scanning electron microscope (SEM) observations, fatigue loading was stopped every 1000 cycles (near final rupture observations frequency is higher).

Focusing the graphite nodules, the damage usually follows a sort of "onion-like" sequence, with the damage that became more and more evident with the cycles number (Fig. 3). Seldom, a crack in the nodule center is observed, probably corresponding to the nucleation site, but the main damaging micromechanism is the one shown in Fig. 3.

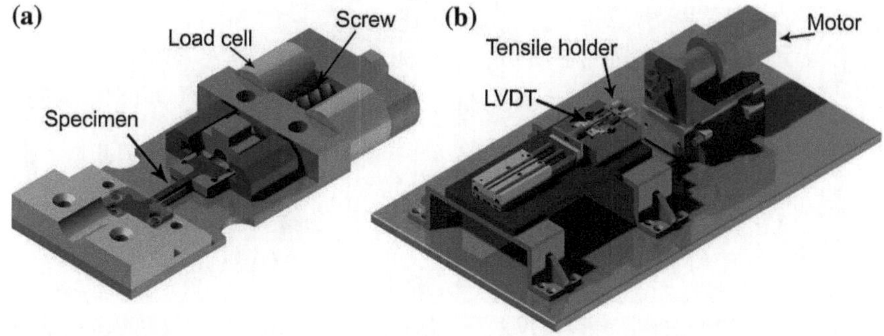

Fig. 2 **a** Removable holder with microtensile specimen; **b** fatigue testing machine

2.2 Methods: Image Analysis

As already pointed out in the Introduction, image analysis may help in the identification and quantification of the effects of damage. At a first sight, its effects appear evident but an automatic detection results difficult due to the presence of scratches and dust. Moreover different kind of damage effects may be present in the same specimen, each of them requiring a different identification procedure. In this chapter the interest is focused on the effects that present the shape of thin curvilinear rectangular, whereas a darker kernel, mainly positioned in the center of the damaged specimen, will not be analyzed. The operation that may help in damage identification is the segmentation; as well known, it is the partition of the image into regions homogeneous with respect to a chosen property, [8]. For the data of this application the objects of interest are the darkest elements of the image, therefore a segmentation with respect to the gray level is required.

The elements of interest are generally not neatly separated one each other and from the background, see Fig. 4 as an example. Therefore before proceeding with the segmentation step a suitable preprocessing is advisable.

First the original data is filtered by a 2-D statistic filter: the image is partitioned into square domains of chosen size and each element in the domain is replaced by the m-order element in the sorted set of neighbors identified by the nonzero elements in the same region. The result is a more uniform image, thus helping in avoiding isolated and small region detection.

The obtained image wasn't yet suitable for the segmentation, and it was necessary to enhance the contrast by a contrast-limited adaptive histogram equalization; again the image is partitioned in tiles, whose contrast is enhanced in order to obtain an histogram of each tile as much as possible similar to a chosen distribution. In the present application the uniform distribution was assumed. This operation was performed without enhancing the darker kernel damage. Finally a gamma correc-

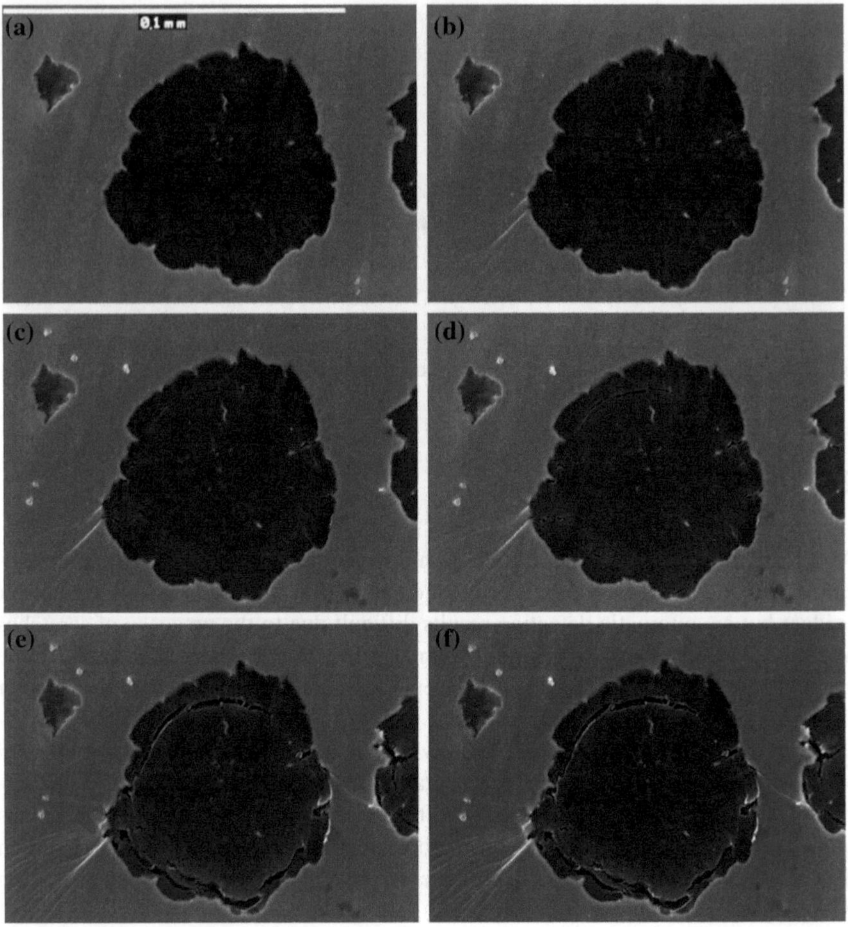

Fig. 3 Graphite nodule damaging evolution. SEM in situ surface analysis corresponding to the following loading cycles: **a** 1; **b** 14100; **c** 38300; **d** 40100; **e** 46000; **f** 48100 cycles

tion operation was useful for illumination problems due to the image acquisition procedure. The processed data was segmented by using the Otsu method, [13]. This method was chosen for its effectiveness, even if, as pointed out in [7], also the discrete level set method [6] yielded satisfactory results. The Otsu method is based on the assumption that the histogram of the data is bi-modal and therefore two classes of pixels are considered, the object and the background. The optimal threshold is obtained by minimizing the intra-class variance:

$$\sigma_{\omega}^{2}(t) = \omega_{1}(t)\,\sigma_{1}^{2}(t) + \omega_{2}(t)\,\sigma_{2}^{2}(t)$$

Fig. 4 Particular of the damaged image of Fig. 3c

where σ_i^2 are the variances of the classes and the weights ω_i represent the probabilities of the two classes separated by the threshold t.

An n-level segmentation, with $n = 8$, was needed; the damage was identified among the objects with the lowest gray level.

The same procedure was used for all the data, also for the calibration image, that is the image without the damaging micromechanisms; the presence of non regular illumination and of the degradation elements (scratches and dust) already discussed above, along with the roughed surface structure, implied that the proposed segmentation procedure yielded the identification of spurious region also for the calibration data. By using a corresponding elements analysis it is possible to cut out the same spurious regions that were identified in all the images. The corresponding elements analysis is based on comparing the regions identified after the n-levels segmentation and cutting all the regions similar to the ones present in the calibration one. For these elements some useful information are available, such as their centroids, their area and their eccentricity. A distance function was introduced: it is sufficient to take into account the position of the detected objects. Therefore, if in the damaged specimen the same false detection of the calibration image were present along with the effects of the damage, these objects were eliminated from the damaged specimen.

On the identified damaged regions useful information were available. In the next Section a possible characterization of damage is proposed.

3 Methods: Damage Evaluation

Focusing the damage evolution in graphite nodules, after the first fatigue cycle no damage is observed. During the fatigue test, damage is more and more evident. The main observed damaging micromechanisms can be classified as follow:

- the initiation and growth of circumpherential cracks inside the graphite nodules (a sort of "internal debonding"), more or less corresponding to the interface

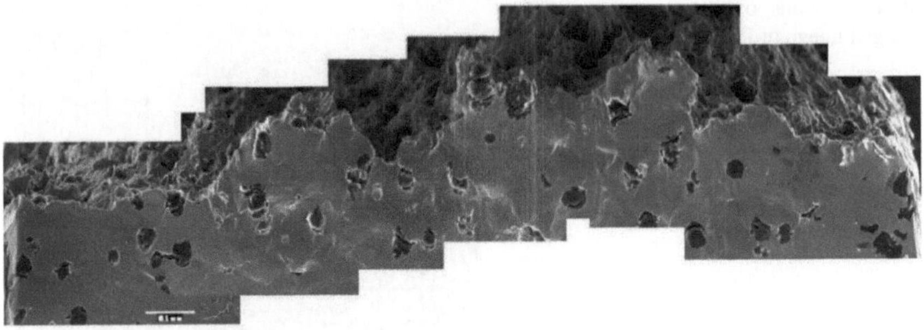

Fig. 5 SEM observation of the specimen lateral surface (near crack surface)

between the graphite obtained directly during solidification and the graphite obtained by means of solid diffusion through the austenite shell, [12];

- always focusing the graphite nodules, seldom microcraks nucleate and growth corresponding to the nodule center with the increase of the loading cycles;
- focusing the ferritic matrix, slip bands emission is often observed corresponding to the interface graphite nodules—matrix (Fig. 3b), becoming more and more evident with the loading cycles increasing. Microcracks can initiate corresponding to these sites and the final rupture is obtained due to the growth of these cracks and their "coalescence".

Unfortunately, all the observed nodules were far from the fracture surface. However, some observations of the lateral surface near crack surface were performed after the final rupture (Fig. 5) and it is possible to confirm that the micromechanisms observed in graphite nodules (Fig. 3) increase their importance up to the end of the fatigue test (final rupture).

In order to evaluate the damage evolution, the following quantities were considered and analyzed: the area and the eccentricity of the nodule, representing its global deformation, and the percentage of the obtained damage after the segmentation procedure, with respect to the initial total graphite nodule area. Moreover it may be useful the evaluation of the evolution of some of the larger damaged regions, in terms of area and eccentricity.

4 Numerical Results and Comments

In this subsection the presented image analysis procedure is applied to two sets of data along with the damage quantitative evaluation.

The first set of data are the ones proposed in Fig. 3. To visualize the preprocessing effects, the images relative to each step applied at the data of Fig. 3e) are shown. For the second order statistic filter a 6×6 domain was assumed, replacing each element of the domain with the element (of the same region) with the lowest gray level, (Fig. 6b). The contrast-limited adaptive histogram equalization operated on small regions of the image, and a 4×4 tile was assumed. Each tile's contrast is enhanced to obtain, as much as possible, a uniform histogram (see Fig. 6c). To avoid non desired enhancement of the dark kernel the contrast enhancement limit was kept low, equal to 0.016. Finally, it could be useful a γ-correction operation, with $\gamma = 0.9$ (Fig. 6d).

The described image preprocessing phase is crucial to enhance the damage effects that are of interest in this context and to reduce the other consequences of the experimental loading procedure. Once the image has been suitably preprocessed an eight levels segmentation is needed to identify the damage. The eight levels segmentation by the Otsu method was obtained hierarchically (Fig. 6e); the objects with the lowest gray level and an eccentricity greater than 0.7 were identified as the damaged elements (Fig. 6f).

The same analysis was performed for all the images of Fig. 3; some false detections were still present but they were cut off by the corresponding analysis, comparing all the detected objects in Figs. 3(b–f) with the ones detected in the calibration image of Fig. 3a.

The nodule damaging may be quantified by analyzing the variations in its area, in pixel value, and the total variation of the damaged areas inside the nodule (Fig. 7, Total). It is interesting also to analyze the evolution of the area of some of its damaged regions, (Fig. 7, areas 1–4) and of the eccentricity (Fig. 8).

The same image analysis was performed on the second set of data; they were relative to a damage caused by the same loading cycles of the specimen of Fig. 3, see Fig. 9.

The analysis on the calibration image suggested a preprocessing phase with a second order statistic filter with a 4×4 domain. For the contrast-limited adaptive histogram equalization an 8×8 tile was assumed. In this case, being the data of this set darker than in the previous example, a more significant γ-correction operation was requested, with $\gamma = 0.4$. Anyway a suitable preprocessing may help the identification, even if the segmentation procedure appears robust with respect to the particular value chosen for the described filtering operations; for this set of data a four-levels segmentations was sufficient. A corresponding analysis was performed, comparing the objects identified in the calibration image with the ones found in the damaged data. The evolution of total and local damage is shown in Fig. 10, whereas in Fig. 11 it is shown the evolution of the eccentricity versus the fatigue loading cycles.

Considering the evolution of the total damaged areas in Figs. 7 and 10, it is evident the increase of the internal damage in graphite nodules, even corresponding to lower values of the loading cycles, where only some slip lines are evident in

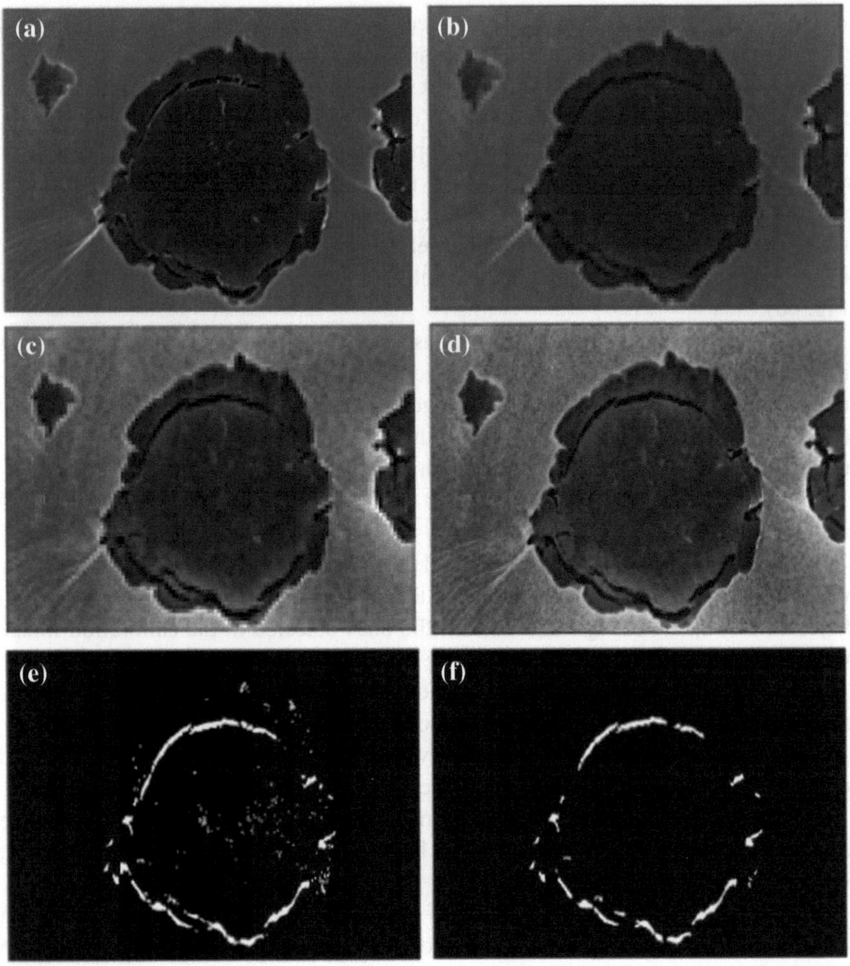

Fig. 6 Damage analysis of the image of Fig. 3c; **a** original data, **b** filtered image; **c** contrast-limited adaptive histogram equalization; **d** γ-correction; **e** eight-levels segmented image; **f** damage identification

the ferritic matrix (and they become more and more evident with the loading cycles number increase, Figs. 3 and 9). Damaging rate strongly increase after 40,000 cycles. Focusing the different investigated area, it is worth noting that the damaging growing kinetics differ depending on the investigated area position, but all the investigated areas are characterized by a strong damaging rate increase after 40,000 cycles up to the specimen rupture. Furthermore, cracks do not nucleate for the same cycles number: considering Fig. 6 – Area 1, crack nucleates only after 38,300 cycle, when

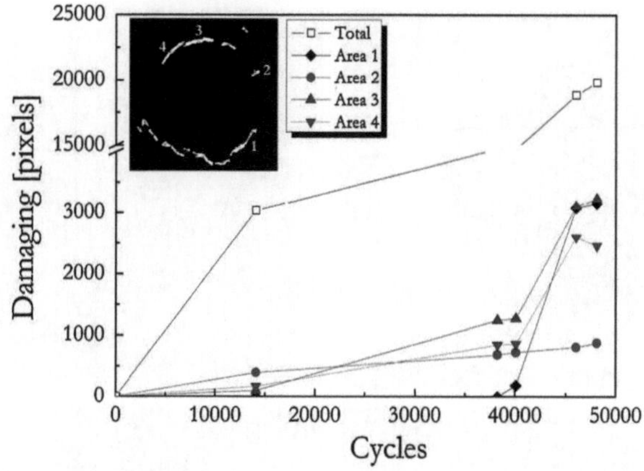

Fig. 7 Damage evolution with fatigue cycles of nodule in Fig. 3

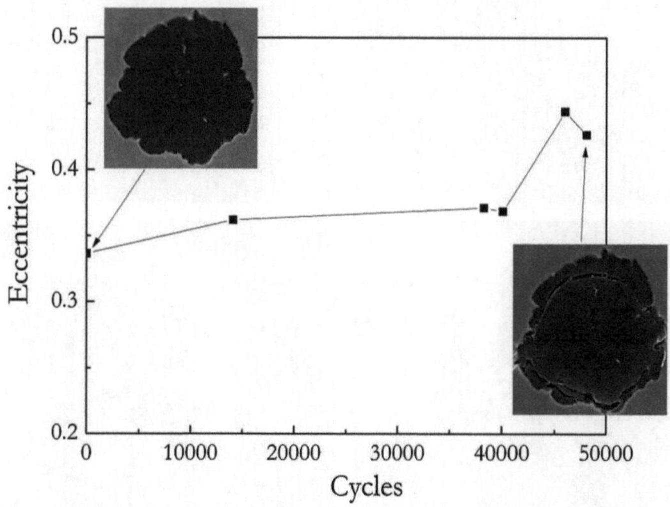

Fig. 8 Eccentricity evolution with fatigue cycles of nodule in Fig. 3

all the other damaged areas are well developed. Finally, some investigated areas are characterized by a reduced damaging decrease from the damaging values obtained after 46,000 and the values obtained after 48,100 cycles (rupture). This is due to the "elastic recovery" after the specimen rupture and is connected with the followed experimental procedure: in fact, for 46,000 cycles the specimen is analyzed by means of a SEM with a tensile loading, on the contrary, for 48,100 cycles, the specimen is broken and the observation is performed without an applied tensile load. This phenomenon is not observed in all the investigated areas, probably due to their position and orientation with respect to the loading direction.

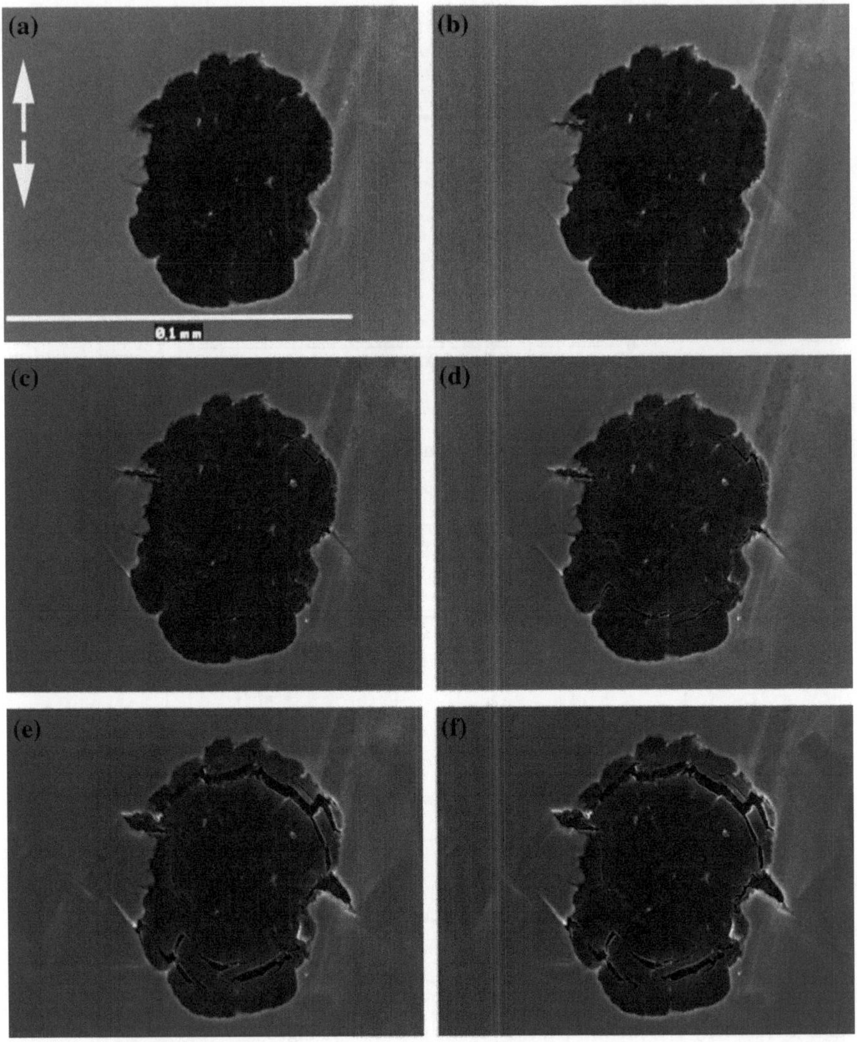

Fig. 9 Graphite nodule damaging evolution. SEM in situ surface analysis corresponding to the following loading cycles: **a** 1; **b** 14100; **c** 38300; **d** 40100; **e** 46000; **f** 48100 cycles (arrows show the loading direction)

Considering the eccentricity evolution (Figs. 8 and 11), it is evident that its increase with the loading cycles is more evident after 40,000 cycles, with a behavior that is analogous to the damaging evolution. Furthermore, both investigated nodules show the final reduced eccentricity decrease, due to the "elastic recovery" after the specimen rupture.

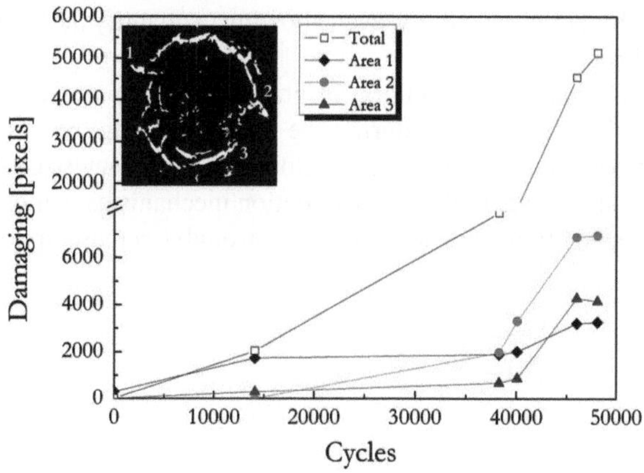

Fig. 10 Damage evolution ith fatigue cycles of nodule in Fig. 9

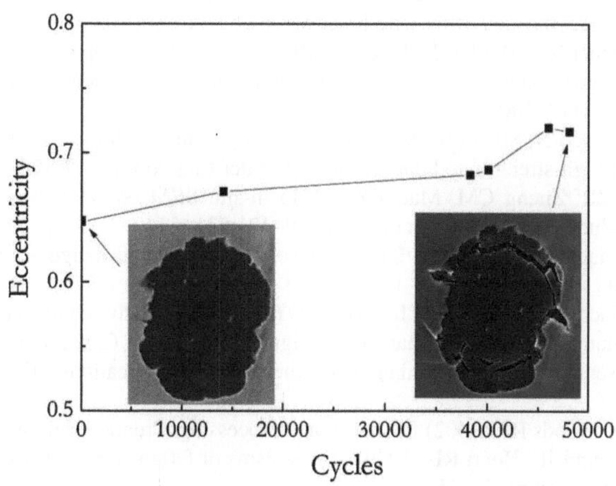

Fig. 11 Eccentricity evolution with fatigue cycles of nodule in Fig. 9

5 Conclusions

The aim of this work was the quantitative analysis of the damage development in a ferritic ductile iron during a fatigue test, focusing the role played by the graphite nodules and optimizing an image analysis based procedure able to obtain an objective evaluation of damage without the supervision of an operator.

On the basis of the experimental and numerical results, the following conclusions can be summarized:

- adopted image analysis technique performances allow to analyze the damaging development in ferritic ductile cast irons, considering the cracks initiation and propagation inside the graphite nodules; it is possible to assess that the procedure is characterized by a high sensitivity, even allowing to quantify the “elastic recovery” after the final rupture;

- the ferritic DCI damaging evolution in graphite nodules seems to be the more evident damaging mechanisms during the fatigue loading; cracks initiation is a continuous process and the damage development is characterized by two stages, at least: a first stage ‘where the crack initiation mechanisms is more evident’ and a second stage, where the crack growth rate strongly increase up to the specimen final rupture.

References

1. Berdin C, Dong MJ, Prioul C (2001) Local approach of damage and fracture toughness for nodular cast iron. Eng Fract Mech 68:1107–1117
2. Cavallini M, Di Bartolomeo O, Iacoviello F (2008) Fatigue crack propagation damaging micromechanisms in ductile cast irons. Eng Fract Mech 75:694–704
3. Chantier I, Bobet V, Billardon R, Hild F (2000) A probabilistic approach to predict the very high-cycle fatigue behaviour of spheroidal graphite cast iron structures. Fatigue Fract Eng Mater Struct 23:173–180
4. Costa N, Machado N, Silva FS (2008) Influence of graphite nodules geometrical features on fatigue life of high-strength nodular cast iron. J Mater Eng Perform 17:352–362
5. Dai PQ, He ZR, Zheng CM, Mao ZY (2001) In-situ SEM observation on the fracture of austempered ductile iron. Mater Sci Eng A 319–321:531–534
6. De Santis A, Iacoviello D (2007) Discrete level set approach to image segmentation. SIViP 1(4):303–320
7. Di Cocco V, Iacoviello F, Rossi A, Iacoviello D (2012) Quantitative characterization of ferritic ductile iron damaging micromechanisms: fatigue loadings. In: Computational modelling of objects represented in images: fundamentals, methods and applications- III. Taylor & Francis, Oxford.
8. Gonzalez RC, Woods RE (2002) Digital image processing. Prentice Hall, New Jersey
9. Greno GL, Otegui JL, Boeri RE (1999) Mechanisms of fatigue crack growth in austempered ductile iron. Int J Fatigue 21:35–43
10. Iacoviello F, Di Cocco V, Cavallini M (2010) Ductile cast irons: microstructure influence on fatigue crack propagation resistance. Frattura ed Integrità Strutturale 13:3–16
11. Jeckins LR, Forrest RD (1993), Properties and selection: iron, steels and high performance alloys. In: ASM handbook ductile iron, vol 1. Metal Park (OH), ASM. International, p 35.
12. Labrecque C, Gagne M (1998) Review ductile iron: fifty years of continuous development. Can Metall Quart 37:343–378
13. Otsu NA (1979) Threshold selection method from gray-level histograms. IEEE Trans Syst Man Cybe 9:62–66
14. Rabold F, Kuna M (2005) Cell model simulation of void growth in nodular cast iron under cyclic loading. Comput Mater Sci 32:489–497
15. Šamec B, Potrc I, Šraml M (2011) Low cycle fatigue of nodular cast iron used for railway brake discs. Eng Fail Anal 18:1424–1434
16. Shirani M, Härkegård G (2011) Fatigue life distribution and size effect in ductile cast iron for wind turbine components. Eng Fail Anal 18:12–24
17. Stokes B, Gao N, Reed PAS (2007) Effects of graphite nodules on crack growth behaviour of austempered ductile iron. Mater Sci Eng A 445–446:374–385 .

18. Tokaji K, Ogawa T, Shamoto K (1994) Fatigue crack propagation in spheroidal-graphite cast irons with different microstructures. Fatigue 16:344–350
19. Yang J, Putatunda SK (2005) Near threshold fatigue crack growth behavior of austempered ductile cast iron (ADI) processed by a novel two-step austempering process. Mater Sci Eng A 393:254–268

Adaptive Sampling and Reconstruction for Sparse Magnetic Resonance Imaging

Laura Ciancarella, Danilo Avola and Giuseppe Placidi

Abstract An adaptive acquisition sequence for Sparse 2D Magnetic Resonance Imaging (MRI) is presented. The method combines random sampling of Cartesian trajectories with an adaptive 2D acquisition of radial projections. It is based on the evaluation of the information content of a small percentage of the k-space data collected randomly to identify radial blades of k-space coefficients having maximum information content. The information content of each direction is evaluated by calculating an entropy function defined on the power spectrum of the projections. The images are obtained by using a non linear reconstruction strategy, based on the homotopic L_0-norm, on the sparse data. The method is tested on MRI images and it is also compared to the weighted Compressed Sensing. Some results are reported and discussed.

Keywords Magnetic resonance imaging (MRI) · Compressed sensing (CS) · L_1-norm · Radial adaptive acquisition · Homotopic L_0-norm.

1 Introduction

Magnetic Resonance Imaging (MRI) has become a major non invasive imaging modality over the past 25 years, due to its ability to provide structural details of human body, like Computed Tomography, and additional information on physiological status and pathologies, like nuclear medicine. The reconstruction of a single image usually involves collecting a series of trajectories. The measurement of a trajectory is a

L. Ciancarella · D. Avola · G. Placidi (✉)
Department of Life, Health and Environmental Sciences, University of L'Aquila,
Via Vetoio Coppito, 67100 L'Aquila, Italy
e-mail: giuseppe.placidi@univaq.it

P. Di Giamberardino et al. (eds.), *Computational Modeling of Objects Presented in Images*, Lecture Notes in Computational Vision and Biomechanics 15,
DOI: 10.1007/978-3-319-04039-4_7,

sampling process of a function evolving with time in a 2D or 3D space domain, referred to as "k-space". The raw data from this sequence of acquisitions are then used to reconstruct an image by using the Fast Fourier Transform after gridding [8, 13].

The most popular k-space trajectories are straight lines from a Cartesian grid, in which each k-space line corresponds to the frequency encoding readout at each value of the phase encoding gradient (Spin Warp Imaging [6]). The lines in the grid are parallel and are equally separated. Although the acquisition of Cartesian trajectories allows easier image reconstruction, recent advances in MR hardware allow other acquisition patterns, such as spirals [12], or radial trajectories (Projection Reconstruction [9]). PR, for example, has many advantages over the conventional Cartesian k-space trajectory, because of its robustness to the motion artifacts, such those due to blood flow or respiration.

A fundamental limitation of MRI is the linear relation between the number of acquired trajectories and net scan time: minutes are often required to collect a complete data set. Such duration can be too high when dynamic processes have to be observed at high temporal resolution, such as in fMRI studies [2]. The acquisition time for each trajectory is limited by the slow natural relaxation processes, which are beyond the control of the acquisition sequence, and have to be respected. Therefore, the only way to speed up acquisition is to reduce the trajectories, that is by using undersampling.

Undersampling is the violation of the Nyquist's criterion where images are reconstructed by using a number of data lower than that theoretically required to obtain a fully-sampled image. One of these methods [16] presented a k-space adaptive acquisition technique for MRI from projections. The method defined the entropy function on the power spectrum of the collected projections, to evaluate their information content, thus driving the acquisition where data variability is maximum. The choice of the projections was made during the acquisition process; this allowed the reduction of acquisition time, by reducing the scanned directions. A modified Fourier reconstruction algorithm, including an interpolation method [15], was used to reconstruct the image from the sparse set of projections. Other authors [3, 5, 7, 11, 20] presented the theory of Compressed Sensing (CS) and the details of its implementation for rapid MRI. They demonstrated that if the underlying image exhibits sparsity in some transform domain, then the image can be recovered from randomly undersampled frequency domain data, providing that an appropriate nonlinear recovery scheme is used. Most of the CS applications used the L_1-norm minimization as reconstruction method. Recently, to improve image quality while reducing the number of collected data even below that required by L_1-norm reconstruction, an alternative non linear reconstruction formulation has been proposed [18, 19] based on homotopic approximation of the L_0-norm. Besides, nonlinear reconstruction can be also improved by increasing samples in the central part of the k-space (low frequency terms contain more energy than high frequency terms, as demonstrated in weighed CS [10, 21]).

In this Chapter an adaptive acquisition sequence and reconstruction is presented. It is based on some significant characteristics of CS (random sampling of spectral coefficients and L_0-minimization), combined with a radial adaptive acquisition criteria. Numerical simulations are reported and compared with weighted CS to show its performances.

2 Compressed Sensing and the Reconstruction Problem

Being the proposed method a joint usage of a radial adaptive acquisition criterion into a Compressed Sensing strategy, the following section presents an overview on CS theory and non linear reconstruction.

Let f be an image, the theoretical image, of interest defined on the domain Ω and suppose there exists a transformation, Ψ, such that the $\| \Psi f \|_0 \;= S << |\Omega|$, i.e. the signal Ψf is sparse in a transform Ψ domain. The key idea of Compressed Sensing is to exploit this a priori knowledge to the fullest degree and to assert conditions under which a signal can be exactly reconstructed from a limited set of measurements of the order of S, certainly lower than $|\Omega|$. When the unknowns are more than the acquired measurements, the problem to recover f becomes underdetermined, that is admitting infinite solutions. One choice for finding a solution u from this infinite set is to use the L_0-norm by solving:

$$u = \min_u \| \Psi u \|_0 \quad s.t. \quad \Phi u = \Phi f$$

where the zero quasi-norm, $\| \|_0$ is a measure of functional cardinality (i.e. the number of nonzero coefficients on the sparse representation) and Φ denotes the undersampled Fourier transform, corresponding to one of the chosen k-space undersampling schemes. The constraint $\Phi u = \Phi f$ requires to consider images producing the same observed measurements. This problem yields a unique solution by finding the sparsest vector u in the solutions space. For images with S nonzero coefficients in Ψ, the sparsest vector recovery with L_0 reconstruction is possible with only $2S$ observed measurements [4], substantially lower than that required by Nyquist's criterion ($|\Omega|$). Despite the obvious potential for drastic reductions in net scan time, the L_0 minimization problem requires a combinatorial search through all $\binom{|\Omega|}{S}$ potential solutions to recover a S-sparse signal on Ω. It is a non-deterministic polynomial-time hard (NP hard) problem, intractable for any practical application. Another approach is to choose the L_2-norm to find the solution with minimum energy:

$$u = \min_u \|\Psi u\|_2^2 \quad s.t. \quad \Phi u = \Phi f.$$

However, this solution may contain significant artifacts such as aliasing and blurring in practical situations, thus resulting in an image of low diagnostic value.

Following that, several authors [3, 5, 11] demonstrated that if one relaxes the L_0-norm to the L_1-norm, a sparse image f can be exactly recovered by using the following convex optimization problem:

$$u = \min_u \|\Psi u\|_1 \quad s.t. \quad \Phi u = \Phi f.$$

In most medical imaging applications including MRI, signals are rarely noise-free and it is desirable to investigate how measurement error affects the stability of the reconstruction program. To include the presence of experimental noise into the reconstruction process, the convex optimization is reformulated as follows:

$$u = \min_u \|\Psi u\|_1 \quad s.t. \quad \|\Phi u - \Phi f\|_2^2 < \varepsilon$$

where ε controls the fidelity of the reconstruction to the k-space measured data Φf, whose choice is dependent on the noise level in the collected data (it is usually set below the expected noise level). Though this approach cannot generally be achieved at the true minimum sampling rate associable with the L_0 case, it offers the ability to sample below the Nyquist rate and performs the recovery with a computationally tractable procedure. Numerical experiments [3] suggested that, for a good reconstruction with L_1-norm, the number of measured k-space samples, Φf, should be roughly $3S \leq \Phi f \leq 5S < |\Omega|$ (an increase of Φf towards 5S would improve the reconstruction).

On the other hand, the reconstruction problem proposed by Trzasko et al. [18, 19] attacked directly the ideal L_0-norm minimization problem. This method minimizes iteratively continuous approximations of the L_0-norm by the use of a suitable non convex semimetric penalty function ρ (i.e. positive definite and symmetric about the origin, no decreasing over R^+) in the minimization:

$$\min_u \lim_{\tau \to 0} \sum_{\Omega} \rho(|\Psi u|, \tau) \; s.t. \; \|\Phi u - \Phi f\|_2^2 < \varepsilon$$

where $\tau > 0$.

The functional commonly employed to satisfy the above equation is the Geman-McClure function (used also in our experiments):

$$\rho(|u|, \tau) = \frac{|u|}{|u| + \tau}.$$

It is said to be homotopic with the L_0-norm in the sense that it can be continuously deformed into the desired measure. Although the method has no guarantee of achieving a global minimum, the homotopic L_0 minimization problem typically allows accurate image reconstruction by using a number of samples which is considerably lower than that usable by L_1-norm minimization and arbitrarily close to the theoretical minimum number associated with direct L_0 minimization (2S measurements).

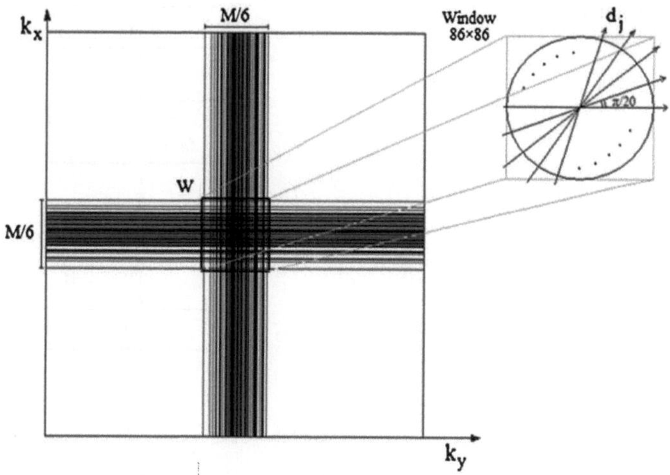

Fig. 1 The starting data set for the adaptive acquisition (*left panel*). The entropy function is measured for a set of 20 equispaced radial projections inside the window W (*right panel*)

3 The Proposed Method

Consider the k-space image support as a M × M matrix. In a first phase, the acquisition process consists in collecting a set of random Cartesian trajectories, having a Gaussian distribution in a central region of the k-space whose width is M/6, both along the rows and along the columns (Fig. 1). Each trajectory is completely sampled but the number of collected trajectories, both along the rows and the columns, is lower than M/6. Lines are collected by randomizing the phase-encoding gradient and the columns are collected by reversing the phase-encoding gradient with the frequency-encoding gradient (also in this case, the randomization process involves phase-encoding).

The square central region *W*, whose size is M/6 × M/6, provides the foundation for the proposed adaptive sampling (Fig. 2).

In fact, we consider an equispaced set of 20 radial projections in the window *W*, whose angular separation was $\pi/20$ (Fig. 1, right insert).

The entropy function of the *j*th direction is defined as:

$$E_j = \frac{1}{q_j} \sum_{i=1}^{q_j} v_i \log v_i \;\; \forall \, \mathrm{j} = 1, \ldots, 20$$

where q_j is the number of measured coefficients in *W* falling along the *j*th radial projection and v_i is the power of the *i*th coefficient allowing to the *j*th projection. Once calculated the entropy of each projection, the average value is chosen as a threshold value T. A "blade" composed by 9 parallel lines of k-space coefficients is

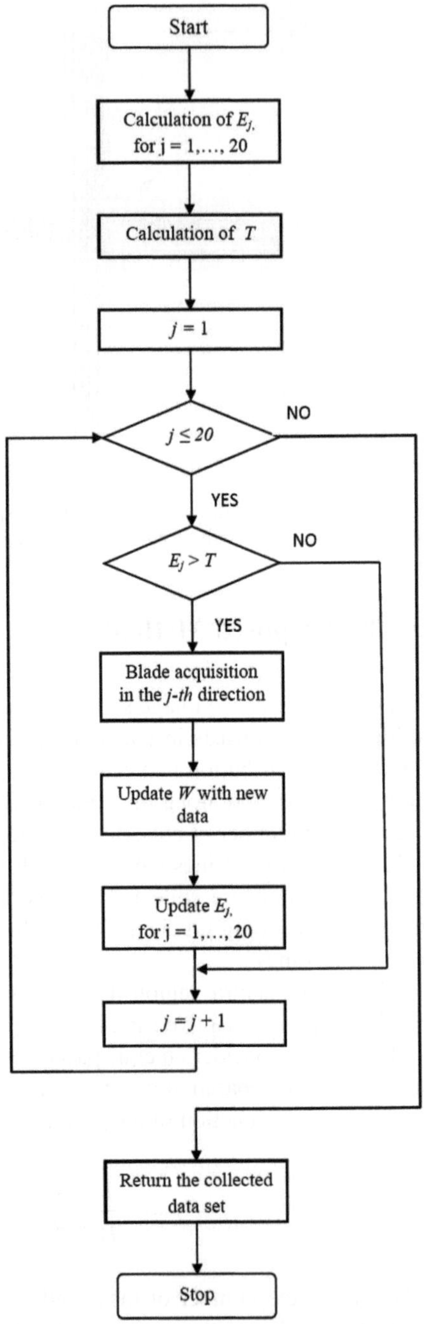

Fig. 2 The adaptive acquisition method

collected around the projections whose entropy is above T (the acquisition resembles a sort of PROPELLER [1, 14]).

Since these adaptive data are not completely regular, the image can be recovered by using a non-linear reconstruction method. The method is suitable for nonlinear L_0-norm reconstruction, in line with the theory of CS [17]. It is important to note that the radial directions involved into the entropy calculation are confined inside the window *W*, while the blades of coefficients are collected into the whole image support.

4 Experiments

To evaluate the performance of proposed method, simulations on different MRI images were performed. The considered images were complete 512×512 images with different orientations and weighting parameters. To simulate MRI acquisition, the Fast Fourier Transform (FFT) of each image was performed and the obtained coefficients were treated as the k-space experimentally collected data, assuming the image and the whole k-space data set are not known a priori (we found this procedure useful to compare the undersampled reconstructed images with the complete, theoretical, image).

The Gaussian distribution function, used in the weighted random undersampling of Cartesian trajectories, was chosen with zero mean and standard deviation $\sigma = 0.1$. The σ value has been found experimentally, with the goal to concentrate the most of coefficients at lower frequency within the window *W* used for the entropy calculation (Fig. 1). The obtained results were compared both with the completely sampled original image and with the image reconstructed by using CS undersampling weighted with a Gaussian distribution function having zero mean and $\sigma = 0.1$. The σ value has been optimized experimentally: $\sigma < 0.1$ produced severe losses of resolution (small details were lost), because the mask resulted too concentrated on the central part of the k-space; $\sigma > 0.1$ produced severe artifacts due to undersampling. In what follows three of these simulations are reported and discussed: the results of each simulation have been compared both visually and numerically, by using the *peak signal-to-noise ratio* (PSNR), with the complete image. Images of enlargements of small details and difference between the original and reconstructed images are also shown.

In the first reported simulation (Fig. 3), the proposed acquisition method was preliminary applied three times. This was done to demonstrate the reproducibility of the proposed method. In fact, the starting point of the adaptive method is a set of randomly collected data: if this data set is too sparse, the resulting adaptively collected data set is strongly dependent upon the k-space initial positions. In this case, different results could occur for different starting sets.

As can be observed in Fig. 4, though a certain variability due to the initial random choice, the corresponding images, reported in Fig. 5, were very similar each other, both visually and in PSNR values.

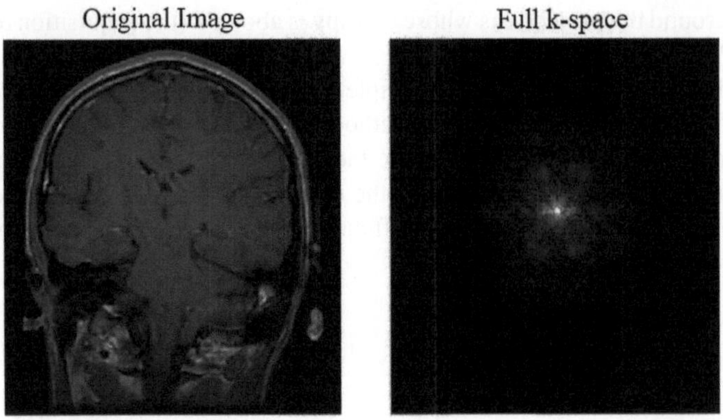

Fig. 3 A complete MRI image and its k-space spectrum

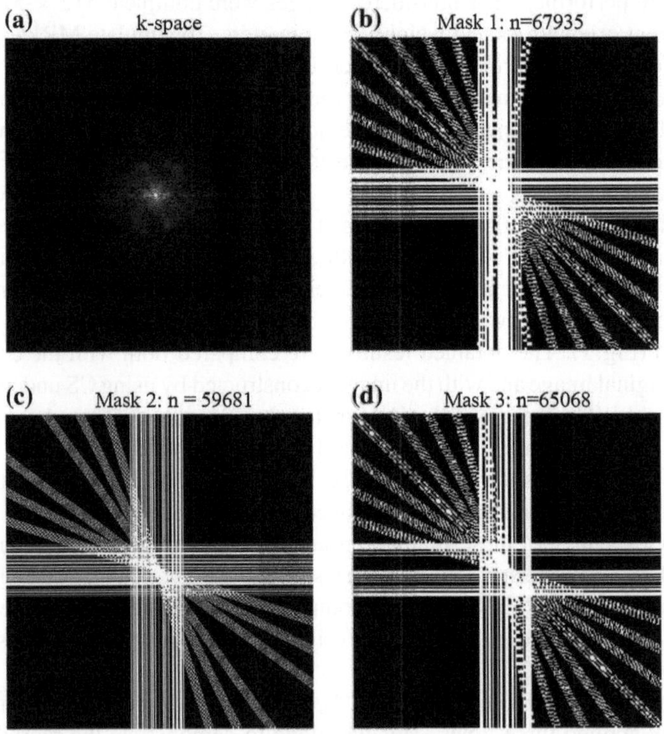

Fig. 4 Complete k-space spectrum of the image reported in Fig. 3 (**a**) and three different sampling masks (**b**), (**c**) and (**d**) obtained with three different applications of the proposed method. The number of collected data, n, is slowly different for the three cases

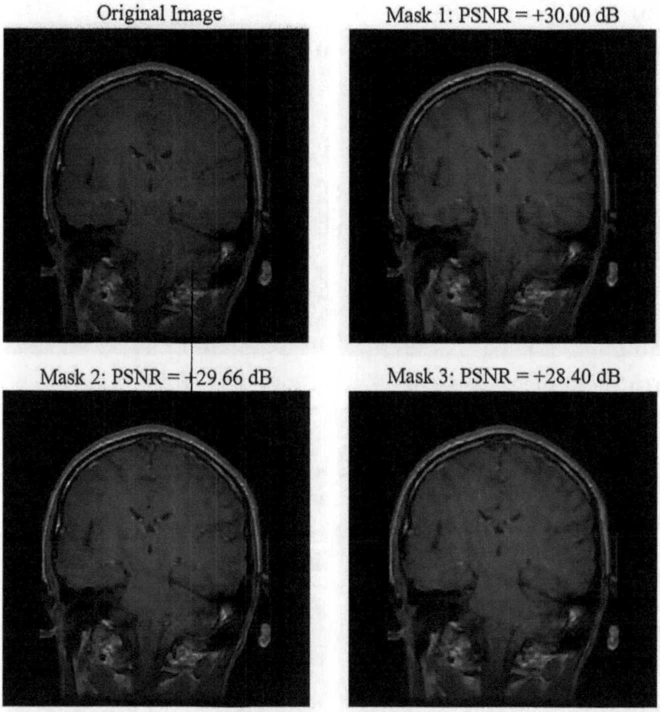

Fig. 5 Images reconstructed by using the three masks reported in Fig. 4. In particular, the original image (a) is compared with the images obtained with mask 1 (Fig. 4b), mask 2 (Fig. 4c), and mask 3 (Fig. 4d), respectively

Based on PSNR values, the worst-case result was considered with the mask #3 (Fig. 5, PSNR = +28.40 dB, n = 65,068). This result was compared with the weighed CS result. The comparison is reported in Figs. 6, 7, and 8. In particular, CS allowed better PSNR value, but the proposed method conserved better resolution, as can be observed in Fig. 7, and produced incoherent artifacts, as can be seen in Fig. 8.

In the second reported simulation (Fig. 9a), the sampling mask shown in Fig. 9b, is obtained for the proposed method (73,566 samples are acquired). The corresponding weighted CS result is reported in Fig. 9c. In this case, the adaptive method overcame weighted CS both visually and in PSNR. This is also evident by looking at the enlargement (Fig. 10). The better conservation of the image edges with our method is evident also from the difference images. In fact, the difference image referred to the weighted CS maintained a huge part of useful information (Fig. 11).

In a third simulation (Fig. 12) the undersampled set (composed by 20 % of the total measurements) has been used for three nonlinear reconstruction strategies: minimum energy, L_1-norm reconstruction and the homotopic L_0 minimization. Figure 13 reports the reconstructed images for each of the reconstruction methods. Both visually

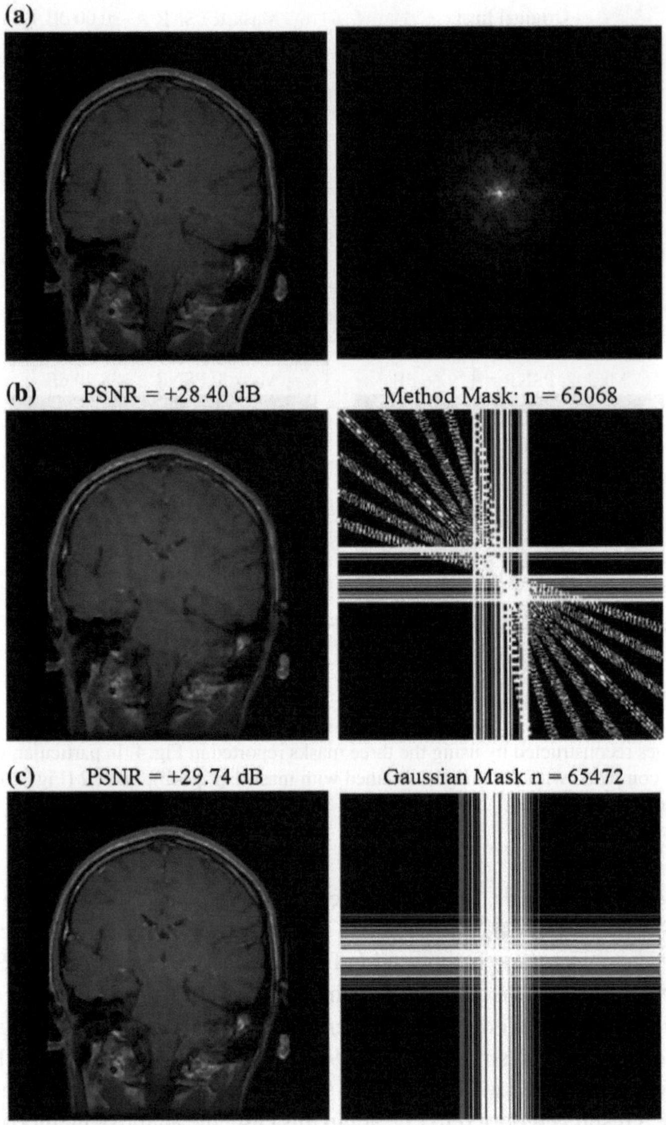

Fig. 6 Visual comparison between the original image (**a**), the reconstructed image with proposed method (**b**), and the reconstructed image with weighted CS (**c**). On the *right part* the used corresponding masks are reported (for the complete image the whole k-space spectrum is reported)

and from the PSNR values, it can be noted how the reconstruction with the homotopic L_0 minimization is more detailed than the reconstruction obtained by the L_1-norm (Fig. 13).

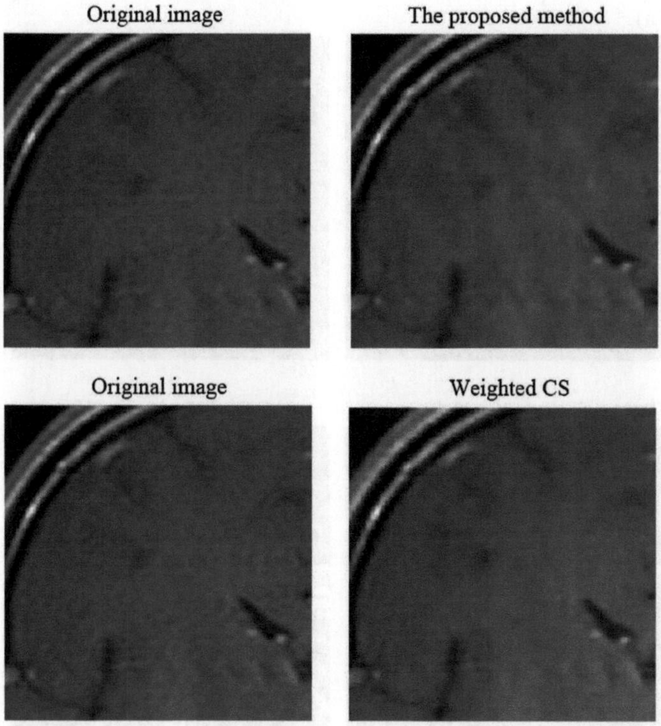

Fig. 7 Enlargement of a particular for the original image (*left column*), for proposed method (*right top*), and for the weighted CS (*right bottom*)

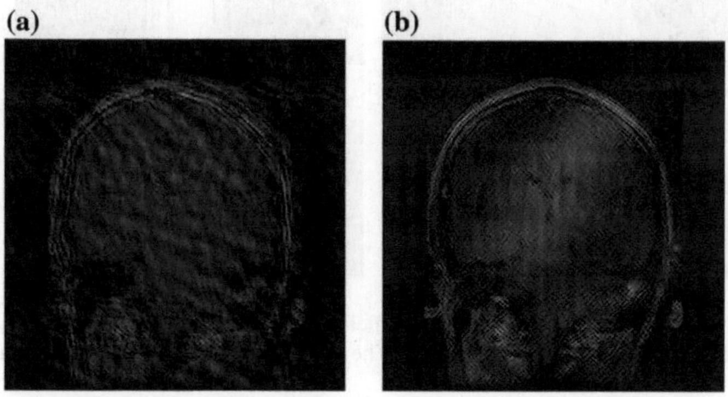

Fig. 8 Difference between the original image and the reconstructed image with the proposed method (**a**) and with the weighed CS (**b**). Differences are shown in an expanded *gray-scale*

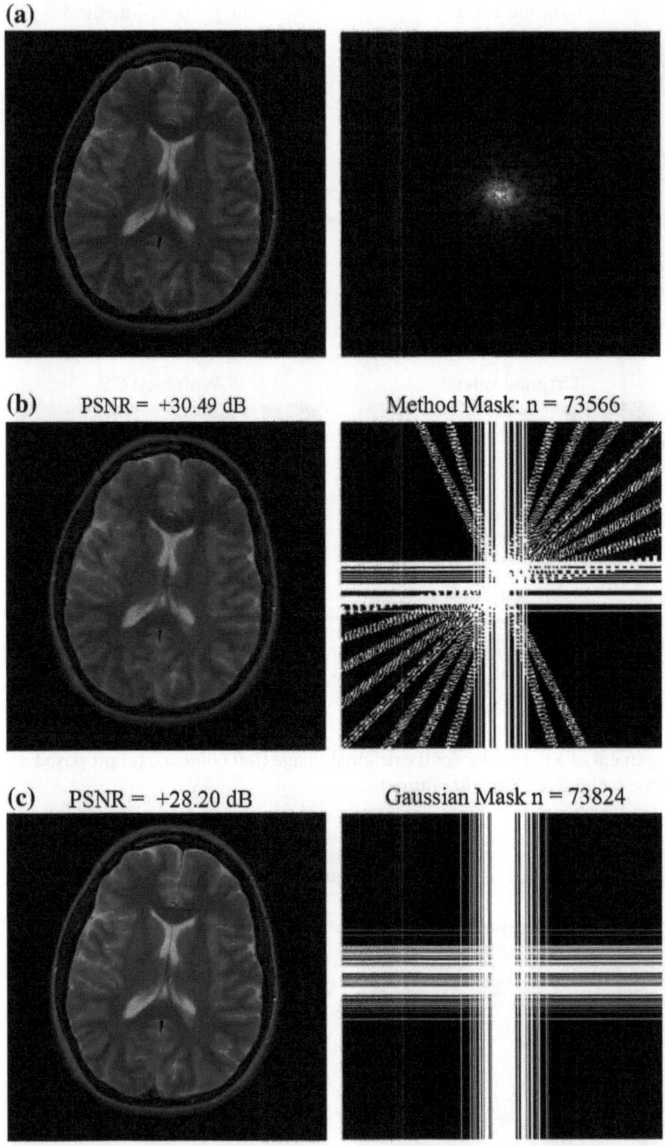

Fig. 9 Test image and its power spectrum coefficients (**a**). Reconstruction obtained by using the proposed method (**b**), and the weighted CS (**c**). The corresponding masks are reported on the *right*

5 Conclusions and Future Work

In the present work, an adaptive acquisition method for MRI has been described, that makes it possible to reduce the total acquisition time, with minimum loss of resolution if used with a homotopic L_0 non-linear reconstruction. It combined two

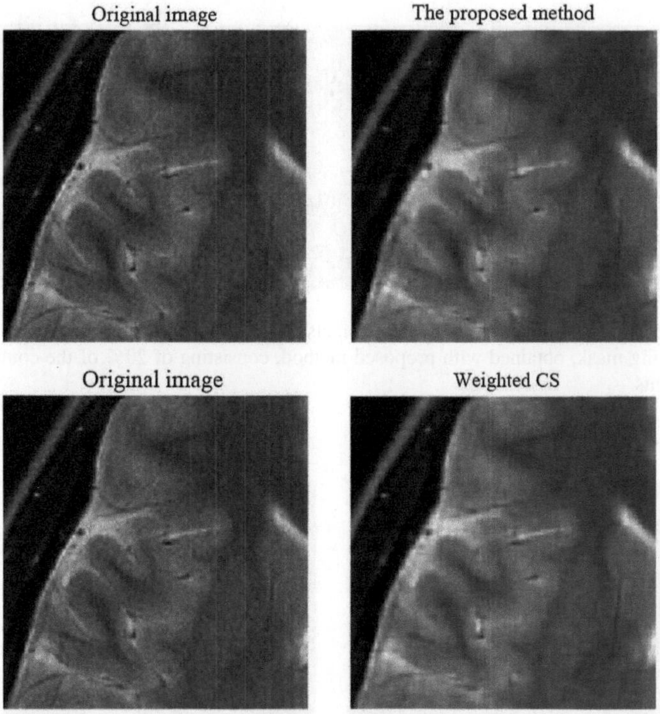

Fig. 10 Enalrgements of a particular for the original image (*left column*), for proposed method (*right top*), and for the weighted CS (*right bottom*)

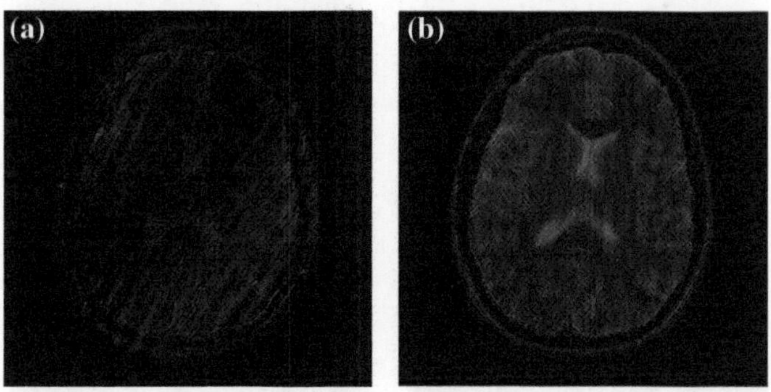

Fig. 11 Difference between the original and the reconstructed image with the proposed method (**a**) and with the weighed CS (**b**). Differences are shown in an expanded *gray-scale*

acquisition techniques: Spin Warp and Adaptive Projection Reconstruction.

The method was tested on different MRI images and three of them were reported. The proposed adaptive technique allowed good quality reconstruction, though a very sparse set of "most informative" data was used. The proposed method given better

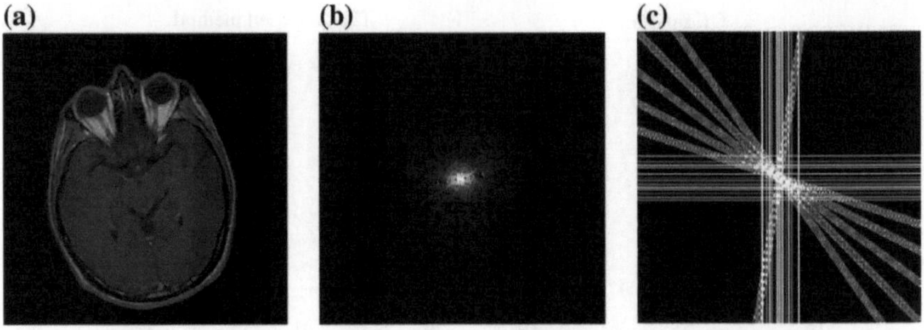

Fig. 12 **a** MRI image with size 512 × 512 pixels, **b** its complete k-space spectrum and (**c**) the undersampling mask, obtained with proposed method, consisting of 20 % of the complete set of measurements

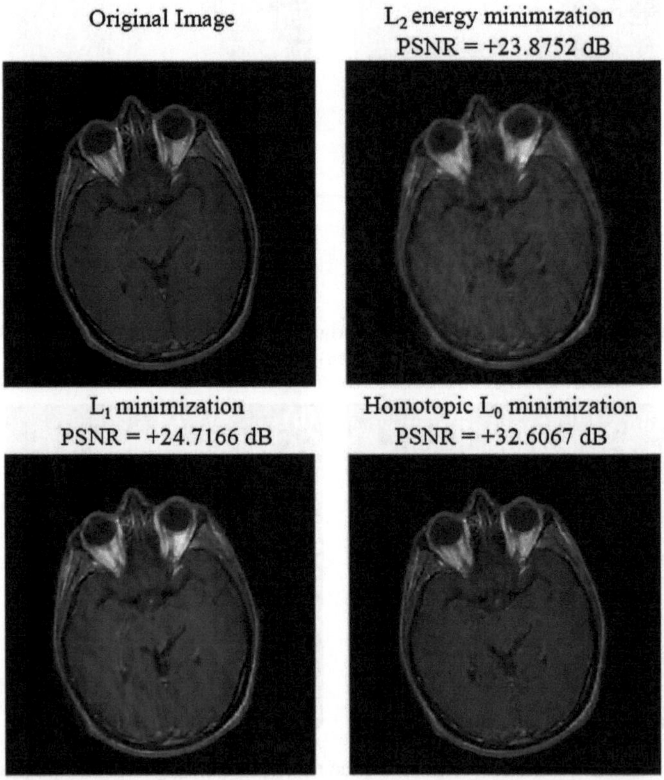

Fig. 13 Images reconstructed by the same data set but with different nonlinear methods. In particular, the original image is compared with those obtained by L_2 energy minimization, L_1 minimization and homotopic L_0 minimization, respectively

results compared with weighted CS. Besides it furnished a criterion to estimate the near optimal number of data to obtain a good reconstruction for the given image: this was impossible for CS that, being it a blind method, required the number of collected data had to be fixed in advance, independently of the image shape.
The values of the peak signal-to-noise ratio and the visual comparison confirmed the proposed method was slightly better than CS.
Moreover, the use of homotopic L_0-norm minimization made possible to obtain better reconstructions than by simple L_1-norm.

In the future we aim to evaluate the performance of the proposed method on experimentally collected MR data.

Acknowledgments We gratefully acknowledge Abruzzo Region for the financial con-tribution to the project through the European Social Fund (FSE). In addition, we acknowledge Dr. Joshua Trzasko, for having pro-vided useful details to implement the homotopic L0-norm minimiza-tion, and the other members of Computer Vision Laboratory and of AAVI Laboratory for their helpful contribution, in particular Mrs Carmelita Marinelli for technical assistance.

References

1. Arfanakis K, Tamhane AA, Pipe JG, Anastasio MA (2005) K-space undersampling in PROPELLER imaging. Magn Reson Med 53:675–683
2. Bernstein MA, King KF, Zhou XJ (2004) Handbook of MRI pulse sequences. Elsevier, USA
3. Candès EJ, Romberg J, Tao T (2006) Robust uncertainty principles: exact signal reconstruction from highly incomplete frequency information. IEEE Trans Inf Theory 52(2):489–509
4. Candès EJ, Tao T (2005) Decoding by linear programming. IEEE Trans Inf Theory 51(12):4203–4215
5. Donoho DL (2006) Compressed sensing. IEEE Trans Inf Theory 52:1289–1306
6. Edelstein WA, Hutchison JM, Johnson G, Redpath T (1980) Spin warp NMR imaging and applications to human whole-body imaging. Phys Med Biol 25:751–756
7. Elad M (2010) Sparse and redundant representations: from theory to applications in signal and image processing. Springer, New York
8. Jackson JI, Meyer CH, Nishimura DG, Macovski A (1991) Selection of a convolution function for fourier inversion using gridding. IEEE Trans Med Imaging 10(3):473–478
9. Lauterbur EC (1973) Image formation by induced local interactions: examples employing nuclear magnetic resonance. Nature 242:190–191
10. Lustig M (2008) SPARSE MRI. Ph.D Thesis, Stanford University
11. Lustig M, Donoho D, Pauly JM (2007) Sparse MRI: the application of compressed sensing for rapid MR imaging. Magn Reson Med 58:1182–1195
12. Meyer CH (1998) Spiral echo-planar imaging. echo-planar imaging. Springer, Berlin
13. O'Sullivan J (1985) A fast sinc function gridding algorithm for fourier inversion in computer tomography. IEEE Trans Med Imaging 4(MI-4):200–207
14. Pipe J (1999) Motion correction with PROPELLER MRI: application to head motion and free-breathing cardiac imaging. Magn Reson Med 42:963–969
15. Placidi G, Alecci M, Colacicchi S, Sotgiu A (1998) Fourier reconstruction as a valid alternative to filtered back projection in iterative applications: implementation of fourier spectral spatial EPR imaging. J Magn Reson 134:280–286
16. Placidi G, Alecci M, Sotgiu A (2000) ω-Space adaptive acquisition technique for magnetic resonance imaging from projections. J Magn Reson 143:197–207

17. Placidi G (2012) MRI: essentials for innovative technologies. CRC Press Inc, Boca Raton, pp 111–160
18. Trzasko JD, Manduca A (2009) Highly undersampled magnetic resonance image reconstruction via homotopic L_0 - minimization. IEEE Trans Med Imaging 28:106–121
19. Trzasko JD, Manduca A (2008) A fixed point method for homotopic L_0—minimization with application to MR image recovery.In: Proc SPIE 6913, Medical Imaging 2008: Phys Med Imaging, 6913F, pp 1–11
20. Usman M, Prieto C, Schaeffter T, Batchelor PG (2011) k-t group sparse: a method for accelerating dynamic MRI. Magn Reson Med 1176(4):1163–1176
21. Wang Z, Arce GR (2010) Variablc dcnsity compressed image sampling. Trans Image Process 19(1):264–270. http://overcode.yak.net/15?width=1600&size=XS

Driver's Hand Detection and Tracking Based on Address Event Representation

Antonio Ríos, Cristina Conde, Isaac Martín de Diego and Enrique Cabello

Abstract This chapter presents a novel biologically-inspired system capable of detecting and tracking the hands of the driver during the driving task. The system needs neither marks nor special device in the hands, so a totally natural driving is allowed. Visual information acquisition has been made using an innovative dynamic vision sensor (DVS) that discards the frame concept entirely, encoding the information in the form of Address-Event-Representation (AER) data. This representation allows the information transmission and processing at the same time. An algorithm for detecting and tracking hands using this information in real time is presented. This method has been designed to work with infra-red visual information, avoiding the dependence of the illumination conditions. The proposed system has been integrated in a highly realistic car simulator and several tests have been carried out. Detailed experiments showing the improvement of using AER representation are presented. The presented work is the first approach to introduce AER technology in an automotive environment.

Keywords Address event representation · Hands tracking · Bio-inspired system

1 Introduction

DRIVER'S distraction or inattention is the main cause of accidents. It is estimated that 25 or 30 % of car accidents are caused by this. In fact, lots of fatalities happen every year because of driver's recklessness (Klauer 2010) [16]. This situation is reported both in the United States and in Europe [17]. Furthermore, to study driver's distractions is a very complex subject, because of the huge number of factors involved

A. Ríos (✉) · C. Conde · I. M. de Diego · E. Cabello
Face Recognition and Artificial Vision Group, Universidad de Rey Juan Carlos,
Madrid, Spain
e-mail: jarios86@gmail.com

P. Di Giamberardino et al. (eds.), *Computational Modeling of Objects Presented in Images*, Lecture Notes in Computational Vision and Biomechanics 15,
DOI: 10.1007/978-3-319-04039-4_8,

in the distraction-related accidents [25]. An accident is made up of three main elements: the vehicle, the road, and the driver. Of these three elements, human factor is the one that has received the least attention in the past. Vehicle manufacturers have increased security measures, both actively and passively. Roads have improved their quality: there are new layers of asphalt, a better signalling and a more appropriate driving design. In recent years different approaches that deal with supervising driver's task by means of computer vision techniques have been presented (Klauer 2012). In most of these works driver behaviour is analysed taking into account the head pose or the eye detection. Nevertheless, despite hands play one of the most important roles when driving [15], neither body nor hands activity have been usually taken into consideration. In recent years, In-Vehicle Information Systems (IVIS) have become increasingly popular. These new devices can also be distracting elements that have been incorporated to the vehicle. The IVIS systems are used: to make the driver feel more comfortable inside the vehicle (air conditioning, heater, radio or DVD), to help the driver communicate (mobile phone) and to organize the chosen route (GPS, navigation systems). These systems can be integrated into the vehicle or they can be placed as nomadic devices in almost every part of the vehicle environment. The main requirement of the user for the position of these devices was that "they should be within the length of a hand". As the number of IVIS in the vehicle increases, the risk of distraction also rises. The main characteristic of these IVIS systems is that they are adjusted manually. Besides that, they can be tuned or manipulated when driving.

In this chapter, it is presented an artificial vision system capable of monitoring and detecting the hands position on the steering wheel in teal time. To do this, it has been used a DVS which encodes the information as AER events. The AER protocol allows asynchronous massive interconnection of neuromorphic processing chip. This protocol was first proposed in Caltech, in 1991, to solve the problem of massive interconnectivity between populations of neurons located in different chips [21]. It uses mixed analogic and digital principles and exploits pulse density modulation for coding information. The state of the neurons is a continuous time varying analogic signal.

AER is based on the transmission of neural information in the brain, by an electrical spike. Figure 1 explains the principle behind the AER. The emitter chip contains an array of cells (e.g., artificial retina chip used in this chapter) where each pixel shows a state that changes with a slow time constant (in the order of milliseconds). Each pixel includes an oscillator that generates pulses of minimum width (a few nanoseconds). Each time a pixel generates a pulse (called "event"), it communicates with the periphery and its address is placed on the external digital bus (the AER bus). Handshaking lines (Acknowledge and Request) are used for completing the communication (Fig. 2).

In the receiver chip the pulses are directed to the pixels or cells whose address was on the bus. This way, pixels with the same address in the emitter and receiver chips will "see" the same pulse stream. The receiver cell integrates the pulses and reconstructs the original low frequency continuous-time waveform.

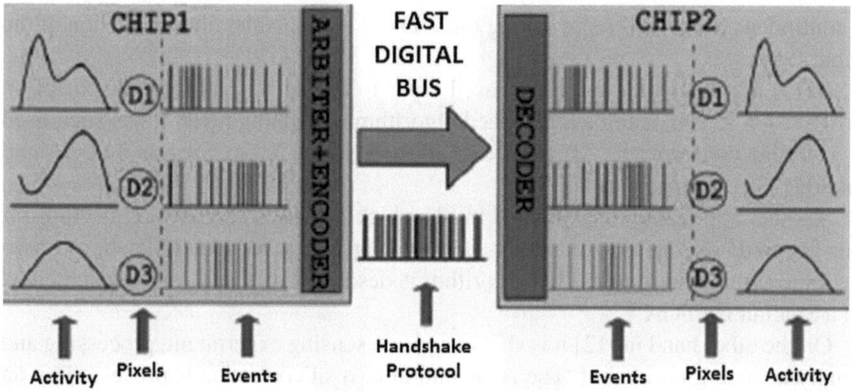

Fig. 1 AER communication scheme [7]

Fig. 2 AER handshake protocol

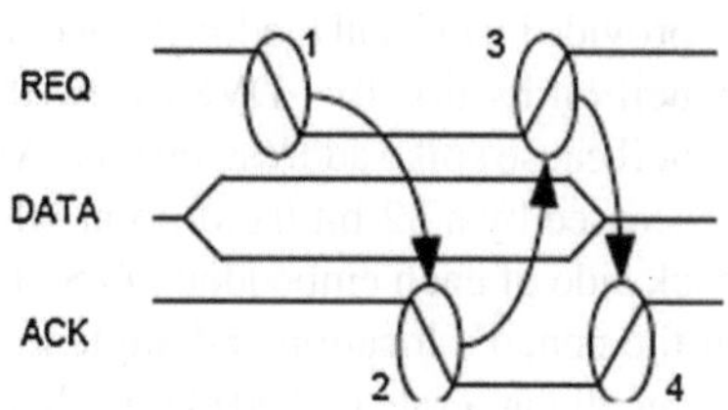

Transmitting the pixel addresses allows performing extra operations on the images while they travel from one chip to another. For example, inserting memories (e.g., EEPROM) allows transformations of images.

Considering AER from a computer vision point of view, it can be understood as a progressive image transmission technique [24]. AER sends the most relevant information first. In usual computer vision systems it is necessary to wait until the whole image is received before starting to apply image processing algorithms. In some specific environments with a poor bandwidth and with fast response demanding this delay may be critic. This is the situation in automotive environments. In computer vision applications for automotive scenarios there are some important technical restrictions [8]: buses are very slow, there are strict technical prerequisites and priorities signals that cannot be interrupted. These hard conditions can be satisfied by AER. AER is a method that allows the events processing at the time they are received, avoiding the bus bandwidth saturation and its interference with other more important signals. This is one of the principal AER advantages.

There is many other application fields of the AER technology in the area of artificial vision and several works have been published, but all of them are laboratory applications not tested in real environments. In [2] it is presented a 2-D chip convolution totally based on pulses, without using the concept of frames. The information is represented by a continuous flow of self-timed asynchronous events. Such events can be processed on the fly by event-based convolution chips, providing at their output a continuous event flow representing the 2-D (32 × 32 pixels) filtered version of the input flow.

In [9] it is presented an AER based layer to correct in real time the tilt of an AER vision sensor, using a high speed algorithmic mapping layer. It has been used a co-design platform (the AER-Robot platform), with a Xilinx Spartan 3 FPGA and an 8051 USB microcontroller.

Another application is explained in [7] which proposes cascade architecture for bio-inspired information processing. Using this architecture, a multiple object tracking algorithm is presented. This algorithm is described in VHDL and implemented in a Spartan II FPGA.

On the other hand in [12] it is shown a visual sensing experiment, processing and finally actuating on a robot. The AER output of a silicon retina is processed by an AER filter implemented in a FPGA to produce a mimicking behaviour in a humanoid robot. The visual filter has been implemented into a Spartan II FPGA.

Another example of visual-motor control is presented in [3], where a DVS is used to provide fast visual feedback for controlling an actuated table to balance an ordinary pencil on its tip. Two DVSs view the pencil from right angles. Movements of the pencil cause spike address-events (AEs) to be emitted from the DVSs. These AEs are processed by a 32-bit fixed-point ARM7 microcontroller (64 MHz, 200 mW) on the back side of each embedded DVS board (eDVS). Each eDVS updates its estimation of the pencil's location and angle in a bi-dimensional space for each received spike (typically at a rate of 100 kHz). This task is done by applying a continuous tracking method based on spike driven fitting to a model of the vertical rod-like shape of the pencil. Every 2 ms, each eDVS sends the pencil's tracked position to a third ARM7-based controller, which computes pencil location in the three-dimensional space and runs a linear PD-controller to adjust X-Y-position and velocity of the table to maintain the pencil balanced upright. The actuated table is built using ordinary high-speed hobby servos.

Additional AER-based image processing algorithms have been presented in different works like [5, 22, 23].

The work presented in this chapter is an application of AER technology designed for working in real world conditions in an automotive context, which takes a further step in bringing this technology to more complex environments.

If the analysis of the state of the art is done regarding classical computer vision techniques applied for driver monitoring, several works have been presented, like [4, 15]. Video systems usually produce a huge amount of data that likely saturate any computational unit responsible for data processing. Thus, real-time object tracking based on video data processing requires large computational effort and is consequently done on high-performance computer platforms. As a consequence, the design of video-tracking systems with embedded real-time applications, where the algorithms are implemented in Digital Signal Processor is a challenging task.

However, vision systems based on AER generate a lower volume of data, focusing only on those which are relevant in avoiding irrelevant data redundancy. This makes possible to design AER-tracking systems with embedded real-time applications, such as the one presented in this chapter, which indeed, it is a task much less expensive. Several examples are shown in [3, 7].

The chapter will be structured as follows. In Sect. 2, it is explained the DVS and the labelling events module. In Sect. 3, hands-tracking algorithm is described. The experimental results of the presented algorithm on real tests are shown in Sect. 4. Finally, in Sect. 5 conclusions are presented.

2 Hardware Components Description

The data acquisition is implemented by two devices: the sensor and the USBAER-mini2 DVS, generating the information encoded in AER format.

The DVS sensor (silicon retina) contains an array of pixels individually autonomous with real-time response to relative changes in light intensity by placing address (event) in an arbitrary asynchronous bus. Pixels that are not stimulated by any change of lighting are not altered, thus scenes without motion do not generate any output.

The scene information is transmitted event to event through an asynchronous bus. The location of the pixel in the pixel array is encoded in the so-called address of events. This address, called AE (Address Event), contains the *(x,y)* coordinates of the pixel that generated the event. The DVS sensor used considers an array of 128×128 pixels, so 7 bits are needed to encode each dimension of the array of pixels. It also generates a polarity bit indicating the sign of contrast change, whether positive (light increment) or negative (light decrement) [11].

As shown in (Fig. 3), the direction AE consists of 16 bits, 7 bits corresponding to the previously mentioned coordinates *(x,y)* , one bit of polarity and a bit NC.

The AE generated is transmitted to USBmini2 on a 16-bits parallel bus, implementing a simple handshake protocol. The device USBAERmini2 is used to label each event that is received from the DVS with a timestamp. This is relevant to maintain the time information in this asynchronous approach. The main elements of the USBAERmini2 device are FX2 and FPGA modules. The FX2's 8051 microcontroller is the responsible of setting the "endpoints" of the USB port, in addition to receive and interpret commands from the PC (Fig. 4).

On the other hand the CPLD is responsible of "handshaking" with the AER devices, connected to the ports, and of reading and writing events in the FIFO's FX2 module.

CPLD module has a counter that is used to generate the "timestamp" to label the events. Using only 16 bits is not enough, because only $2^{16} = 65536$ timestamps could be generated, which is the same as 65 ms when using a tick of 1 μs. This is clearly not sufficient. But if more bits are considered, like 32 bit timestamps, it consumes too much bandwidth, as the higher 16 bits change only in rarely occasions. So as optimal solution, and to preserve this bandwidth, a 15 bit counter is used on the device side, and another 17 bits (so-called wrap-add throughout) are later added by the host software for monitoring events [1].

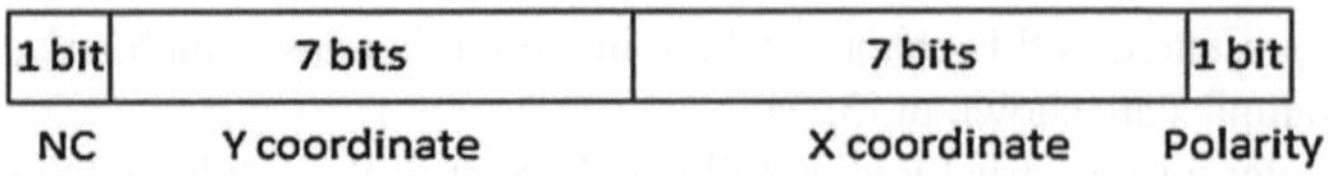

Fig. 3 AE address structure

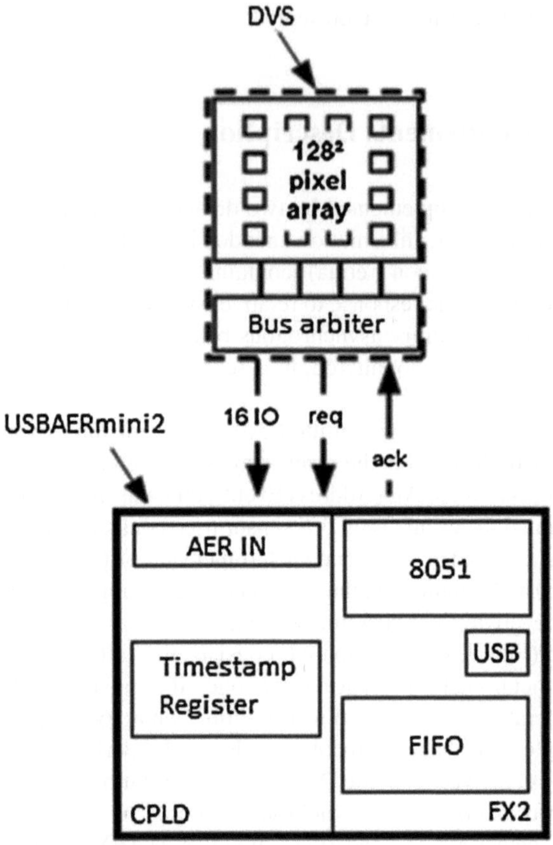

Fig. 4 System architecture

Both devices plus three infrared lights conform the system black box, which is shown in Fig. 5. The whole system has been conveniently package for easy installation of the system in different vehicles and in order to avoid bumps. Infrared illumination was used in order to avoid damaging the driver's visibility and interfere in the driving task. Besides that, it makes the system much more independent of lighting conditions (day or night). A visible light filter was added to the DVS lens to allow only infrared information acquisition.

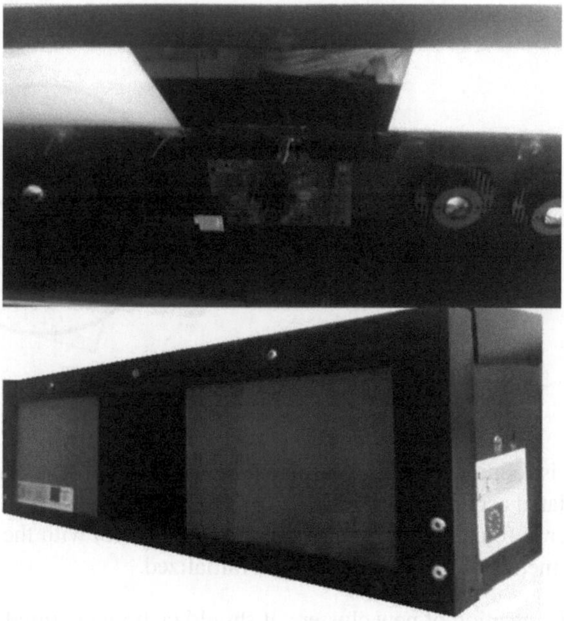

Fig. 5 Portable packaged system

3 Hands Tracking Algorithm

The developed algorithm is absolutely based in AER information, considering its intrinsic characteristics. The proposed algorithm performs a permanent clustering of events and tries to follow the trajectory of these clusters. The algorithm focuses on certain user-defined regions called regions of interest (ROI), which correspond to certain parts of the front compartment of a vehicle (wheel, gearshift, …). These different ROIs are customizable, allowing the user to define several shapes, sizes or number of regions. The events received are processed without data buffering, and can be assigned to a cluster or not, based on a distance criterion. If the event is assigned to a cluster, it will update the values of the cluster, such as position, distance, and number of events [14].

The algorithm can be described in detail as follows:

(a) Every time there is a new event belonging to one ROI, a cluster from the list of clusters is selected, being the one whose distance between the cluster centre to the event is less than a value Dv (see Fig. 6). This condition can be written as:

$$D = |x - x_e| < D_v$$

where x_e is the event position and x is the centre cluster position.

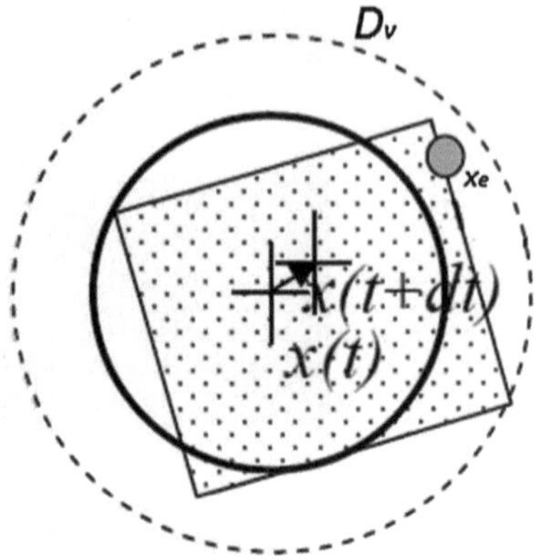

Fig. 6 Continuous clustering of AE

(b) If a cluster is found where the above condition is true, all features of the cluster list are updated accordingly.
(c) If no cluster is found, a new one is created (if possible) with the centre x_e and all the parameters of this new cluster are initialized.

Regarding the creation of new clusters, it should be borne in mind that the maximum number of clusters is limited to two (number of hands presented in the scene).

The cluster update process is sketched in Fig. 5. As it was previously indicated, x_e is the coordinate of an AE produced by the edge of a moving cluster. Let *x(t)* be the original cluster centre, then the new centre-coordinate $x(t + dt)$ is calculated as:

$$x(t + dt) = x(t) \cdot \alpha + x_e \cdot (1 - \alpha)$$

where $0 < \alpha < 1$ is an heuristically fixed parameter of the algorithm, and *dt* is the timestamp difference between the current and the last AE's that were assigned to the cluster. This approach shifts the clusters center by a certain distance controlled by α, which is usually chosen near 1 to obtain a smooth tracking.

Basin on the cluster location, the cluster speed has been calculated too. It gives valuable information about the movement presented in the scene. The speed calculation is performed similar to location; ensure soft changes in the velocity vector. An abrupt movement indicates noise, so it is not considered:

$$v(t + dt) = v(t) \cdot \alpha + v \cdot (1 - \alpha).$$

As it has been previously explained, the algorithm focuses just on certain R.O.I. The region with a more complex movement, corresponding to the wheel, was deeply analysed and a specific situation that could generate some mistakes was covered.. This region of interest has the shape of a circular ring and when the driver uses one hand to manipulate the wheel, the system detects two hands, generating a mistake (see Fig. 7). This is very common driver behaviour, so a specific module was added to the algorithm to manage this situation.

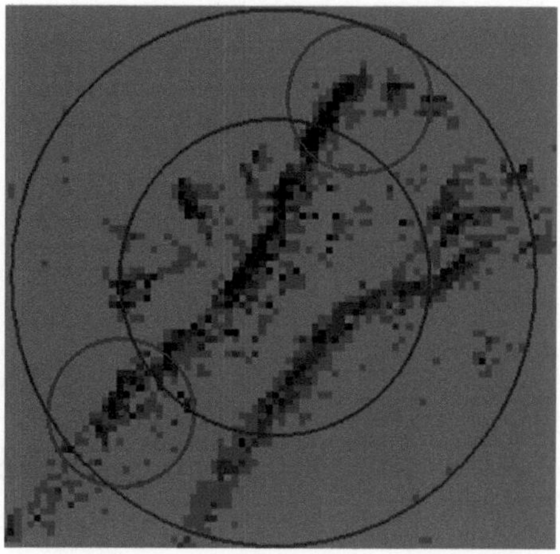

Fig. 7 Wrong detection situation

The added module considered geometrical information in the scene, calculated only with AE. As shown in Fig. 7, when the forearm is inserted fully into the ROI, there are two oblique parallel lines. To detect this situation it has been used a pattern recognition approach based on AER convolution. Notice that the AE convolution cannot be the same as the classical frame convolution, because the whole information of the image is not available at each time, just the events sequentially generated by the DVS. The AER convolution is based on the idea of a matrix *Y* of integrators (neurons). Every time an event is received, a convolution kernel is applied to those events and its neighbours in the array *Y*. When a neuron (a cell of *Y*) reaches a threshold, it generates an event and is reset [13, 18]. These neurons can be understood as bins that receive the modified events after the kernel is applied, generating a new event when this bin is "full".

Two convolution kernels, basing on the geometry of the objects to be detected in the scene, have been used simultaneously, one for each arm (left "//", right "\\"). When either arm appears on the scene, it will be registered a maximum in the average output of the convolutioned events of the corresponding kernel that matches with the arm presented. A minimum (with respect to previous output) would be obtained in the case of the convolution kernel that does not match. However, the output of the two convolution kernels, in the usual driving situation (both hands on the wheel), is very similar, not registering any maximum or minimal output.

Looking at the average of both convolutions, it is possible to identify the situation in which either arm is in scene and know with which arm it is been driving. So basing on the output of this module, the problematic situation to be avoided can be detected. Moreover, it can be identified what arm is presented: left or right. The presence of just one arm in the scene is normal during short period times, but when it is detected during a long time, a risky situation for the driver can be supposed and corresponding alarm actions could be applied.

This behaviour can be observed in Fig. 8. When the driving situation is normal, the mean number of events convolutioned is similar in the case of both kernels, so

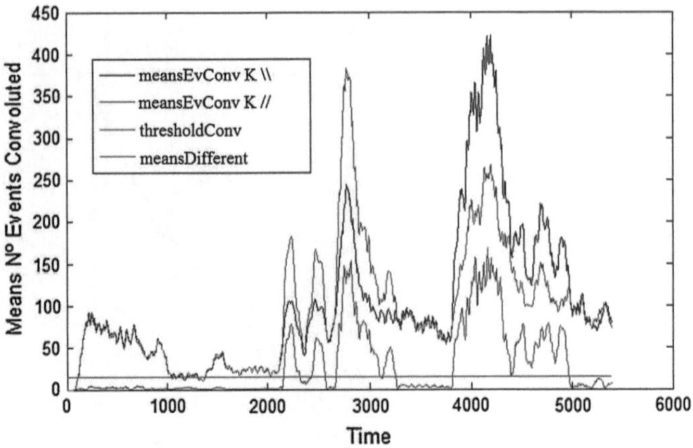

Fig. 8 Difference between the two convolutions outputs

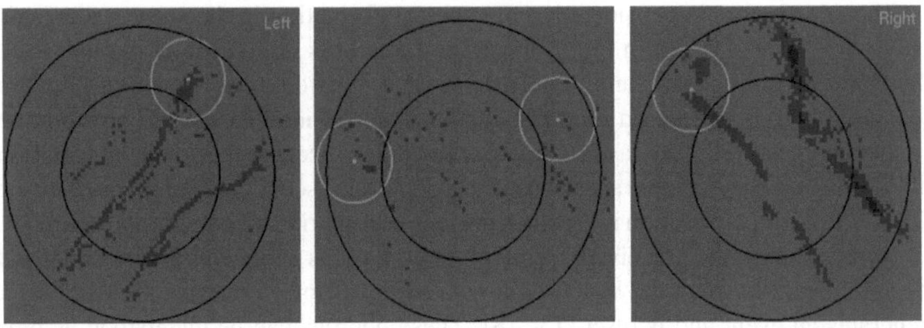

Fig. 9 From *left to right*: *left forearm* on scene, normal driving situation (both hands on the wheel), *right forearm* on the scene

that their difference is practically zero. When a forearm is detected on scene, the convolution kernel that coincides triggers the number of convolutioned events, while the convolution kernel which does not coincide is not able to reach so high levels. Therefore, when the difference between the means of both convolution kernel events exceeds a threshold, we can detect that there is a forearm on the scene and know to which hand belongs (see Fig. 9).

4 Results

Deeply test was done in a highly realistic driving simulator (see Fig. 10). Different scenarios, drivers or environments was considered, conforming different test sessions. In each session the following parameters were obtained:

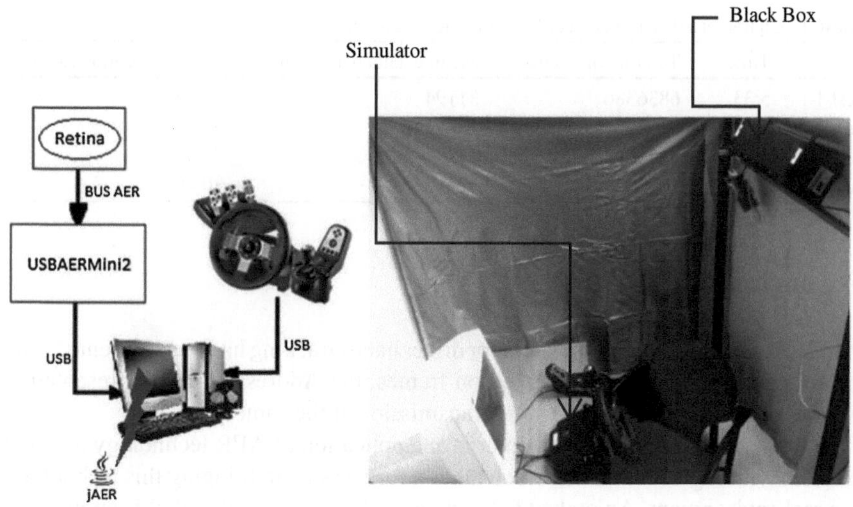

Fig. 10 Simulation scenario

- Total exercise time
- Total number of events generated
- Means motion.

The last parameter represents the average amount of movement detected during the session acquisition. As explained in Sect. 2, the sensor used is a motion sensor so in the case of scenes with high movement, the number of events per second will be high. Thus, the greater number of events generated, the more information you have and the more accurate the calculations and operations of the algorithm are obtained.

Tests have been carried out in a very realistic simulator. In each test it has been considered different types of driving scenarios. In the test one the scene considered is very dynamic, in an urban environment, with lots of curves where the driver has to move his hands at a high speed. The next test, the number two, has been acquired in a rally stage scenario, where the driving task is done faster. In test three, the scenario used was a highway, where the movements made by the driver are very scarce. The latest test has been developed in an urban ride, in which the driver did not found many obstacles and made soft movement.

To calculate the system effectiveness, it has been compared with the ground truth, where the number of hands present in each region is known, calculating the correct location rate of the proposed algorithm. Experimental results are shown in Table 1. It can be observed that in all cases the proposed method obtains a good performance. In the case of tests with a high movement in the scene, the correct location rate is bigger, because much more information is detected by the DVS.

Table 1 Characteristics and correct location rate of each test

	Time	Total n^o of events	Mean events per second	Correct location rate (%)
Test 1	5:33	6836386	31194	89.54
Test 2	5:30	9557951	16872	81.00
Test 3	3:54	4075592	3588	75.46
Test 4	5:50	10993454	12525	80.40

5 Conclusion

In this chapter a bio-inspired system for driver hands tracking has been presented. The information considered is not based on frames, but Address Event Representation (AER), allowing the processing and transmission at the same time.

The work presented in this chapter is an application of AER technology to a real problem with high constrains, which takes a further step in bringing this technology to a real environment. An embedded system could be designed with this application to be used in smart cars. This chapter demonstrates the possibility of using AER systems in automotive environments, detecting the small and fast movements that a high-speed camera is not able to notice.

Experimental results acquired in a realistic driving simulator are presented, showing the effectiveness of AER-processing applied to an automotive scenario.

To maximize the capacity and speed of AER is necessary to implement this system on a hardware platform. For this, as has been proposed future work the implementation of the system presented in this chapter on a hardware platform. This requires designing the algorithm presented in this chapter in a hardware description language such as VHDL for subsequent loading in a programmable logic device such as an FPGA. For the detection of patterns can be made use of convolution processor chips based entirely on AER described in [2] so that the system will be designed entirely under EAR technology.

Currently there are more powerful vision sensors like those presented in [19] that can be used for future work spoken of. Already exits new applications of these new retinas like that presented in [20].

Other future-work plans, it will be carried out a comparison between both systems, the based AER and the based on frames, to get results, concerning the processing speed, amount of relevant information generate, efficiency… to improve the system performance that is proposed in this chapter when little data is generated.

Acknowledgments Supported by the Minister for Science and Innovation of Spain project VULCANO (TEC2009-10639-C04-04).

References

1. Berner R (2006) Highspeed USB 2.0 AER interface, Diploma thesis, Institute of Neuroinformatics UNI–ETH Zurich, Department of architecture and computer technology, University of Seville, 14 April 2006
2. Camunas-Mesa L, Acosta-Jimenez A, Zamarreno-Ramos C, Serrano-Gotarredona T, Linares-Barranco B (2011) A 32 x 32 pixel convolution processor chip for address event vision sensors with 155 ns event latency and 20 Meps throughput. IEEE Trans Circuits Syst I Regul Pap 58(4):777–790
3. Conradt J, Berner R, Cook M, Delbruck, T (2009) An embedded AER dynamic vision sensor for low-latency pole balancing. In: IEEE 12th international conference on computer vision workshops (ICCV workshops), pp 780–785
4. Crespo R, Martín de Diego I, Conde C, Cabello E (2010) Detection and tracking of driver's hands in real time. In: Progress in pattern recognition, image analysis, computer vision, and applications, vol 6419. pp 212–219
5. Delbruck T (2008) Frame-free dynamic digital vision. In: Symposium on secure-life electronics, advanced electronics for quality life and society, pp 21–26
6. Union E (2004) Aide - adaptive integrated driver-vehicle interface. European project fp6 (ist-1-507674-ip). http://www.aide-eu.org/index.html
7. Gómez- Rodríguez F, Miró-Amarante L, Diaz-del-Rio F, Linares-Barranco A, Jimenez G (2010) Real time multiple objects tracking based on a bio-inspired processing cascade architecture. In: Proceedings of IEEE international symposium on circuits and systems (ISCAS), pp 1399–1402
8. IEEE (2004) Standard for motor vehicle event data recorders (mvedrs). http://grouper.ieee.org/groups/1616a/
9. Jimenez-Fernandez A, Fuentes-del-Bosh JL, Paz-Vicente R, Linares-Barranco A, Jiménez G (2010) Neuro-inspired system for real-time vision sensor tilt correction. In: Proceedings of 2010 IEEE international symposium on circuits and systems (ISCAS), pp 1394–1397, 30 May 2010–2 June 2010
10. Klauer S, Guo F, and Sudweeks J (2010) An analysis of driver inattention using a case-crossover approach on 100-car data: final report. National highway traffic safety administration. U.S. Department of transportation, Technical representative
11. Lichtsteiner P, Posch C, Delbruck T (2008) A 128x128 120 dB 30 mW asynchronous vision sensor that responds to relative intensity change. IEEE J Solid-State Circuits 43:566–576
12. Linares-Barranco A, Gomez-Rodriguez F, Jimenez-Fernandez A, Delbruck T, Lichtensteiner P (2007) Using FPGA for visuo-motor control with a silicon retina and a humanoid robot. ISCAS 2007. In: IEEE international symposium on circuits and systems, pp 1192–1195, 27–30 May 2007
13. Linares-Barranco A, Paz-Vicente R, Gómez-Rodríguez F, Jiménez A, Rivas M, Jiménez G, Civit A (2010) On the AER convolution processors for FPGA. In: Proceedings of IEEE international symposium on circuits and systems (ISCAS), pp 4237–4240
14. Litzenberger M, Posch C, Bauer D, Belbachir AN, Schön P, Kohn B, Garn H (2006) Embedded vision system for real-time object tracking using an asynchronous transient vision sensor. In: Digital signal processing workshop 12th–signal processing education, workshop 4th September 2006, pp 173–178
15. McAllister G, McKenna SJ, Ricketts IW (2000) Tracking a driver's hands using computer vision. In: Systems, man, and cybernetics, 2000 IEEE international conference on, vol 2, pp 1388–1393
16. Nations U (2010) Decreasing driver distraction. International telecommunication union. ITU-T technology watch report, Technical representative. http://www.itu.int/dmspub/itut/oth/23/01/T230100000F0002PDFE.pdf
17. NTHSA (2005) Drowsy driver detection and warning system for commercial vehicle drivers: field proportional test design, analysis and progress. In: National highway traffic safety administration, Washington, DC, Technical representatives. http://www.nhtsa.dot.gov/

18. Pérez-Carrasco JA et al (2010) Fast vision through frameless event-based sensing and convolutional processing: application to texture recognition. IEEE Trans Neural Networks 21:609–620
19. Serrano-Gotarredona T, Linares-Barranco B (2013) A 128 128 1.5 % Contrast Sensitivity 0.9 % FPN 3 μs Latency 4 mW asynchronous frame-free dynamic vision sensor using transimpedance preamplifiers. IEEE J Solid-Stated Circuits 48(3):827–838
20. Serrano-Gotarredona T, Park J, Linares-Barranco A, Jiménez A, Benosman R, Linares-Barranco B (2012) Improved contrast sensitivity DVS and its application to event-driven stereo vision, Telluride
21. Sivilotti M (1991) Wiring considerations in analog VLSI systems with application to field-programmable networks, Ph.D. dissertation, computer science division, California institute of technology, Pasadena
22. Serrano-Gotarredona R et al (2009) A 45k neuron, 5m synapse, 12g connects/s aer hardware sensory processing learningactuating system for high-speed visual object recognition and tracking. IEEE Trans Neural Networks 20(9):1417–1438
23. Serrano-Gotarredona R et al (2008) On real-time aer 2-d convolutions hardware for neuromorphic spike-based cortical processing. IEEE Trans Neural Networks 19(7):1196–1219
24. Tzou K (1987) Progressive image transmission: a review and comparison of techniques. Opt Eng 26(7):581–589
25. Zhang H, Schreiner C, Zhang K, Torkkola K (2007) Naturalistic use of cell phones in driving and context-based user assistance. In: Proceedings of the 9th international conference on Human computer interaction with mobile devices and services, ser. MobileHCI '07. New York, ACM, pp 273–276

Determination of In-Plane and Off-Plane Surface Displacements with Grids Virtually Applied to Digital Images

Valerio Lux, Emanuele Marotta and Pietro Salvini

Abstract Digital image devices have experienced an enormous increment in their capabilities, associated with a significant reduction in the economic effort. In particular, the increasing number of pixel made available for each picture allows developing software that is able to perform precise surface characterizations. In the present chapter the interest is oriented into two directions. The firs one concerns detecting the geometric features of surfaces through digital image comparison. The method does not require stereo image processing but it is based on a single camera vision. The base of this first part of the work regards the displacements of a grid virtually applied on the surface. To this goal the real printed grid case is firstly discussed. The grid virtually attached to the pictures identifies a finite element mesh associated to the comparing images. The second part aims to evaluate surface strains experienced on the specimen surface. The algorithm performs the analysis of the two comparing images, before and after the application of loads. Two different strategies are proposed: a partial grouping of pixels by equation averaging; the use of Hu's invariants applied to sub-images.

Keywords Strain measurements · Digital image correlation · Finite elements

1 Introduction

Image interpretation and processing is a fundamental analysis in most of medical applications [5]. The main objective is to help the analyst in the interpretation of the results while introducing quantitative data. In some cases, the attention is focused on surface detection, while in other contexts, the observation is dedicated to morphological changes or surface extension (strain or deformations).

V. Lux · E. Marotta · P. Salvini (✉)
Department of Industrial Engineering, Università di Tor Vergata, Roma, Italy
e-mail: salvini@uniroma2.it

P. Di Giamberardino et al. (eds.), *Computational Modeling of Objects Presented in Images*, Lecture Notes in Computational Vision and Biomechanics 15,
DOI: 10.1007/978-3-319-04039-4_9, © Springer International Publishing Switzerland 2014

Considering rigid body detection and surface out of plane measurements, this item has been extensively studied by many researchers [11]. In many cases the objective is directed towards the recognition of objects, whatever is their spatial positioning and minimal surface deformation. This is often accomplished by methods that make use of patterns of key points [9].

For the reconstruction of surface deformations many efforts have been done by researchers, in both 2D and 3D approach, some of these methods have been compared in [14]. The general achievements show that many benefits are gained if the entire acquired image is simultaneously considered; this is to say non-considering each subset individually. In this optics, some smoothing can be achieved by B-spline regularization [3] or by finite element formulation for the acquisition of the deformation field [7] by DIC.

In the present chapter the attention is firstly devoted on the capability to extract the geometric shapes of a surface, originally flat. This means that the interest is not only directed towards object recognition, but to new surface characteristics for the identification of its off-plane displacements. In the present case the tests consider the displacement of a sheet of paper, easily deformed in the out of plane orientation but experiencing minor surface strains. Within the paper, it is demonstrated that using an effective image, sufficiently variegated (such as a speckle image or any other non-uniform and non-periodical picture) is equivalent to a regularly meshed grid [1]. This equivalence is achieved by mapping the picture through a regular or non-regular mesh of quadrilateral sub-images (elements). These non-superimposed sub-images are managed as four node bilinear membrane elements, well known in finite element analysis. Each element of the grid maintains its peculiarity because it is characterized by a different color content and distribution (sub-image).

Another aspect, that makes use of the same image recognition methods, regards the capability to extrapolate the strains experienced by mating surfaces using non-invasive methods. The most promising methods involve photographic techniques, such as digital image correlation [4, 12–14]. Usually the strain and motion analysis procedures make use of a sequence of pictures that follows the whole strain progress [2]. In this chapter a method that requires only two images is proposed; the first is taken when no loads are applied, the second one when all loads and resulting deformations are settled. This method can thus be applied in principle when a limited number of images are available, as the initial and the final image only.

There exist 2-D digital Correlation techniques as well as 3-D ones [10]. Here we deal with 2-D technique which is based on the use of a single camera. Most of the techniques are based on sub-image correlations. This means that the local correlation imposed on a sub-image does not have an influence on all other correlations performed on sub-images far away from the previous one. In this chapter, according to former approaches [1, 3], we discuss a technique that solves the displacement fields as a whole, so that the continuity conditions is fulfilled in the whole processed image.

When consistent displacements are faced, the correlation techniques meet considerable difficulties to keep precision, as discussed in [12].

The displacement field solution generally needs the handling of a very high number of equations; this can even attain the order of the number of pixels recorded into the image. Therefore, a technique directed to reduce the number of equations while increasing the efficiency is discussed.

2 Out of Plane Surface Deformation

The geometric model adopted is the simple equivalent pinhole camera. According to this assumption, being *f* the distance between the pinhole and the image sensor, the following ratios can be written:

$$X' = -\frac{f}{Z}X; \qquad Y' = --\frac{f}{Z}Y; \qquad Z' = -f \tag{1}$$

The negative sign is generally changed by considering the image projected between the viewing point and the object (Fig. 1).

In the pinhole assumption, the complex dioptric lens system is substituted by an ideal single lens, infinitesimally thin, thus the optical system agrees with the following assumptions [15]:

- all parallel light rays are concentrated on the focus;
- no refraction is induced to all rays passing through the lens center;
- all non-centered rays are deviated in correspondence of the middle plane.

Other assumed hypotheses, adopted when dealing with digital images are:

the optical axis is perfectly orthogonal to the sensor plane and centered on it;
the sensor gauge is organized by a two perfectly orthogonal cell disposition.

2.1 *Identification of Grid Images*

In this section we assume that the image is simply constituted by a regular square grid. In the next section the association of a grid to a general image is discussed. Figure 2 shows the projection of a simple square on the CCD plane that is reversed, as usually. The geometry projected on the plane is given by the four vectors connecting the observation point to the square corners.

Once the image is digitally acquired, each vector **v** associated to a point is known in its direction, while its magnitude remains unknown. All unknowns are represented by the moduli associated to the respective vectors. According to this logic, all vectors **U** are computed as differences of vectors **V** (Fig. 2). In the following, the vectors **V** will be addressed making use of respective unit vectors: $\mathbf{V} = \mathrm{m} \cdot \mathbf{v}$.

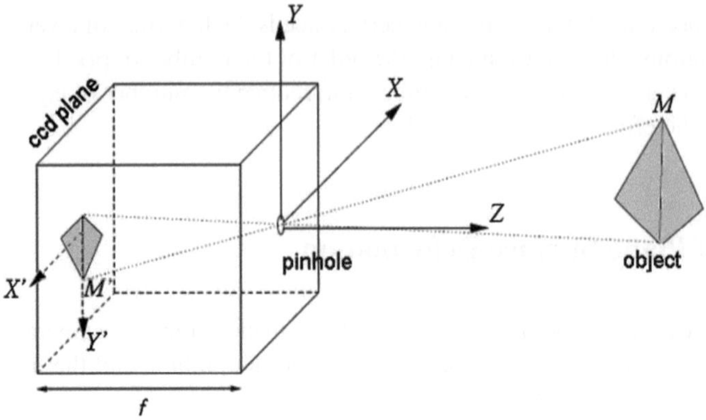

Fig. 1 Scheme of pinhole camera view

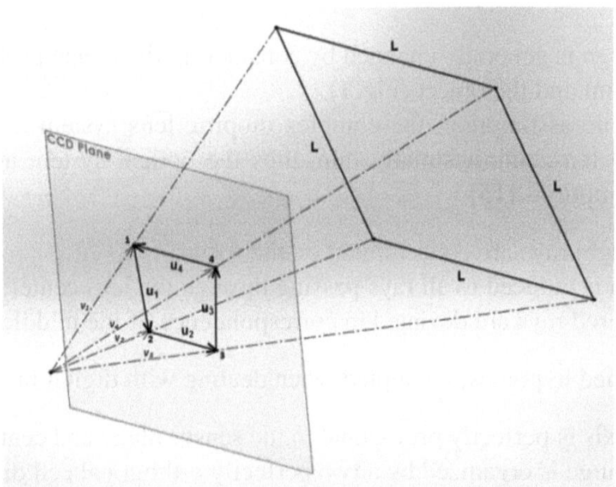

Fig. 2 Vectors identifying the positioning of element nodes

Making reference to the 3 × 3 grid represented in Fig. 3, the first element gives the following equations:

$$\begin{aligned} \mathbf{U_1} &= \mathbf{V_5} - \mathbf{V_1} = m_5\mathbf{v}_5 - m_1\mathbf{v}_1 \\ \mathbf{U}_2 &= \mathbf{V}_6 - \mathbf{V}_5 = m_6\mathbf{v}_6 - m_5\mathbf{v}_5 \\ \mathbf{U}_3 &= \mathbf{V}_2 - \mathbf{V_1} = m_2\mathbf{v}_2 - m_1\mathbf{v}_1 \\ \mathbf{U}_4 &= \mathbf{V}_6 - \mathbf{V}_2 = m_6\mathbf{v}_6 - m_2\mathbf{v}_2 \end{aligned} \tag{2}$$

Being the grid formed by equal squares, several conditions can be imposed to each of them - note that not all of them are independent - represented in Table 1.

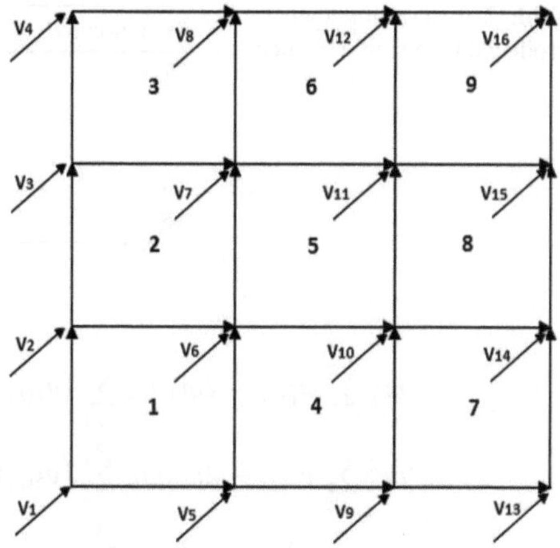

Fig. 3 Nomenclature of a 3 × 3 grid

Table 1 Vector and scalar conditions for a square grid

Geom. condition	Vector eq.	Number of scalar eqs
$U_2 \parallel U_3$	$U_2 \times U_3 = 0$	3
$U_1 \parallel U_4$	$U_1 \times U_4 = 0$	3
$U_1 \perp U_2$	$U_1 \cdot U_2 = 0$	1
$U_2 \perp U_4$	$U_2 \cdot U_4 = 0$	1
$U_3 \perp U_4$	$U_3 \cdot U_4 = 0$	1
$U_1 \perp U_3$	$U_1 \cdot U_3 = 0$	1
$\lvert U_1\rvert = L$	$U_1 \cdot U_1 = L^2$	1
$\lvert U_2\rvert = L$	$U_2 \cdot U_2 = L^2$	1
$\lvert U_3\rvert = L$	$U_3 \cdot U_3 = L^2$	1
$\lvert U_4\rvert = L$	$U_4 \cdot U_4 = L^2$	1

The equations given in the previous Table 1 generates, using the modules as the unknowns, the following 14 equations (first two are vector equations):

$$\begin{aligned} m_1m_5(\mathbf{v}_5 \times \mathbf{v}_1) - m_1m_6(\mathbf{v}_6 \times \mathbf{v}_1) - m_2m_5(\mathbf{v}_5 \times \mathbf{v}_2) - m_2m_6(\mathbf{v}_6 \times \mathbf{v}_2) = \mathbf{0} \\ m_1m_2(\mathbf{v}_1 \times \mathbf{v}_2) - m_1m_6(\mathbf{v}_1 \times \mathbf{v}_6) - m_2m_5(\mathbf{v}_5 \times \mathbf{v}_2) + m_5m_6(\mathbf{v}_5 \times \mathbf{v}_6) = \mathbf{0} \end{aligned} \tag{3}$$

$$\begin{aligned} m_1m_5(\mathbf{v}_1 \cdot \mathbf{v}_2) - m_1m_6(\mathbf{v}_1 \cdot \mathbf{v}_6) - m_5m_5(\mathbf{v}_5 \cdot \mathbf{v}_5) + m_5m_6(\mathbf{v}_5 \cdot \mathbf{v}_6) = 0 \\ -m_2m_6(\mathbf{v}_2 \cdot \mathbf{v}_6) + m_2m_5(\mathbf{v}_2 \cdot \mathbf{v}_5) - m_5m_6(\mathbf{v}_5 \cdot \mathbf{v}_6) + m_6m_6(\mathbf{v}_6 \cdot \mathbf{v}_6) = 0 \\ m_1m_2(\mathbf{v}_1 \cdot \mathbf{v}_2) - m_1m_6(\mathbf{v}_1 \cdot \mathbf{v}_6) - m_2m_2(\mathbf{v}_2 \cdot \mathbf{v}_2) + m_2m_6(\mathbf{v}_2 \cdot \mathbf{v}_6) = 0 \\ m_1m_1(\mathbf{v}_1 \cdot \mathbf{v}_1) - m_1m_2(\mathbf{v}_1 \cdot \mathbf{v}_2) - m_1m_5(\mathbf{v}_1 \cdot \mathbf{v}_5) + m_2m_5(\mathbf{v}_2 \cdot \mathbf{v}_5) = 0 \end{aligned} \tag{4}$$

Table 2 List of unknowns produced by a single element

Unknowns			
1	m_1^2	6	m_2m_6
2	m_1m_2	7	m_2m_5
3	m_1m_6	8	m_5^2
4	m_1m_5	9	m_5m_6
5	m_2^2	10	m_6^2

$$\begin{aligned}
m_1^2\sum_{i=1}^{3}\nu_{1(i)}^2 - 2m_1m_3\sum_{i=1}^{3}\left(\nu_{1(i)}\nu_{5(i)}\right)^2 + m_5^2\sum_{i=1}^{3}\nu_{5(i)}^2 &= L^2\\
m_5^2\sum_{i=1}^{3}\nu_{5(i)}^2 - 2m_5m_6\sum_{i=1}^{3}\left(\nu_{5(i)}\nu_{6(i)}\right)^2 + m_6^2\sum_{i=1}^{3}\nu_{6(i)}^2 &= L^2\\
m_2^2\sum_{i=1}^{3}\nu_{2(i)}^2 - 2m_2m_1\sum_{i=1}^{3}\left(\nu_{2(i)}\nu_{1(i)}\right)^2 + m_1^2\sum_{i=1}^{3}\nu_{1(i)}^2 &= L^2\\
m_6^2\sum_{i=1}^{3}\nu_{6(i)}^2 - 2m_6m_2\sum_{i=1}^{3}\left(\nu_{6(i)}\nu_{2(i)}\right)^2 + m_2^2\sum_{i=1}^{3}\nu_{2(i)}^2 &= L^2
\end{aligned} \tag{5}$$

All above equations give a non-linear (quadratic) system of equations where the unknowns are vector magnitudes. If one considers all possible combinations of products of unknowns as unknowns themselves, they turn to be 10 for a single element, with 14 equations each. As an example, for the element n. 1 of Fig. 3, the 10 unknowns are listed in Table 2.

The full system of equations is therefore over-determined and the solution can be found solving all the quadratic unknowns involved. After the full solution, each vector magnitude is computed by the root square of the quadratic unknowns. Furthermore, the mixed product of the unknowns can be used to check the accuracy of the solution gained.

2.2 *Virtual Image Embedded on a Picture*

If an image is present on a surface, this can be associated to a virtual grid. The point is to guarantee that the grid follows the changes of the image, due to movements of the surface that can be considered as a combination of rigid and deformable displacements.

This can be accomplished by considering the grid as a mesh of bilinear finite elements, whose movements guarantee the continuity of the surface. Each element contains a part of the initially flat image; this information is maintained in a natural coordinate system as shown in Fig. 4.

Such reference approach is particularly suitable to compare elements that are initially irregular or become irregular due to large displacements on the image. Therefore, each sub-image is interpolated though a cubic spline approach. By this

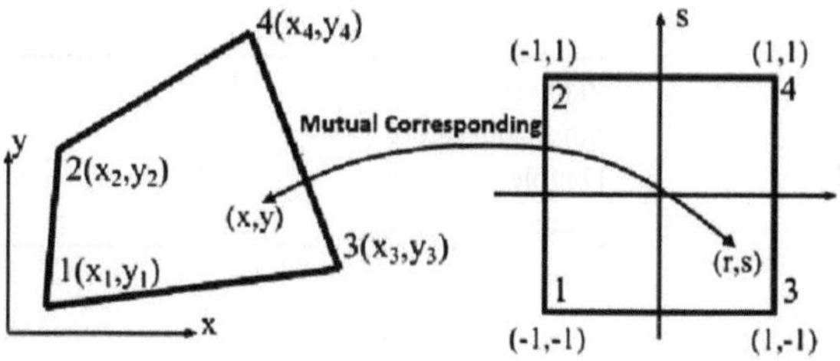

Fig. 4 Physical/Natural coordinate systems

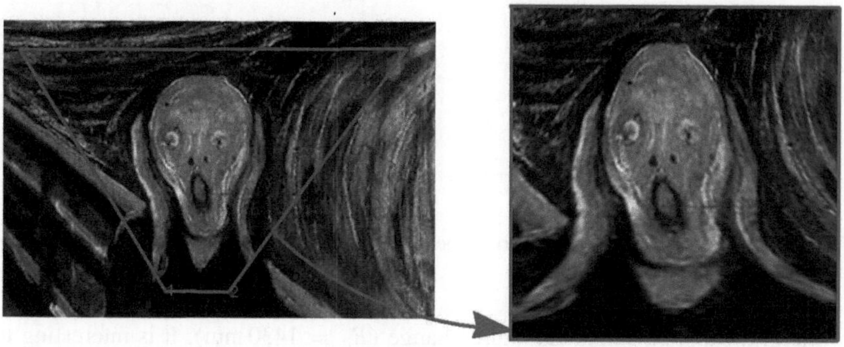

Fig. 5 Change from physical to natural coordinates

procedure, each element is always square-represented and keeps the same image content. In Fig. 5 is shown an example of how interpolation deforms the image.

2.3 Results on Out of Plane Deformation

The data here presented, apart the very next subsection, refers to all effective pictures taken with a focal distance equal to 29 mm, corresponding to a printed paper positioned at 1500 mm from the ideal lens center. All images have been obtained with an aperture equal to 1/8 to increase overall focus depth.

2.3.1 Test of the Procedure on Exact Grids

The theoretical correctness of the procedure presented has first of all been investigated through the application on a simulated grid (no pictures does effectively exist) that has been deformed applying one or two finite curvatures. We can see that the reconstruction is perfectly accurate (no digital error on pixel definitions is present since pixel positions are recorded with 12 digit precision) only if the local orientation

Table 3 Noise effect on accuracy for various curvatures

	No noise (%)	Added noise (%)
Plane grid	~1e-10	4.06
Single curvature	~1e-10	4.87
Double curvature	23.13	24.21
D.curv. refined el.	13.61	15.93

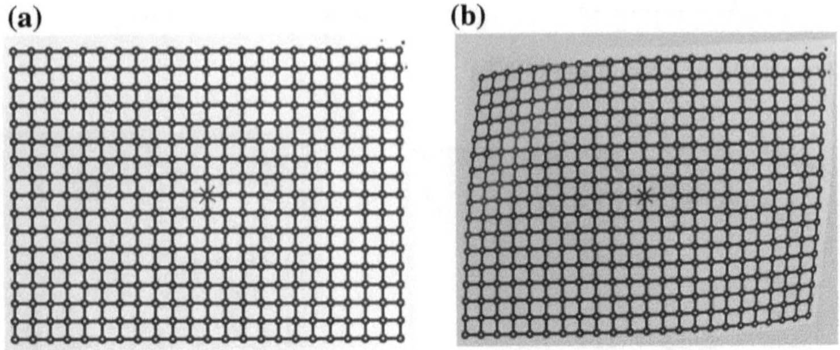

Fig. 6 Digital pictures of the printed grid, **a** before and **b** after off-plane deformation

of the grid causes a single curvature change ($R_c = 1430\,\text{mm}$). It is interesting to highlight that the application of a small noise (1 % of the diagonal length of a single element) reduces considerably the precision if the results are very accurate, but does not appreciably changes the behavior if discrepancies are already encountered when data are not affected by noise.

From the above reasons, it is clear that the assumption of square grid to maintain its shape is very strong, difficult to obtain when double curvature are present. This means that the size of the elements of the grid should be taken as small as the curvature increases. As a matter of fact, the last row in Table 3 shows much better results in this case, as expected (double curvature keeping the same equivalent value than single curvature case).

2.3.2 Tests on Pictures of Printed Grids

The grid is printed on a sheet of paper that is first photographed in a plane orthogonal to the focal axis, and the second picture considers the sheet deformed in various ways, such as the one shown in Fig. 6.

Four cases are here presented; (i) it concerns a $5 - 10 - 15°$ rigid rotation of the paper on a vertical axis as to generate a prospective view; (ii) it regards a simple half-fold oriented as the vertical axis in the center, and folded at a corner; (iii) the paper leaned on a cylinder (diameter = 450 mm) with a vertical axis; (iv) the paper applied on the same cylinder with the sheet base inclined of 30°.

In Fig. 7 two operating ways are compared: the black lines show the results when the over-determined solution is performed on all squares at the same time, the blue

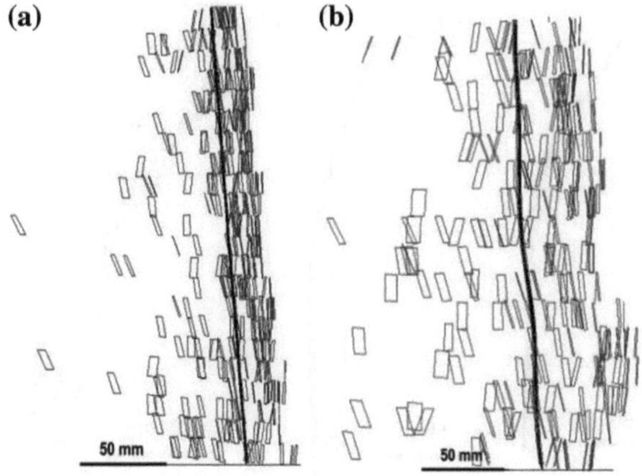

Fig. 7 Comparison of overall result and square dispersion for; **a** printed grid, **b** virtual grid on speckle image

Table 4 Angle identified when varying the point of view

Angle (°)	Grid method results (°)	Speckle method	
		16 × 16 el. (°)	37 × 37 el. (°)
5	4.64	3.96	4.50
10	9.72	8.23	8.69
15	14.86	9.64	11.68

lines consider the solution performed at each square, individually. The whole solution is much better than the second, since pixel errors compensate.

Table 4 shows the errors introduced when varying sheet inclination.

The results show that a rigid displacement on one of the grid axes can be managed by the method in the average by both images (grid or speckle above discussed) (Fig. 8).

The two cases of folds considered (ii) reveal a particular behavior of the algorithm. As a matter of fact, the mean square method tends to compensate the errors so that there is the tendency to keep flat in one direction. Referring to Fig. 9a and b the dispersion is illustrated when the fold is located in the center or in the corner, respectively. The maximum determined fold displacement respects the values imposed in the test within a 2 % error. Figure 10b results seem to be erroneously similar to the previous case, as the top views show. It is clear that the identification algorithm is affected by eventual curvatures non-aligned with the grid. In practice, since the algorithm tends to maintain the overall length at each element, it encounters some difficulties while managing elements that change all side-length due to curvatures imposed.

The results performed on cylindrical surfaces confirm the deficiencies previously indicated on double curvature grids. As a matter of fact the comparison between

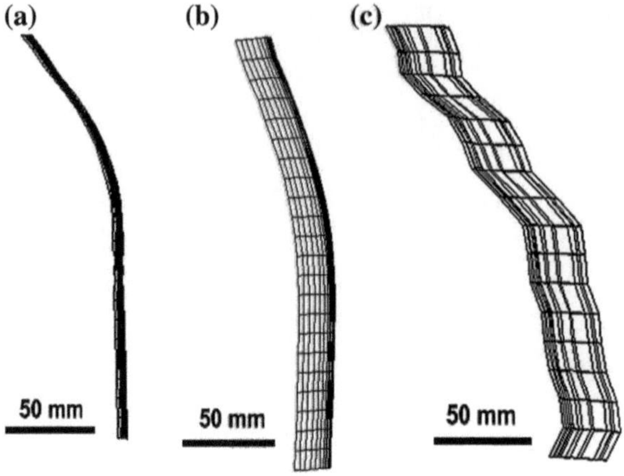

Fig. 8 Top view of the profiles for case (ii): **a** vertical fold **b** corner fold, **c** vertical fold for speckle image

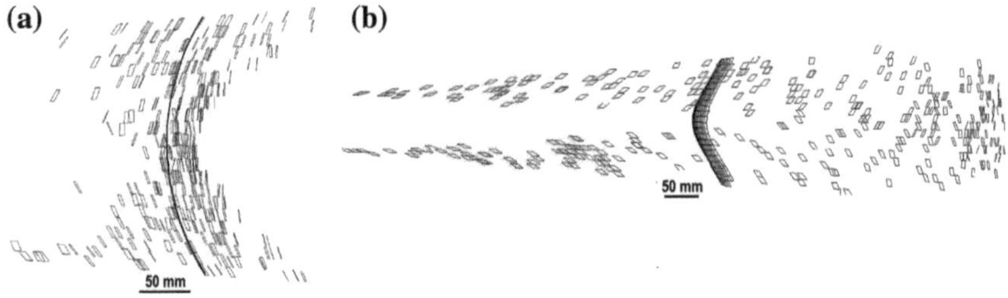

Fig. 9 Dispersion of individually identified elements for: **a** vertical cylinder, **b** inclined cylinder

cases (a) and (b) in Fig. 9 shows a much more evident dispersion of single computed squares (blue) when the sheet base is inclined toward horizon—relative full picture is visible in Fig. 7b. The global results (black lines) of case (a) are quite accurate (error in radius lower than 1 %) while case (b) provides erroneous results.

2.3.3 Tests on a Printed Speckle Picture

Indeed, the application of a virtual grid introduces some additional errors by respect to the printed grid. These errors amplify the deficiencies already evidenced before. The algorithm used to detect the displacement of the virtual grid by means of speckle deformed image is presented in the next session. The convergence is achieved by means of minimum square error search. For example, one can compare the results given in Figs. 10 and 11a and b, respectively. Case (a) identifies the virtual grid imposed on the image to be taken as reference; case (b) in Fig. 10 shows good identification that can also be seen in Fig. 7b through square dispersion. On the

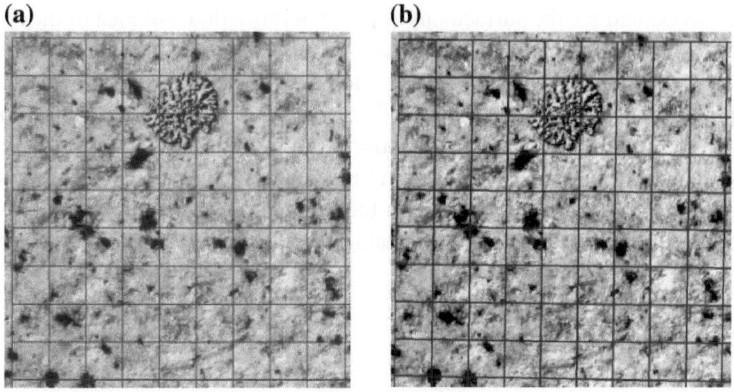

Fig. 10 Virtual node locations before and after 5° inclination

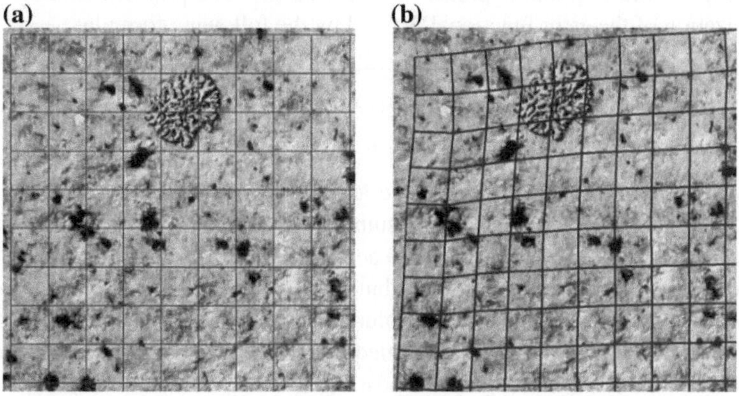

Fig. 11 Virtual node locations before and after application on inclined cylinder

contrary, one can see that the corner correspondence on Fig. 11a, b is very poor, particularly at the left top corner where the deformations are the highest, according to results presented in Fig. 9b.

2.3.4 Discussion on Out of Plane Deformations

It is evident that algorithm proposed here shows some difficulties when applied to structures that deforms with effective double curvatures. As a matter of fact, when double curvatures are present, the side lengths cannot be computed accurately by simple node distances. A better computation should accounts of effective surface distance through an iterative procedure that takes into account of geometry on curved surfaces. From another point of view, the advantage of the method is that no regularization conditions are required to the identifying surface, so that no simplified shape is accounted for the surface out of plane deformation. An idea of the solution accuracy can be reached from the dispersion of the results when computation regards each square element individually. When the dispersion is high the global results is correspondently worse. Use of speckle image instead of a printed grid is possible and a theoretical increment of information is available. However, the differential method, discussed hereinafter, requires a limitation of the displacements introduced in the image to keep consistency. When the strain are less than 50 % of the virtual grid nodes moves correctly, for higher values accuracy problems become evident.

3 Differential Method

The deformation field is calculated by comparing the original image and the deformed one. In this work a global approach is followed [2]. The problem consists in the minimization of the error functional defined by the following formula:

$$\mathrm{E} = \sqrt{\sum_{\mathrm{i}} [I_d(x_i, y_i) - I_u(x_i, y_i)]^2} \tag{6}$$

where $I_u I_d$ represent the images before and after deformation. x_i, y_i are the i-th pixel coordinates into the images. The summation comprehends all pixels. To each element a sub-image is associated. At each sub-image (corresponding to a single finite element) the internal spatial distribution is based on the displacements of the four nodes bordering the element. The solution allows finding the node locations that make it possible to overlap the undeformed image onto the deformed one. Once the image is divided into sub-images, it is possible to write the formula (6):

$$\mathbf{E} = \sqrt{\sum_{\mathrm{j}} \left\| \mathbf{S}_j(\mathbf{x}) - \mathbf{S}_{j0}(\mathbf{x}_0) \right\|^2} \tag{7}$$

where $\mathbf{S}_j, \mathbf{S}_{j0}$ are the j-th sub-image, while $\mathbf{x}$ and $\mathbf{x}_0$ represent the final and initial nodal coordinates, respectively. The rate of change between $\mathbf{x}$ and $\mathbf{x}_0$ is non-linear; for this reason it is not possible to directly find the solution, but an iterative procedure is needed. The algorithm consists in the linearization of the non-linear least squares problem. It is based on Taylor series expansion, truncated to its first order, of the sub-image when varying the generic nodal coordinate:

$$\mathbf{S}_j(X') = \mathbf{S}_0(X_0) + \sum_{\mathrm{k}} \frac{\partial \mathbf{S}_0}{\partial \mathrm{x_k}} (x_k - x_{k0}) \tag{8}$$

For the sake of clarity, the same is written in matrix formulation, evidencing the Jacobian matrix:

$$\begin{bmatrix} \frac{\partial \mathbf{S}_{1,0}}{\partial \mathrm{X}_1} & \frac{\partial \mathbf{S}_{1,0}}{\partial \mathrm{X}_2} & \cdots & \frac{\partial \mathbf{S}_{1,0}}{\partial \mathrm{X}_M} \\ \frac{\partial \mathbf{S}_{2,0}}{\partial \mathrm{X}_1} & \frac{\partial \mathbf{S}_{2,0}}{\partial \mathrm{X}_2} & \cdots & \frac{\partial \mathbf{S}_{2,0}}{\partial \mathrm{X}_M} \\ \vdots & \vdots & \cdots & \vdots \\ \frac{\partial \mathbf{S}_{N,0}}{\partial \mathrm{X}_1} & \frac{\partial \mathbf{S}_{N,0}}{\partial \mathrm{X}_2} & \cdots & \frac{\partial \mathbf{S}_{N,0}}{\partial \mathrm{X}_M} \end{bmatrix} \cdot \begin{Bmatrix} x_1 - x_1' \\ x_2 - x_2' \\ \vdots \\ x_M - x_M' \end{Bmatrix} = \begin{Bmatrix} \mathbf{S}_{1,0} - \mathbf{S}_{1,j}{}' \\ \mathbf{S}_{2,0} - \mathbf{S}_{2,j}{}' \\ \vdots \\ \mathbf{S}_{N,0} - \mathbf{S}_{N,j}{}' \end{Bmatrix} \tag{9}$$

or the equivalent $\mathbf{J} \cdot \Delta\mathbf{x} = \Delta\mathbf{s}$. Each term of the Jacobian matrix is composed by a number of elements that coincides with the number of pixels contained in the sub-image. Therefore, the matrix shows considerable dimensions. The computation is based on centered first derivate, evaluated by considering the pixels around each node. For this reason, the Jacobian matrix of the reference image is computed by respect to all possible node displacements. As mentioned before, the Jacobian matrix is composed of partial derivatives. Each matrix derivative is calculated by the four central point derivatives by respect to the unknowns as:

$$\frac{\partial \mathbf{F}(x)}{\partial x} = \frac{1}{12h}\left[\mathbf{F}(x-2h) - 8\mathbf{F}(x-h) + 8\mathbf{F}(x+h) - \mathbf{F}(x+8h)\right] \tag{10}$$

where h denotes the discretization step. For example, the term $\mathbf{F}(x\text{-}2h)$ represents the sub-image when a node is moved back $2h$. The choice of the parameter h is crucial. The solution requires the minimization of the error (7) through an iterative procedure. As a matter of fact the inversion of the Jacobian matrix is required (9):

$$\Delta\mathbf{x} = \mathbf{J}^{-1} \cdot \Delta\mathbf{s} \tag{11}$$

The Jacobian matrix is a sensitivity matrix; however, its costly inversion must be performed just once. When the displacements of all nodes have been computed, it is easy to gain the internal strains, known by means of the nodal displacements of each element. This is made possible through the pre-multiplication of the vector of element nodal displacements by the matrix **B** (obtain by appropriate derivative of Q4 shape functions) [16] if first order approximation is accepted, or more sophisticated expressions if first order simplification is not applicable.

3.1 Convergence Enhancement

In this section, the optimal choice of the number of internal points, to achieve a quick convergence of the results, is discussed. A criterion to reduce the equations and to speed-up the solution process is introduced. As an example, for a high-definition 3000 × 4000 pixel image, meshed through almost 10000 elements having eight degrees of freedom each, a 240 billion of equations results. In this chapter two possible techniques have been developed; the first considers possible grouping of pixels belonging to confined areas, the second one makes use of Hu's invariants to discriminate each sub-image.

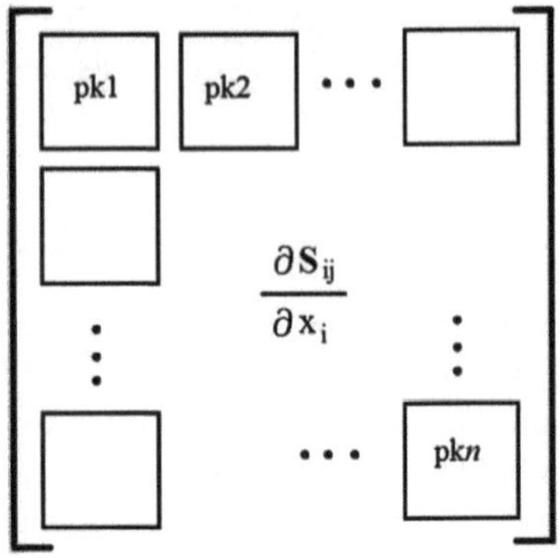

Fig. 12 Grouping technique representation

3.1.1 Method I: Grouping Technique

The technique of grouping is helpful to reduce the number of equations to solve. As cited before, the Jacobian presents a considerable dimension; in fact each term of the matrix is a partial derivative of the sub-image. The grouping method introduced in this chapter, handles the single partial derivative of the sub-image. These are divided into sub-areas, and a sum of the values inside them is considered, as shown in Fig. 12.

By this way, the number of equations is reduced, and the iterative calculation speeds up. The size of the grouping is important, and must be wisely chosen. A considerable grouping amount is required for saving computational time, the data information, is reduced making it difficult to gain convergence in the iteration process.

3.1.2 Method II: Hu's Invariants

Here we refer to moments as scalar quantities able to characterize a scalar field and possibly to point out some significant features. In statistics moments are widely used to describe the shape of a probability density function; in classic rigid-body mechanics to account of the mass distribution of a body, forming the inertia tensor. In mathematical terms, the moments are projections of a function onto a polynomial basis [6, 8]. General moments M_{pq} of an image *I(x,y)*, where *p*, *q* are non-negative integers and $r = p + q$ is called the order of the moment, are defined as:

$$M_{pq} = \iint p_{pq}(x, y) \cdot I(x, y) \cdot dx\ dy \tag{12}$$

Where $p_{00}(x, y), p_{10}(x, y), \ldots, p_{pq}(x, y)$, are polynomial basis functions defined in the domain. In this chapter moments of the the image are used, consequently the function *I(x,y)* is an image characterized by two coordinates *x,y* and a color value (e.g. RGB uses three values between 0 and 255 each).

A geometric moment of a discretized image is defined as a moment having the standard power basis $p_{pq}(x, y) = x^p y^q$. Therefore, it results:

$$m_{pq} = \sum_x \sum_y x^p \cdot y^q \cdot I(x, y) \tag{13}$$

Moreover Hu's invariants are built up through a combination of geometrical moments that show the characteristics of non-changing their values when some geometrical transformations are applied. Hu's invariants are originally seven, but other invariants could be computed. However, higher image invariants would increase considerably their magnitude, so that they cannot be managed together with the first seven.

Only the first invariant moment has an intuitive meaning: polar moment of inertia.

In this section Hu's invariants are used to characterize each sub-image. Even using this technique, the solution requires the inversion of the Jacobian matrix; in this case the Jacobian is not calculated through image differences, but differences on Hu's invariants. The image is meshed into sub-images by a grid; each sub-image is represented be its set of Hu's invariant moments. Hu's invariants are seven, but here, to increase the discriminant power, the computed invariants are doubled: they are computed on the sub-image itself and on its negative.

The invariant moments are insensitive to translations, rotations and scaling transforms. In an index compact notation they are:

$$\begin{aligned}
\varphi_1 &= m_{20} + m_{02} \\
\varphi_2 &= (m_{20} - m_{02})^2 + 4m_{11}^2 \\
\varphi_3 &= (m_{30} - 3m_{12})^2 + (3m_{21} - m_{03})^2 \\
\varphi_4 &= (m_{30} + m_{12})^2 + (m_{21} - m_{03})^2 \\
\varphi_5 &= (m_{30} - 3m_{12})(m_{30} + m_{12})\left[(m_{30} + m_{12})^2 - 3(m_{21} + m_{03})^2\right] + \\
&\quad + (3m_{21} - m_{03})(m_{21} + m_{03})\left[3(m_{30} + m_{12})^2 - (m_{21} + m_{03})^2\right] \\
\varphi_6 &= (m_{20} - m_{02})\left[(m_{30} + m_{12})^2 - (m_{21} + m_{03})^2\right] + \\
&\quad + 4m_{11}(m_{30} + m_{12})(m_{21} + m_{03}) \\
\varphi_7 &= (3m_{21} - m_{03})(m_{30} + m_{12})\left[(m_{30} + m_{12})^2 - 3(m_{21} + m_{03})^2\right] + \\
&\quad - (m_{30} + 3m_{12})(m_{21} + m_{03})\left[3(m_{30} + m_{12})^2 - (m_{21} + m_{03})^2\right]
\end{aligned} \tag{14}$$

3.2 Natural Coordinate System Applied on Elements

Both methods require the image comparison to minimize the error. To this goal it is useful referring to the natural coordinate system used in the isoparametric element formulation [16].

Their characteristics are particularly suitable because, in the natural coordinate system, all the elements, as well as in the reference picture as in the deformed one, have the same shape and dimensions (a simple square as shown in Fig. 4).

For the isoparametric four-node element, all internal points are mapped through natural coordinates *r,s* in the following manner:

$$\begin{cases} x(r,s) = \frac{1}{4}(1-r)(1-s)x_1 + \frac{1}{4}(1-r)(1+s)x_2 + \\ \quad + \frac{1}{4}(1+r)(1-s)x_3 + \frac{1}{4}(1+r)(1+s)x_4 \\ y(r,s) = \frac{1}{4}(1-r)(1-s)y_1 + \frac{1}{4}(1-r)(1+s)y_2 + \\ \quad + \frac{1}{4}(1+r)(1-s)y_3 + \frac{1}{4}(1+r)(1+s)y_4 \end{cases} \tag{15}$$

As a matter of fact, one of the difficulties encountered in both methods regards the change of the edges during displacement, now overtaken by using elements having a fixed domain shape, whatever is the image content. By this change of reference, an interpolation is required between the pixels in each element (only on sub-images of whole picture) and the values assumed in the *r-s* coordinate system. According to the isoparametric formulation, the same interpolation used to locate any internal point is adopted to evaluate internal displacements. The use of *r-s* coordinate system allows also to manage non-regular shaped elements. And to modify the number of unknowns considered.

3.3 Comparison Between Grouping Technique and Hu's Invariant

In this section a comparison is proposed: (i) full pixel computation; (ii) grouping technique by varying packaging dimension; (iii) Hu's invariant moments. All techniques have been applied on the same reference image. This image shows the surface of a granite (Fig. 13). The use of this image is due to his particular distribution of color that is a natural sort of speckle. The image is divided in 3×3 elements and 16 nodes; the dimension of a single element is 100×100 pixels. The original image is digitally deformed by $\varepsilon_x = 0.02$ and $\varepsilon_y = 0.01$. The (i) results (no enhancement) are obtained when the number of packets (a packet contains adjacent pixel grouped together) id equal to 10000 (number of pixels in each sub-image).

Several tests are performed progressively decreasing the number of packets. The lowest number of packets considered is 9, while the maximum numbers is 10000, representing the solution without any enhancement technique. Both convergence time and final error of the displacements are compared. All computations are performed on an internal processor Intel® Core *i7-2600* K having 3.4 GHz.

The error is calculated through a ratio: the numerator is the sum of the displacement differences between the identified final nodal position and the theoretical one (known due to strain imposed); the denominator is the sum of the differences between the theoretical position and the initial one.

In Fig. 14 errors and convergence times are normalized by respect to the highest values encountered. Note that this relative definition of error penalizes the lower displacements and this must be kept in mind when comparing different deformation magnitudes.

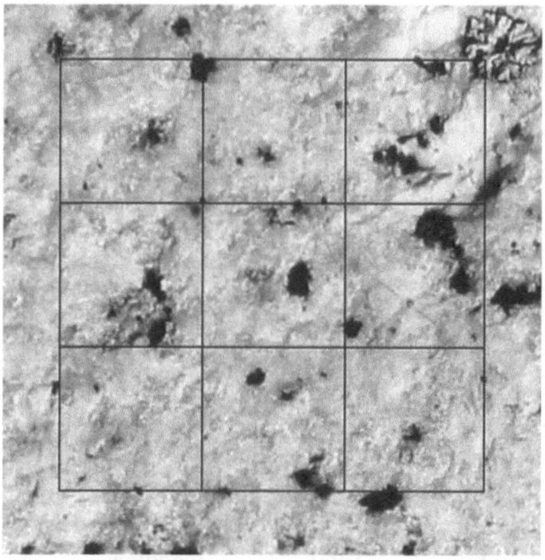

Fig. 13 Reference undeformed image 500 × 500 pixel

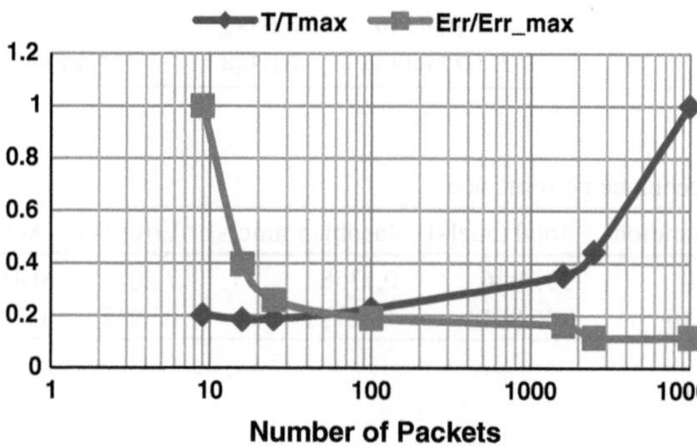

Fig. 14 Cpu Time versus error for the grouping technique for the grouping technique

As expected, the maximum errors are obtained with the minimum number of packets; the worst convergence time is obtained when no enhanced technique is used. Increasing the number of packets decreases the error convergence, but increases the calculation time and vice versa. It is possible to detect a crossing point of minimum error-time curves (Fig. 14, Table 5). It is interesting to highlight that the red curve (squares) identifies a well-defined knee, demonstrating that a strong grouping is possible while shortly affecting accuracy.

The results obtained with the method of Hu's invariant moments are s hown in Table 6. This method does not show at the present time particularly good outcomes. The invariants allow to greatly reducing the number of equations of the system, but they do not ensure acceptable results both in terms of computing time and precision of the solution. Even the use of non-speckle images helped to gain accurate results.

Table 5 Grouping technique performace

Number of packs	Iterations	Total times[s]	Jacobian Time[s]	Error[%]	Average Error [pixel]
4			Not convergence		
9	12	0,8886	0,0243	8,1729	0,2311
16	11	0,8166	0,0242	3,7483	0,1060
25	10	0,8252	0,0242	2,6902	0,0760
100	12	0,9963	0,0256	1,5607	0,0441
1600	13	1,5676	0,0531	1,4710	0,0416
2500	13	1,9551	0,0728	1,0258	0,0290
No enhancement	17	4,4014	0,2526	1,0848	0,0306

Table 6 Hu's invariant moments technique performance

Number invariants utilized	Iterations	Total time[s]	Jacobian time[s]	Error[%]	Average error[pixel]
14	236	20,7042	0,0367	10,0316	0,2837
12	236	20,7139	0,0382	10,0397	0,2840
10	258	22,6446	0,0384	22,3302	0,6316

Table 7 Grouping technique performance

Number of packs	Iterations	Total time[s]	Jacobian time[s]	Error[%]	Average error[pixel]
25	26	39,7946	0,1358	7,2077	0,4189
No enhancement	410	926,9013	10,2175	6,7912	0,3947

However, at strain values of the order of some percent, the Hu's invariant method works acceptably. The increase of the convergence time is mainly due to the increment in the number of iterations required to converge (Table 7).

Further tests have been performed using the grouping technique. In particular, some tests considered large strains applied, (over 30 %). It is interesting to observe that the grouping technique is able to manage also this amount of image differences, even when the non-enhanced technique is unable to reach convergence. Thus, the use of packets helps to speed up the solution time, but it is also skillful to organize information so that the convergence capability is stronger than before. As an example, in the case analyzed and proposed in Fig. 13, presenting a strong deformation reaching 0.35 in both principal directions, calculated with 25 packages, the method returns a solution with an error close to 0.56 % and 9.84 s of convergence time, whereas when non-using packages the solution does not converge at all (Fig. 15).

To validate the grouping technique, another example is performed: the image used is not a speckle, but a generic image (canvas paint in Fig. 16). In this case the deformations are not of the same magnitude of the preceding ones, but they are set to $\varepsilon_x = 0.03$ and $\varepsilon_y = 0.01$; much more elements are used to mesh the image.

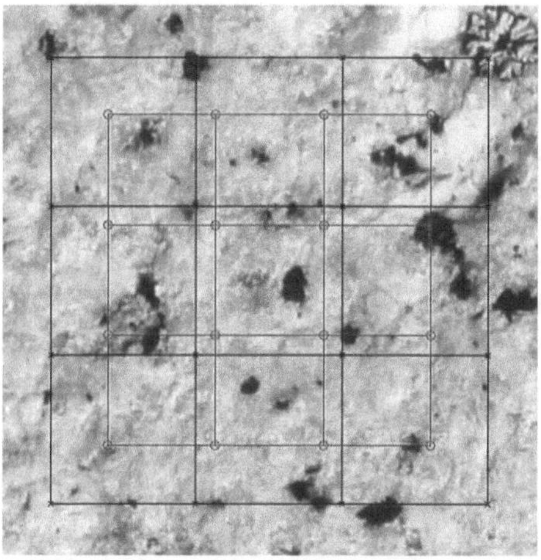

Fig. 15 Example large deformed image and grid solution obtained by grouping technique

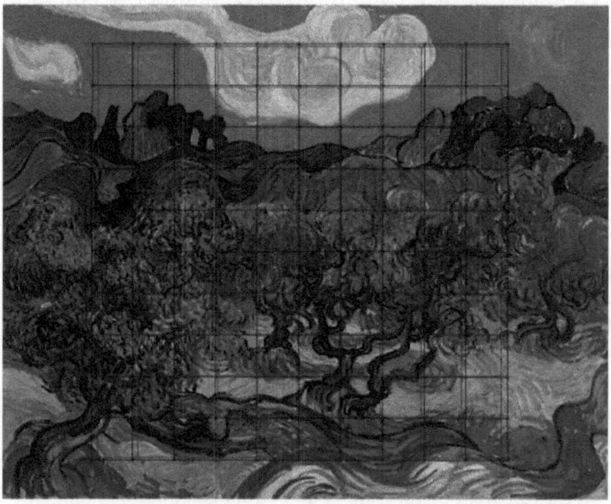

Fig. 16 Example deformed image and grid 10 × 10 solution obtained by grouping technique

In particular a grid of 10 × 10 elements, having 50 × 50 pixels each is used. The study was performed both with a number of packets equal to 25, and without any convergence enhancement technique.

This latter example shows once again the convenience of the use of packets, both in terms of accuracy and computational time. This convenience is stronger and stronger when increasing the number of sub-images managed. Incidentally, it is shown that the use of packets is profitable on non-speckled images.

4 Conclusions

In this work it has been discussed a discretization technique that is able to account of off-plane displacements of a surface as well as in-plane deformations. For both circumstances a differential method to determine the displacement field is presented. In the chapter two different procedures to reduce the number of equations are discussed. The first method consists on the grouping of the Jacobian matrix. Despite the reduction of the number of equations, the system is always over-determined, the solution converges with an error decreasing while increasing the number of packets. This method is robust and reliable and allows convergence even when very high deformations occur.

A possible use is to apply this procedure as a preliminary calculation in order to approach the exact solution, then refining the results by omitting packets grouping. The second method uses Hu's invariants for the assembly of the Jacobian matrix. The number of the equations is reduces to the number of Hu's invariant moments. This second method designed to enhance the convergence is not as reliable as the previous one; as a matter of fact, even though the number of equations is lower than in the grouping method, the iterations required increase significantly. Furthermore, the increase in the total time is not accompanied by accuracy growth.

References

1. Amodio D, Broggiato GB, Salvini P (1995) Finite strain analysis by image processing: smoothing techniques. Strain 31(3):151–157
2. Broggiato GB, Cortese L, Santuci G (2006) Misura delle deformazioni a campo intero attraverso l'elaborazione di sequenze di immagini ad alta risoluzione. In: XXXV Convegno Nazionale AIAS
3. Cheng P, Sutton MA, Schreier HW, McNeill SR (2002) Full-field speckle pattern image correlation with B-spline deformation function. Exp Mech 42(3):344–352
4. Cofaru C, Philips W, Van Paepegem W (2010) Improved Newton-Raphson digital image correlation method for full-field displacement and strain calculation. Appl Opt 49:33
5. Dougherty G (2009) Digital image processing with medical applications. Cambridge University Press, Oxford
6. Flusser J, Suk T, Zitová B (2009) Moments and moment invariants in pattern recognition. Wiley, New York
7. Hild F, Roux S (2008) A Software for "Finite-element" displacement field measurements by digital image correlation. Internal report n. 269, LMT-Cachan, UniverSud Paris
8. Hu MK (1962) Visual pattern recognition by moment invariants. IRE Trans Info Theory IT-8:179–187
9. Lowe DG (2004) Distinctive image features from scale-invariant keypoints. Int J Comput Vis 60(2):91–110
10. Lu H, Zhang X, Knauss WG (1997) Uniaxial, shear, and poisson relaxation and their conversion to bulk relaxation: studies on poly(methyl methacrylate). Polym Compos 18(2):211–222
11. Pilet J, Lepetit V (2007) Fast non-rigid surface detection. Registration and realistic augmentation. Int J Comput Vis 76(2):109–122
12. Lagattu F, Brillaud J, Lafarie-Frenot M (2004) High strain gradient measurements by using digital image correlation technique. Mater Charact 53(2004):17–28

13. Sutton MA, Cheng MQ, Peters WH, Chao YJ, McNeill SR (1986) Application ofan optimized digital correlation method to planar deformation analysis. Image Vis Comput 4(3):143–150
14. Sutton MA, McNeill SR, Helm ID, Schreier HVr, Chao YJ (2000) Photomeehanics. In: Rastogi PK (ed) Advances in 2D and 3D computer vision for shape and deformation measurements. Topics in applied physics, vol 77. Springer, New York, pp 323–372
15. Sutton MA, Orteu JJ, Shreier HW (2009) Image correlation for shape. Motion and deformation measurements, basic concept, theory and applications. Springer, New York
16. Zienkiewicz OC, Taylor RL (1967) The finite element method, McGraw-Hill, New York

Can Numerical Modelling Help Surgeons in Abdominal Hernia Surgery?

Belén Hernández-Gascón, Estefanía Peña, Gemma Pascual, Juan M. Bellón and Begoña Calvo

Abstract The absence of universally and accepted guidelines to select the most appropriate surgical mesh for each patient and type of defect in hernia surgery could complicate surgeons decisions when choosing the surgical mesh and deciding which is the best orientation of the mesh in the abdomen. An interdisciplinary work between clinicians and engineers may lead to great advances in medical protocols through the development of computational methodologies which could reduce the long periods of time and high costs involved by experimental research procedures. Numerical simulations of hernia treatment could also allow a better knowledge of the post-operative condition. This work is projected to define a computational methodology based on experimental techniques that would help surgeons in deciding which prosthesis is the most convenient depending on the type of abdominal hernia defect and particularities of the patient so current treatments and procedures could be improved with regard to the quality of patient life.

Keywords Finite element model · Hyperelasticity · Surgical meshes

---

B. Hernández-Gascón · E. Peña · B. Calvo
Aragón Institute of Engineering Research (I3A), University of Zaragoza, María de Luna s/n, Edif. Betancourt, 50018 Zaragoza, Spain
e-mail: belenhg@unizar.es, fany@unizar.es, bcalvo@unizar.es

G. Pascual · J. M. Bellón
Departament of Medical Specialities, University of Alcalá, Campus Universitario Ctra. A-2, Km. 33.600, Alcalá de, Henares, Spain
e-mail: gemma.pascual@uah.es, juanm.bellon@uah.es

B. Hernández-Gascón · E. Peña · G. Pascual · J. M. Bellón · B. Calvo (✉)
Centro de Investigación Biomédica en Red en Bioingeniería, Biomateriales y Nanomedicina (CIBER-BBN), Zaragoza, Spain
e-mail: bcalvo@unizar.es

P. Di Giamberardino et al. (eds.), *Computational Modeling of Objects Presented in Images*, Lecture Notes in Computational Vision and Biomechanics 15,
DOI: 10.1007/978-3-319-04039-4_10,

1 Introduction

Hernia appearance is a frequent disease in the medical field. A hernia is defined as the protrusion of one or several internal organs through an opening in the wall that contains them due to a weakening of the wall. According to statistics, more than 20 millions hernias are estimated to be repaired worldwide [16]. Abdominal surgery for hernia repair is based on the implantation of a surgical mesh in the defect area which aims at reinforcing the damaged wall. This intervention is common in clinical practice and diverse problems that reduce the quality of life of patients may appear in unfavorable cases such as obese patients or patients with large defects. To begin with, fibrosis is one of the most common problems between others such as hernia relapse and bad compliance between tissue and mesh. Nowadays, there is no definitive and universally guideline to select the most appropriate surgical mesh for each patient and type of defect, meaning that the choice of one or another prosthesis, and their orientation in case of anisotropic meshes, is a decision to be taken by the surgeons according to their experience. According to that, biomechanics plays a key role in the success of hernia surgery in the long term and may help advancing our current understanding of hernia repair. Hence, biomechanics plays a fundamental role in better understanding the pathology and outcomes of hernia surgery and a strong link between clinicians and engineers specialized in biomechanics is vital to achieve a quick advancement in surgery.

Numerical modelling throughout computer simulations of biomechanical phenomena are potentially significant to analyze the mechanical response to loads experienced by the abdominal wall. Furthermore, computer simulations can reproduce surgical procedures, for instance, hernia surgery could be modelled and the interaction between medical devices and biological materials can be explored. Traditional mechanical models are not directly applicable to modelling soft tissues but sophisticated and robust numerical schemes that consider constitutive nonlinearities, and couple structural, fluid, chemical and electrical fields, are needed to characterize their mechanical behaviour. For instance, biological tissues have the inherent property of adapting mechanically and chemically to the environment. Hence, in hernia surgery after mesh implantation, cellular changes occurs provoking the growth of new tissue due to the presence of a foreign body.

To the author's knowledge, there is no deep research in abdominal biomechanics. There is few literature about the diagnosis, treatment and analysis of long term results of hernia disease throughout numerical models so a numerical approach to hernia repair is provided in this chapter. However, the main goal is to establish an interdisciplinary framework between clinical practice and biomechanics in order to define some guidelines that may help surgeons to follow the optimum methodology in hernia repair. Specifically, Sect. 2 establishes a methodology to obtain a finite element (FE) model of the human abdomen from magnetic resonance imaging (MRI) from a healthy patient. Posteriorly, this model is used to define a FE model of a herniated human abdomen. Section 3 describes the experimental protocol and results to mechanically characterize the abdominal tissues and surgical meshes used. In

Sect. 4, these experimental results are used to determine the constitutive model of the soft tissues introduced. Section 5 describe the computational modelling of a herniated human abdomen in order to analyze the outcomes of hernia surgery depending on the protocol used to place the surgical mesh and in Sect. 6, an interdisciplinary framework is defined to program patient-specific clinical interventions. Finally, Sect. 7 presents the main conclusions of the study presented in this chapter.

2 Image Reconstruction and FE Model

2.1 Healthy Human Abdomen

Medical images obtained from MRI are used to define a three dimensional model of the human abdomen. Specifically, DICOM files from MRI from a healthy man aged 38 are taken to define a reference model. A manual segmentation of the different slices allows the identification of different anatomical structures that comprise the abdominal wall (see Fig. 1). The procedure was developed using the commercial software MIMICS® and the image resolution allows to differentiate primarily the internal and external surfaces of the abdomen. In addition, different masks identify the linea alba (LA), rectus abdominis (RA) and oblique muscles (OM). The oblique muscles comprises three different muscles: external oblique (EO), internal oblique (IO) and transversus abdominis (TA). Despite being independent anatomical units, their mechanical behaviour do not express separate movements. Hence, the whole thickness comprising the EO, IO and TA is considered a monolayer (composite) and only one anatomical unit is identified. This assumption does not alter the passive mechanical characterization of the abdominal wall.

The segmentation of the different main muscles of the abdomen allows the definition of a three dimensional model. The meshing of the model is obtained using the commercial software ABAQUS®. Specifically, a structured volumetric mesh was made employing a total of 13,200 hexahedral elements. The meshing considers 5 elements throughout the thickness of the wall so, according to the work published by Norasteh et al. [23], approximately 2 elements represent the EO, 2 elements represent the IO and the last one represents the TA. Apart from the abdominal muscles, the abdominal wall is comprised of aponeuroses (denoted by fascias or tendons too) that wrap muscles and are collagenous biological tissues [20]. To begin with, the anterior and posterior rectus sheaths (ARS and PRS, respectively) end in the midline of the abdomen forming the linea alba. The ARS and PRS come from the aponeuroses that wrap the oblique muscles. At the level of the oblique muscles, these fascias are supposed to be part of the composite previously defined. Besides, there is an internal aponeurosis covering the inner abdominal cavity, denoted by fascia transversalis. Numerically, 2,092 membrane elements which represent these aponeuroses are defined in the model. Likewise, some tendinous structures appear inside the rectus abdominis (rectus tendon, RT) and the oblique muscles (oblique

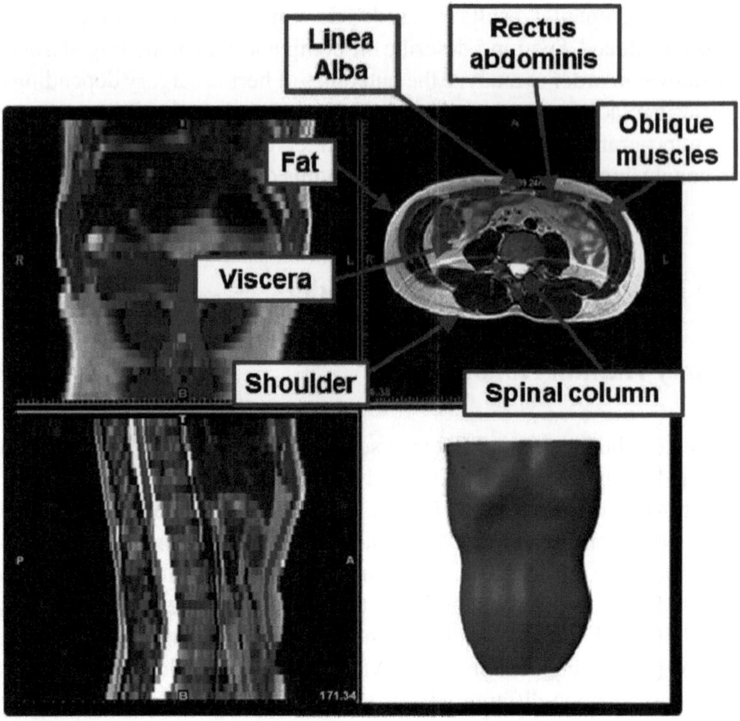

Fig. 1 Magnetic resonance imaging (MRI) from a healthy man aged 38 where the different anatomical structures are identified. The 3D model reconstruction is shown

muscle tendon, OMT) and they are identified in the structured hexahedral mesh (see Fig. 2).

The anatomy of the abdomen includes other anatomical structures that close the abdominal cavity and allows the correct functioning of the different organs: the diaphragm and the pelvis. Those units are also defined in the reference model and 432 shell elements are added to the model using the software FEMAP® (see Fig. 2).

2.2 Herniated and Repaired Human Abdomen

The previous FE model was used to develop a new FE model that represents a herniated human abdomen bearing a large incisional hernia along the linea alba [8]. The procedure followed to generate the large hernia consisted of separating some nodes of the FE model of the healthy abdomen and, after that, an internal pressure was applied and increased until the hernia defect measures 120×200 mm [27] (see Fig. 3).

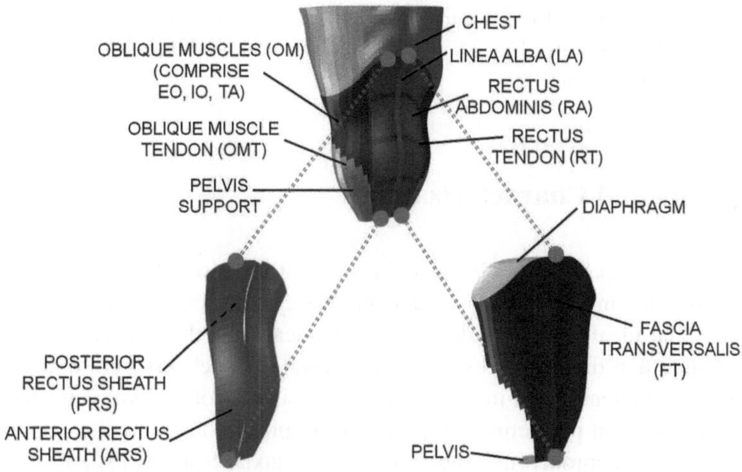

Fig. 2 Finite element model of the healthy human abdomen where the different anatomical structures are identified. Since different structures are superimposed anatomically, they are shown separately and the dotted lines indicate the geometrical correspondence

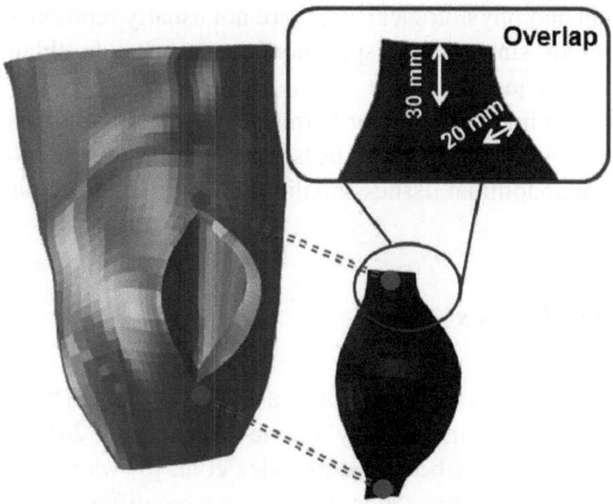

Fig. 3 Finite element model of the herniated human abdomen and the surgical prosthesis. The procedure to place the mesh and the overlap between tissue and mesh is indicated

After the defect is created, the condition just after hernia repair surgery is modelled by placing a prosthesis covering the hernia. The prosthesis is modelled using a total of 165 membrane elements of 1 mm thickness [9] with the software *ANSYS ICEM CFD*® and its placement reproduces the onlay mesh technique [1]. The overlap between the surgical mesh and the abdominal tissues covers 3 elements of the numerical mesh on the lateral edges and 2 elements on the upper and lower sides of the prosthesis (see Fig. 3). The sutures are modelled through matched nodes between mesh and tissue.

3 Experimental Characterization

The laboratory experiments aim at collecting information about the mechanical response and this information is used as the basic input for constitutive modelling of tissues. The ideal goal is to develop mechanical tests that reproduce the physiological state that tissues works in. Experimental data derived from uniaxial tests could not be sufficient for the mechanical characterization of multidimensional material models aimed at predicting the behaviour in physiological loading states [11]. Hence, a faithful approach may be achieved by biaxial testing [13] and it may be even improved with inflation [28] or punching tests [14, 26]. However, having access to some testing equipment is not always possible and numerous studies in the literature report experimental studies based on uniaxial tests [13, 21, 22]. Likewise, experimental testing of soft tissues is somewhat limited since human specimens are not easy to obtain and physiological states are not usually reproduced in traditional testing. Furthermore, since human specimens are not easy to obtain, experimental animal models are frequently used.

Due to in clinical interventions for hernia repair surgical meshes are used, their mechanical behaviour needs to be addressed as well. In this Section experimental uniaxial testing of abdominal tissues and different prostheses are introduced.

3.1 Abdominal Tissues

The laboratory experiments were developed using New Zealand White rabbits, a frequently used animal model in the study muscle behaviour [2, 24]. The experimental protocol followed was described by Hernández et al. [6] who also obtained initial strains. With respect to the linea alba, two zones were differentiated for the study; the first one, located close to the rectus abdominis muscle and the linea alba, was composed of two muscles: the EO and the IO, whereas the second one, located close to the para-spinous muscle, comprised three muscles, namely, the EO, the IO and the TA (see Fig. 4). The experiments were performed without separating muscle layer so results refer to the composite material. For the mechanical testing, one sample in both the longitudinal and transversal directions were harvested from each of the zones of the tissue patch (see Fig. 4). Samples with a width/length ratio around 1/7 were cut in order to preserve the uniaxial tension hypothesis along both, longitudinal and transversal directions. The mechanical characterization was addressed throughout uniaxial tests under displacement control on an INSTRON 3,340 microtester with a 1 [kN] full scale load cell. An initial preconditioning, consisting of three cycles at a

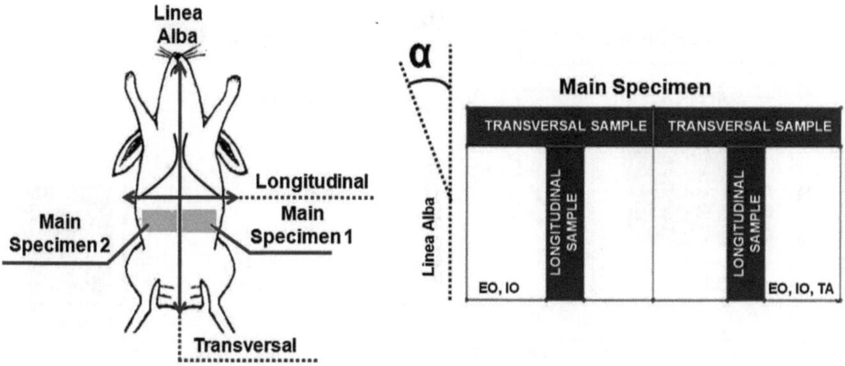

Fig. 4 On the *left*, experimental animal used (New Zealand White rabbit) and specimens extracted to characterize the abdominal muscle behaviour. On the *right*, scheme of the samples cut in the longitudinal and transversal direction. The angle α indicates the direction to define the preferential direction of material anisotropy

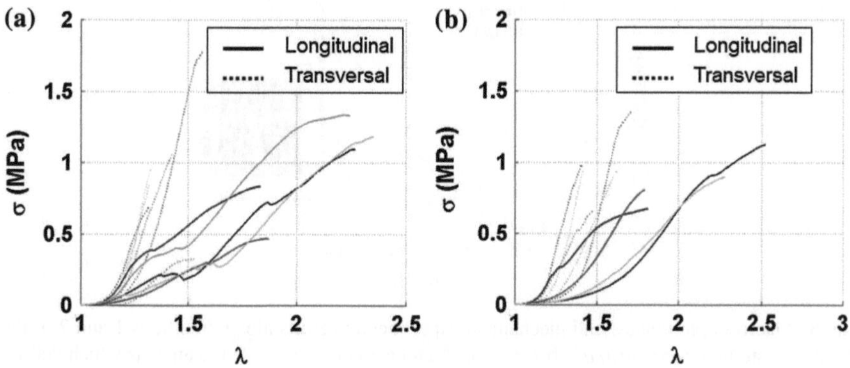

Fig. 5 Cauchy stress-stretch curves obtained from the two studied areas shown in Fig. 4 which are composed of different muscle layers. The curves were truncated before the maximum stress point. *Continuous* and *dotted lines* show the results from the longitudinal and transversal samples, respectively. **a** External and internal obliques. **b** External and internal obliques and trasversus abdominis

nominal strain of 40 %, was imposed to the samples so that the tissue was subjected to physiological loading states. The applied displacement rate was 5 [mm/min] in order to preserve quasi-static testing conditions.

Load and displacements were recorded until sample rupture from the tests to calculate the stretch of the sample as $\lambda = \frac{L_0 + \Delta L}{L_0}$, where L_0 is the initial length between the clamps and ΔL is the clamp displacement. Cauchy stress in the direction of the stretch was computed as $\sigma = \frac{N}{CSA}\lambda$, where N is the applied load and CSA is the cross sectional area. The Cauchy stress-stretch curves are represented in Fig. 5 for the different groups of studied samples (see Fig. 4) [6].

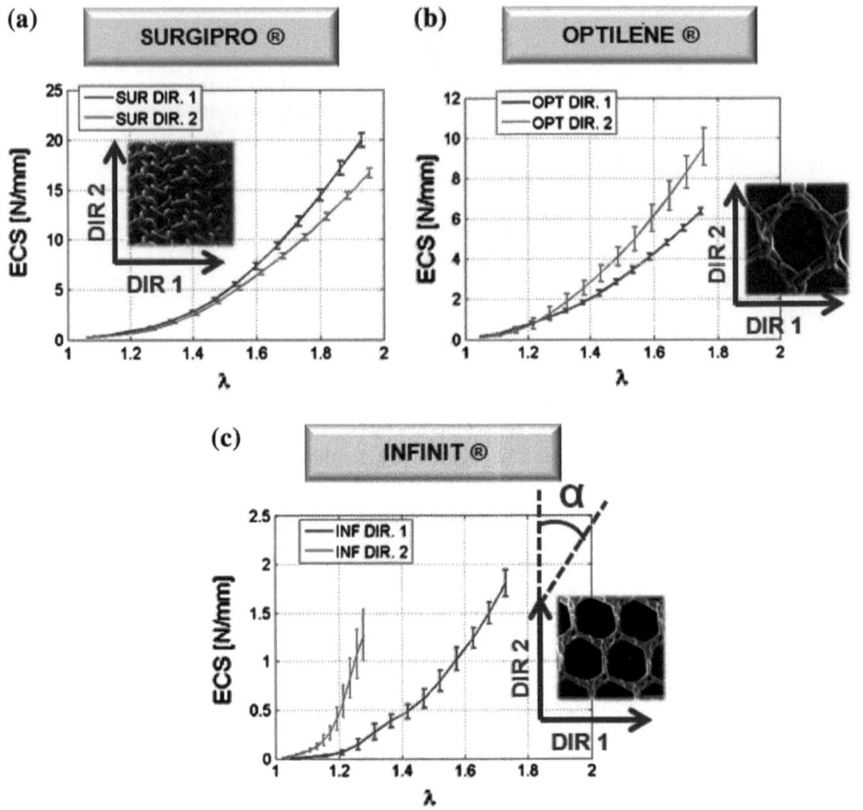

Fig. 6 Macroscopic images and mechanical experimental results along directions 1 and 2 of the prostheses studied: **a** *Surgipro*®, **b** *Optilene*® and **c** *Infinit*® . Note the angle α which defines the preferential direction of anisotropy is shown in **c** [9]

3.2 Surgical Prostheses

Despite the wide variety of surgical meshes offered in the market, only three non-absorbable, biocompatible surgical meshes were tested (see Fig. 6): *Surgipro*® (SUR), a HW (84 g/m^2) polypropylene (PP) monofile mesh with a small pore size (pore surface area $= 0.26 \pm 0.03$ mm^2); *Optilene*® (OPT), a LW (48 g/m^2) PP monofile mesh but with a large pore size (pore surface area $= 7.64 \pm 0.32$ mm^2); and *Infinit*® (INF), a MW mesh (70 g/m^2) with a large pore size composed of a polytetrafluoroethylene (PTFE) monofilament (pore surface area $= 4.05 \pm 0.22$ mm^2). For the mechanical testing, two perpendicular directions (denoted by 1 and 2) were defined to determine the anisotropy of the materials and mesh samples tested were 20 mm wide by 190 mm long (see Fig. 6). The experimental protocol consisted of a uniaxial preload of 2 N and uniaxial loading, both applied with an INSTRON 5,548 microtester with a 50 N load cell [9]. Then a displacement rate of 10 mm/min was maintained until the rupture of the sample. The value of the thickness of the meshes cannot be defined due to its discontinuous cross sectional area including filaments and interspersed empty areas, so Cauchy stress ($\sigma_{Cauchy} = \frac{Force(N)}{Width(mm)Thickness(mm)}\lambda$) can not be computed. Thus, to compare the three meshes, force per unit width multiplied by stretch (Equivalent Cauchy Stress, ECS) was obtained using the expression $\frac{Force(N)}{Width(mm)}\lambda$, where Force(N) is the load applied during the test.

Figure 6 provides the mean ECS versus stretch curves obtained in the mechanical tests for SUR, OPT and INF, respectively. Significant differences were addressed between the three different prostheses; SUR emerged as the stiffest mesh with an isotropic behaviour, OPT mesh showed an anisotropic mechanical response and finally INF mesh emerged as a highly anisotropic prosthesis.

4 Constitutive Modelling

Biological soft tissues are subjected to large deformations with negligible volume changes due to high water content and show an anisotropic mechanical response due to their internal structure. The extra-cellular matrix is composed of a network of collagen, elastin and muscular fibres embedded in a more or less isotropic ground substance. Experimental evidence shows that abdominal muscles subjected to axial tensile stresses have a typical non-linear response, with an initial low stiffness toe region, a linear part with approximately constant stiffness, and a third region corresponding to progressive failure of the composing fibres [6].

Usually, the description of the constitutive behavior of this type of material relies on the identification of an appropriate strain energy density function (SEF) from which stress-strain relations and local elasticity tensors are derived. The laboratory experiments needed to define the SEF that characterize the mechanical response of abdominal tissues and surgical prostheses are those described in the previous sections.

Even though different SEFs have proved to be successful for particular applications and for describing many of the material properties, their use is limited, in most cases, to the range of physiological loads. Hence, the SEFs proposed for both, abdominal tissues and surgical meshes, have been showed a good agreement with the experimental results within the physiological range. However, viscoelastic effects in muscle tissues were despised.

4.1 Anisotropic Hyperelastic Model

A brief review of basic concepts needed to establish the formulation within the large hyperelasticity theory is provided in this Section.

Let consider a continuum body with reference configuration Ω_0 at the initial reference time $t = 0$ and let assume a motion χ which maps this configuration to the current configuration Ω at each time t. Hence, a point $\mathbf{X} \in \Omega_0$ transforms to a point $\mathbf{x} \in \Omega$, where $\mathbf{X}$ and $\mathbf{x}$ define the respective positions of a particle in the reference and current or deformed configurations relative to a global coordinates. The direction of anisotropy given by collagen fibres at a point $\mathbf{X} \in \Omega_0$ is defined by a unit vector field $\mathbf{m}_0(\mathbf{X})$, $|\mathbf{m}_0| = 1$. Then, the stretch of the fibres is defined as:

$$\lambda_{\mathrm{m}}^2 = \mathbf{m}_0 \cdot \mathbf{C}\mathbf{m}_0, \tag{1}$$

The SEF that allows the formulation of the elastic constitutive law for anisotropic materials, Ψ, explicitly depends on both the right Cauchy-Green tensor $\mathbf{C}$ [12, 25, 29] and the fibres direction $\mathbf{m}_0$ in the reference configuration:

$$\Psi(\mathbf{C}, \mathbf{M}) = \Psi_{\mathrm{vol}}(J) + \bar{\Psi}(\bar{\mathbf{C}}, \mathbf{M}) = \Psi_{\mathrm{vol}}(J) + \bar{\Psi}(\bar{I}_1, \bar{I}_2, \bar{I}_4), \tag{2}$$

where $\Psi_{\mathrm{vol}}(J) = \frac{1}{D}(J-1)^2$ and $\bar{\Psi}$ are given scalar-valued functions of $J, \bar{\mathbf{C}} = \bar{\mathbf{F}}^T\bar{\mathbf{F}}$, $\mathbf{M} = \mathbf{m}_0 \otimes \mathbf{m}_0$, respectively, that describe the volumetric and isochoric responses of the material [10, 29]; $\mathbf{F} = \frac{\partial \mathbf{x}}{\partial \mathbf{X}}$ is the standard deformation gradient, $J = \det(\mathbf{F})$, $\bar{\mathbf{F}} = J^{-\frac{1}{3}}\mathbf{F}$, $\bar{I}_1$ and $\bar{I}_2$ are the first and second modified strain invariants of the symmetric modified Cauchy-Green tensor $\bar{\mathbf{C}} = J^{-\frac{2}{3}}\mathbf{C}$ [5]. Finally, the invariant $\bar{I}_4 = \bar{\mathbf{C}} : \mathbf{M} = \bar{\lambda}_{\mathrm{m}}^2 \geq 1$ characterizes the anisotropic behaviour of the material.

We now define the constitutive equation for compressible hyperelastic materials in the standard form, where the Cauchy stress tensor $\boldsymbol{\sigma}$ can then be obtained from the second Piola-Kirchhoff $\mathbf{S}$ [10] as follows:

$$\mathbf{S} = 2\frac{\partial \Psi(\mathbf{C}, \mathbf{M})}{\partial \mathbf{C}} = 2\frac{\partial \Psi_{\mathrm{vol}}(J)}{\partial \mathbf{C}} + 2\frac{\partial \bar{\Psi}(\bar{\mathbf{C}}, \mathbf{M})}{\partial \mathbf{C}}, \tag{3}$$

and the associated decoupled elasticity tensor may be written as

$$\mathbb{C} = \mathbb{C}_{vol} + \bar{\mathbb{C}} = 2\frac{\partial \mathbf{S}_{vol}}{\partial \mathbf{C}} + 2\frac{\partial \bar{\mathbf{S}}}{\partial \mathbf{C}}. \tag{4}$$

The Cauchy stress tensor $\boldsymbol{\sigma}$ and the elasticity tensor in the spatial description $\mathbb{c}$ is $1/J$ times the push-forward of $\mathbf{S}$ or $\mathbb{c}$ respectively [10]:

$$\boldsymbol{\sigma} = J^{-1}\chi_*(\mathbf{S}), \qquad \mathbb{c} = J^{-1}\chi_*(\mathbb{C}). \tag{5}$$

4.2 Strain Energy Functions

Different SEFs are proposed to characterize the mechanical behaviour of both, abdominal tissues and prostheses. However, in both cases, the fitting of the mean curves of experimental data was performed using a Levenberg-Marquardt minimization algorithm [18].

4.2.1 Abdominal Tissues

The three dimensional model defined to model the human abdomen incorporates muscles and aponeuroses. The laboratory experiments were only conducted for abdominal muscles whereas experimental data regarding aponeuroses were taken from the work published by Martins et al. [19].

The isotropic response of both, muscles and aponeuroses, is described using the Demiray's SEF [4]:

$$\bar{\Psi}_{\text{iso}} = \frac{c_1}{c_2}\left[\exp\left(\frac{c_2}{2}[\bar{I}_1 - 3]\right) - 1\right], \tag{6}$$

whereas the anisotropic response is reproduced differently. Specifically, the anisotropic response of muscles is reproduced by Holzapfel's SEF [12], i.e.:

$$\bar{\Psi}_{\text{ani}} = \frac{c_3}{2c_4}\left[\exp\left(c_4[\bar{I}_4 - 1]^2\right) - 1\right], \tag{7}$$

and the anisotropic response of the aponeuroses is described by Calvo's SEF:

$$\begin{aligned}
&\bar{\Psi}_{\text{ani}} = 0 && \bar{I}_4 < \bar{I}_{4_0}\\
&\bar{\Psi}_{\text{ani}} = \frac{c_3}{c_4}(e^{c_4(\bar{I}_4 - \bar{I}_{4_0})} - c_4(\bar{I}_4 - \bar{I}_{4_0}) - 1), && \bar{I}_4 > \bar{I}_{4_0} \text{ and } \bar{I}_4 < \bar{I}_{4_{ref}}\\
&\bar{\Psi}_{\text{ani}} = c_5\sqrt{\bar{I}_4} + \frac{1}{2}c_6\ln(\bar{I}_4) + c_7 && \bar{I}_4 > \bar{I}_{4_{ref}},
\end{aligned} \tag{8}$$

In previous Equations, $\bar{I}_1$ is the first modified strain invariant of the symmetric modified right Cauchy-Green tensor, $\bar{\mathbf{C}}$, and the anisotropic constitutive response is characterized by the invariant $\bar{I}_4 \geq 1$. It was assumed that the strain energy corresponding to the anisotropic terms only contributes to the global mechanical response of the tissue when stretched, that is, when $\bar{I}_4 > \bar{I}_{4_0}$. Furthermore, $c1 > 0$, $c3 > 0$, $c5 > 0$ and $c6 > 0$ are stress-like parameters, $c2 > 0$ and $c4 > 0$ are dimensionless parameters and $c7 > 0$ is an energy-like parameter. The constants that fit the different proposed SEFs are shown in Table 1. The preferential direction of anisotropy obtained by the numerical fitting is included at each integration point of the FE model and that of the aponeuroses is defined according to the literature [20].

4.2.2 Surgical Meshes

To fit the experimental results obtained with prostheses, the isotropic response was reproduced using Eq. 6 and the anisotropic component was addressed using Eq. 7. The corresponding constants are included in Table 1. The angle α that symbolizes the anisotropy of the prosthesis is included at each integration point. It is important to note that since mesh thickness is small, in the constitutive 3D model for materials,

Table 1 Material parameters obtained from prior works [6, 9, 19]

	c_1 [MPa]	c_2 [–]	c_3 [MPa]	c_4 [–]	c_5 [MPa]	c_6 [MPa]	c_7 [MPa]	I_{40} [–]		ε [–]
Set 1* [19]	0.2434	0.8	0.0064	9.63	31.8214	−36.9188	−31.4118	1.0	–	0.1483
	c_1 [MPa]	c_2 [–]	c_3 [MPa]	c_4 [–]					α[°]	ε [–]
Set 2* [6]	0.16832	0.6319	0.01219	5.68158	–	–	–	–	87.8	0.17873
Set 3* [6]	0.10445	6.86123	0.001	0.00491	–	–	–	–	0.0	0.10923
Set 4* [6]	0.16832	0.6319	0.01219	5.68158	–	–	–	–	–	0.17873
Set 5* [15]	0.18	–	–	–	–	–	–	–	–	–
SUR® [9]	2.10163	1.17805	–	–	–	–	–	–	–	0.1467
OPT® [9]	1.25112	1.5	0.28	0.03062	–	–	–	–	0.0	0.0807
INF® [9]	0.25	2.5	0.07804	5.49131	–	–	–	–	0.0	0.3714

Angle α is considered from the craneo-caudal direction and direction 2 for abdominal tissues and surgical prostheses, respectively (see Figs. 4 and 6)
**Set 1* LA, RAT, OMT, FT, ARS and PRS. *Set 2* Oblique muscles. *Set 3* Rectus abdominis muscle. *Set 4* Chest, back and pelvis. *Set 5* Diaphragm and pelvis

normal stresses were assumed to be zero. Therefore, we considered a membrane model according to the algorithm proposed by Klinkel et al. [17]. We computed ECS by Cauchy Stress considering a thickness of 1 mm.

5 Outcomes of Hernia Surgery Depending on Mesh Placement

After the abdomen is opened, initial stresses are released so they do not have to be included in the FE model. The modelling of the herniated and repaired human abdomen to intraabdominal pressures (IAP) due to physiological loads is defined by two independent load steps conducted using $ABAQUS\ v.11^{®}$ software; Firstly, the body mass, including including the weight of the viscera and muscles, and the IAP in the standing position (20 mmHg) [3] are applied to simulate the change from the supine to the standing position. Secondly, the second load step applies the maximum IAP provoked by the physiological motion of standing cough (P = 112.51 mmHg) [3], which is commonly observed in the post-operative course and is considered responsible for negative outcomes after hernia surgery such as hernia formation or relapse. The boundary conditions in displacements that define the problem restrict completely the movement of the nodes corresponding to the ribs on the back of the abdomen and its lower part (denoted by pelvis support, Fig. 2).

The analyses developed in this work is focussed in analyzing what occurs after the two different but common IAP considered, standing and standing cough, since the major adverse effects after hernia surgery take place during extreme load conditions the patient is subjected to. Furthermore, one of the most commons complaints that patients report is abdominal discomfort due to a bad compliance between tissue and mesh. An inadequate stiffness of the mesh is the fundamental reason of this phenomenon. Likewise, this condition may be associated with a non appropriate placement

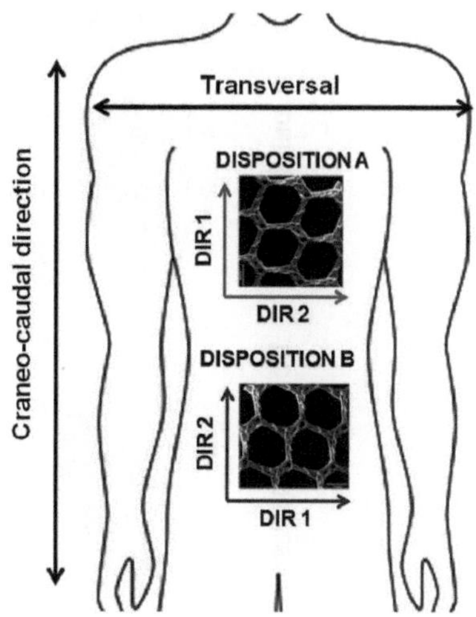

Fig. 7 The hernia defect can be covered with the prosthesis according to disposition *A* or *B*, where the stiffer direction of the mesh (in anisotropic prostheses, OPT or INF) is placed along the transversal and craneo-caudal direction, respectively

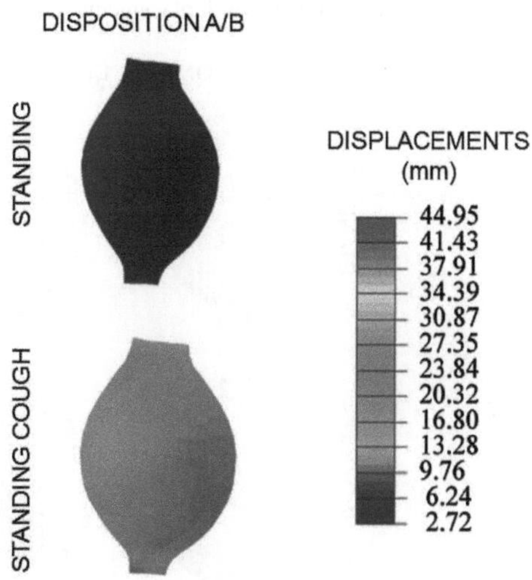

Fig. 8 Displacements (mm) addressed by SUR mesh in the defect area after the standing and the standing cough motion. Note that the results with both dispositions are the same due to the isotropic behaviour of SUR mesh

of the mesh when the prosthesis is anisotropic. Thus, this study also considers how the mesh is placed in the abdomen, i.e whether the stiffest direction is align with the transversal direction (disposition A) or the craneo-caudal one (disposition B) (see Fig. 7).

Results from this study are focussed in addressing the main differences in terms of compliance, i.e our major concern is determining differences in the field of displacements that appear in the prosthesis (see Figs. 8, 9 and 10).

The displacement fields obtained in the numerical simulations address significant differences after both motions studied. Considering the first one, the standing cough, it corresponds to the normal condition of any patient and it does not suppose any

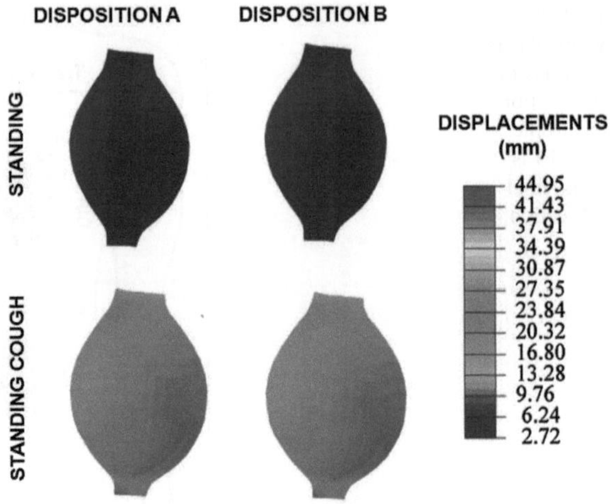

Fig. 9 Displacements (mm) addressed by OPT mesh in the defect area after the standing and the standing cough motion and with placements *A* and *B* defined in Fig. 7

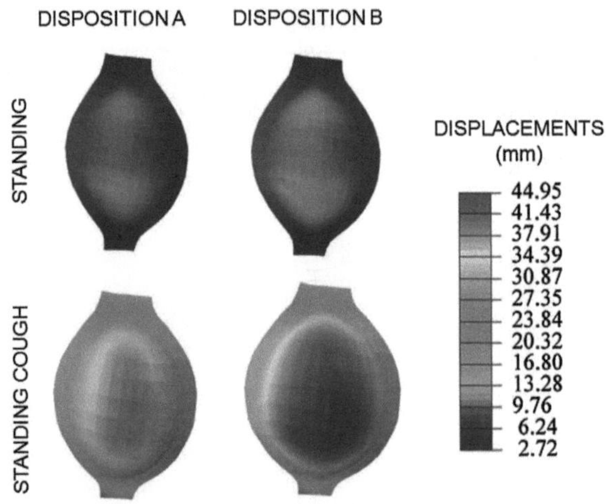

Fig. 10 Displacements (mm) addressed by INF mesh in the defect area after the standing and the standing cough motion and with placements *A* and *B* defined in Fig. 7

extra effort. As a result, the displacement fields reach low values through the mesh and there are not notable differences when using the different studied prostheses. However, it is important to note that the maximum values are addressed with INF mesh and, specifically, the maximum displacements appear in the upper and lower part of the prosthesis (see Fig. 10). This condition may turn in higher distensibility in those areas compared to that of the central zone. Furthermore, the displacements in the area that corresponds to the overlap give an idea of the compliance between tissue and mesh; when placing SUR or OPT in either disposition, displacements show a continuity with respect to the overlap, meaning that the compliance could be appropriate. However, the values reported by INF in the defect area exceed those addressed in the overlap, turning thus probably into a higher distensibility than the required.

Regarding the motion of standing cough, the displacement fields address higher values. Specifically, SUR mesh shows that displacements in the central defect area are lower than those reported in the upper and lower parts and in the overlap. In terms of patient compliance, this condition suggests that this prosthesis could decrease the distensibility of the abdominal wall provoking a poor compliance and could lead to patient discomfort due to the high stiffness of the mesh. With regard to OPT mesh, a more homogeneous displacement field is obtained and results are similar with both dispositions. Lastly, INF mesh addresses significant differences in displacements when placing the mesh using disposition A and B and values exceed notably those reported in the overlap zone. Thus, this prosthesis allows the abdomen to have a superior distensibility than that required. Furthermore, the differences observed between dispositions A and B suggest that the anisotropy of the mesh turns into different abdominal wall compliance. Specifically, the displacement field with disposition B reports higher values. We could thus suggest that the most appropriate disposition of anisotropic prosthesis should align the stiffest direction with the transversal direction of the abdomen.

6 Numerical Framework to Program Patient-Specific Clinical Interventions

The end goal is to establish a methodology to automatize the clinical procedure starting from the capture of medical images to hernia surgery (see Fig. 11). The main outcomes of this methodology is a better planning of the intervention, since patient-specific characteristics are known, and an improved protocol which helps surgeons when deciding which surgical prosthesis is better in each particular case. Therefore, it would be possible to predict for a patient the most adequate surgical mesh, analyzing for example the consequences of different types of mesh for this single patient. For that purpose, the patient-specific geometry should be reproduced with the more detail as possible. Whether a patient only reports some abdominal symptom, the methodology proposed could help in the diagnosis of possible hernia formation [7]. In Sect. 2, we have proposed a methodology to manage medical images in order to define a three dimensional model of the abdomen. Likewise, the mechanics of the different tissues involved in the model were addressed and the preferential directions of anisotropy were taken into account. Although as a first approach we directly created a hernia defect in the abdomen, the same methodology could be applied when the patient has an abdominal hernia. In this case, medical images would allow the direct reconstruction of the model of a herniated abdomen.

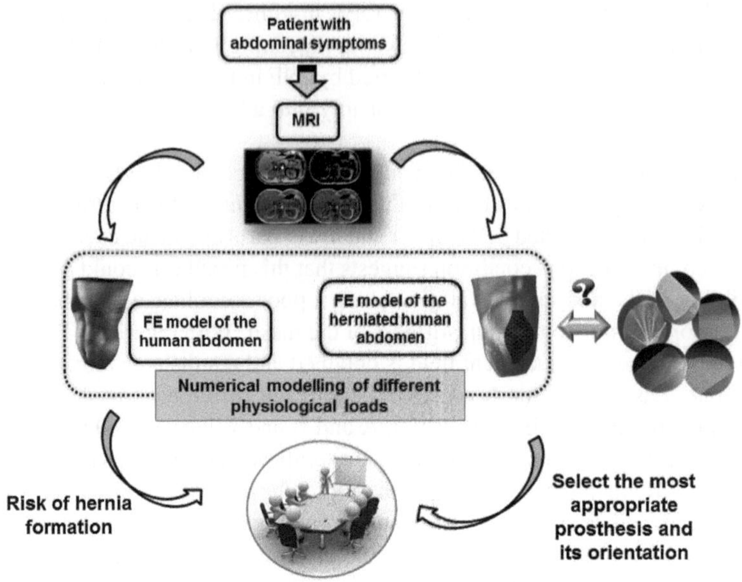

Fig. 11 Scheme of the methodology proposed to improve the outcomes of hernia treatment

7 Conclusions

Finite element biomechanical models of biological tissues can be a powerful tool for the prediction of the effects of physiological loads. Regarding to hernia surgery, there is no universally and accepted guidelines to choose the most appropriate type of prosthesis for each type of patient and defect and post-operative complications are still frequent. Likewise, traditional research has been focussed in experimental procedures that involve high costs and long periods of time so computational techniques aim at improve surgical procedures.

This work proposes a computational methodology to improve surgical treatments related to hernia surgery. The fundamental idea is that medical images can be processed to obtain numerical models which can be posteriorly used to simulate different loading states. The outcomes of the numerical simulation can determine the optimum way to develop hernia surgery and the effect of different types of prosthesis can be analyzed previous to surgery.

In order to feed numerical models, experimental data are needed. Therefore, the basis of the study is found in experimental techniques aimed at characterizing the mechanical response of the different tissues involved in the clinical problem. Firstly, an experimental study of the abdominal muscle mechanics using an experimental animal model, the New Zealand White rabbit, is described and the fundamental relationship between stresses and stretches along two perpendicular directions is obtained. Our findings demonstrate the anisotropic response of the abdominal wall being stiffer in the transversal direction. Furthermore, the understanding of the mechanics of three different commonly used surgical meshes was addressed by the mechanical experimental characterization. Results reveal an isotropic response of SUR mesh, an anisotropic behaviour of OPT mesh and a highly anisotropic response of INF mesh.

The outcomes of hernia surgery after placing the three different surgical meshes studied have allow us to conclude that anisotropic meshes should be placed so that the stiffest direction coincides with the transversal direction of the abdomen. In addition, our findings suggest that INF mesh could provoke excessive displacement in the defect area so its use is not recommended in obese patients or in patients with large defects.

The major limitation of this study is that numerical models are feeded with uniaxial experimental test which are not completely capable of reproducing multiaxial loading states. Thus, further studies are needed to improve the understanding the mechanics of both, abdominal tissues and prostheses. Other improvements required in this first approach to modelling hernia surgery include the consideration of viscoleastic effects, the loss of stiffness due to damage after hernia appearance and the definition of a constitutive model that incorporates the formation of new collagenous tissue over the prosthesis as a response to the placement of a foreign body into the abdomen.

To conclude, numerical simulations of hernia treatment could allow a better knowledge of the outcomes of hernia surgery. In addition, the methodology proposed could allow a better decision to choose the most appropriate prosthesis to improve the quality of patient life, hence helping to improve current treatments and surgical procedures.

Acknowledgments This study was supported by the Spanish Ministry of Economy and Competitiveness through research project DPI2011-27939-C02-01/C02-02, the Spanish Ministry of Science and Innovation through research project DPI2011-15551-E and the Instituto de Salud Carlos III (ISCIII) through the CIBER initiative project ABDOMESH. B. Hernández-Gascón was also funded by a grant (BES-2009-021515) from the Spanish Ministry of Science and Technology.

References

1. Bauer JJ, Harris MT, Gorfine SR, Kreel I (2002) Rives-stoppa procedure for repair of large incisional hernias: experience with 57 patients. Hernia 6:120–123
2. Bellón JM, Rodríguez M, García-Honduvilla N, Gómez-Gil V, Pascual G, Buján J (2009) Comparing the behavior of different polypropylene meshes (heavy and lightweight) in an experimental model of ventral hernia repair. J Biomed Mater Res Part B Appl Biomater 89B(2):448–455
3. Cobb WS, Burns JM, Kercher KW, Matthews BD, Norton HJ, Heniford BT (2005) Normal intraabdominal pressure in healthy adults. J Surg Res 129:231–235
4. Demiray H, Weizsacker HW, Pascale K, Erbay H (1988) A stress-strain relation for a rat abdominal aorta. J Biomech 21:369–374
5. Flory PJ (1961) Thermodynamic relations for high elastic materials. Trans Faraday Soc 57:829–838

6. Hernández B, Peña E, Pascual G, Rodríguez M, Calvo B, Doblaré M, Bellón JM (2011) Mechanical and histological characterization of the abdominal muscle: a previous step to model hernia surgery. J Mech Behav Biomed Mater 4:392–404
7. Hernández-Gascón B, Mena A, Peña E, Pascual G, Bellón JM, Calvo B (2013) Understanding the passive mechanical behavior of the human abdominal wall. Ann Biomed Eng 41(2):433–444
8. Hernández-Gascón, B, Peña E, Grasa J, Pascual G, Bellón JM, Calvo B (2013) Mechanical response of the herniated human abdomen to the placement of different prostheses. J Biomech Eng (135) 051004–8
9. Hernández-Gascón B, Peña E, Melero H, Pascual G, Doblaré M, Ginebra MP, Bellón JM, Calvo B (2011) Mechanical behaviour of synthetic surgical meshes: finite element simulation of the herniated abdominal wall. Acta Biomater 7:3905–3913
10. Holzapfel GA (2000) Nonlinear solid mechanics. Wiley, New York
11. Holzapfel GA (2006) Determination of material models for arterial walls from uniaxial extension tests and histological structure. J Theor Biol 238:290–302
12. Holzapfel GA, Gasser TC, Ogden RW (2000) A new constitutive framework for arterial wall mechanics and a comparative study of material models. J Elast 61:1–48
13. Hwang W, Carvalho JC, Tarlovsky I, Boriek AM (2005) Passive mechanics of canine internal abdominal muscles. J Appl Physiol 98(5):1829–1835
14. Junge K, Klinge U, Prescher A, Giboni P, Niewiera M, Shumpelick V (2001) Elasticity of the anterior abdominal wall and impact for reparation of incisional hernia using mesh implants. Hernia 5:112–118
15. Kauer M (2001) Inverse finite element characterization of soft tissues with aspiration experiments. Ph.D. thesis, Swiss Federal Institute of Technology, Znrich
16. Kingsnorth A, LeBlanc K (2003) Hernias: inguinal and incisional. Lancet 362:1561–1574
17. Klinkel S, Govindjee S (2002) Using finite strain 3D-material models in beam and shell elements. Eng Comput 19(8):902–921
18. Marquardt DW (1963) An algorithm for least-squares estimation of nonlinear parameters. SIAM J Appl Math 11:431–441
19. Martins P, Peña E, Jorge RMN, Santos A, Santos L, Mascarenhas T, Calvo B (2012) Mechanical characterization and constitutive modelling of the damage process in rectus sheath. J Mech Behav Biomed Mater 8:111–122
20. Moore W (2008) Gray's Anatomy celebrates 150th anniversary. The Telegraph (Telegraph Media Group)
21. Nilsson T (1982) Biomechanical studies of rabbit abdominal wall. Part I. - The mechanical properties of specimens from different anatomical positions. J Biomech 15(2):123–129
22. Nilsson T (1982) Biomechanical studies of rabbit abdominal wall. Part II.- The mechanical properties of specimens in relation to length, width, and fibre orientation. J Biomech 15(2):131–135
23. Norasteh A, Ebrahimi E, Salavati M, Rafiei J, Abbasnejad E (2007) Reliability of B-mode ultrasonography for abdominal muscles in asymptomatic and patients with acute low back pain. J Bodywork Mov Ther 11:17–20
24. Pascual G, Rodríguez M, Gómez-Gil V, García-Honduvilla N, Buján J, Bellón JM (2008) Early tissue incorporation and collagen deposition in lightweight polypropylene meshes: bioassay in an experimental model of ventral hernia. Surgery 144:427–435
25. Peña E, del Palomar AP, Calvo B, Martínez MA, Doblaré M (2007) Computational modelling of diarthrodial joints. Physiological, pathological and pos-surgery simulations. Arch Comput Methods Eng 14(1):47–91
26. Podwojewski F, Otténio M, Beillas P, Guérin G, Turquier F, Mitton D (2012) Mechanical response of animal abdominal walls in vitro: evaluation of the influence of a hernia defect and a repair with a mesh implanted intraperitoneally. J Biomech 46(3):561–566
27. Sabbagh C, Dumont F, Robert B, Badaoui R, Verhaeghe P, Regimbeau JM (2011) Peritoneal volume is predictive of tension-free fascia closure of large incisional hernias with loss of domain: a prospective study. Hernia 15(5):559–565

28. Song C, Alijani A, Frank T, Hanna G, Cuschieri A (2006) Mechanical properties of the human abdominal wall measured in vivo during insufflation for laparoscopic surgery. Surg Endosc 20:987–990
29. Weiss JA, Maker BN, Govindjee S (1996) Finite element implementation of incompressible, transversely isotropic hyperelasticity. Comput Methods Appl Mech Eng 135:107–128

Current Research Results on Depth Map Interpolation Techniques

Stefania Colonnese, Stefano Rinauro and Gaetano Scarano

Abstract The goal of this chapter is twofold. Firstly, we provide the reader with a summary of the state-of-the-art depth map interpolation techniques. Secondly, we present recent results making use of markovian priors for depth map interpolation. Specifically, we provide insight into Markovian mathematical models recently presented in the literature, and we show that such priors allow interpolation without making use of contemporaneously acquired luminance views. This feature extends the scope of the interpolation procedure and decouple its performances from those of the luminance/depth images registration stage.

Keywords Depth map · Interpolation · Markov random fields

1 Introduction

Acquisition of images and video is currently often carried out jointly with the acquisition of the so called depth map, or range map, which displays information on the distance of each framed object from the camera. Depth map acquisition techniques may be active or passive, and can be coarsely categorized into two classes: techniques base on time of flight estimation, and techniques based on matching of views from a stereo camera. It is worth noting that active time-of-flight range acquisition suffers of errors which are somewhat complementary to those observed in passive stereo matching. Thus, different simplicity versus accuracy tradeoffs are encountered

S. Colonnese (✉) · S. Rinauro · G. Scarano
DIET, University of Rome "Sapienza", Rome, Italy
e-mail: colonnese@infocom.uniroma1.it

S. Rinauro
e-mail: rinauro@infocom.uniroma1.it

G. Scarano
e-mail: scarano@infocom.uniroma1.it

P. Di Giamberardino et al. (eds.), *Computational Modeling of Objects Presented in Images*, Lecture Notes in Computational Vision and Biomechanics 15,
DOI: 10.1007/978-3-319-04039-4_11,

depending on the particular acquisition device. In most cases, the accuracy of on-the-shelf depth acquisition devices [32] is limited in range as well in spatial resolution, and it must be improved for ever demanding higher quality applications.

This chapter addresses a particular depth map processing problem, namely the upsampling of a low-resolution depth map to reconstruct the unknown high resolution depth map. Our contribution is twofold. Firstly, we provide an unified review of the recent literature on depth map upsampling. Secondly, we apply recent theoretical results on natural image interpolation to the case of depth map upsampling. Specifically, we describe a single pass upsampling procedure based on modeling the unknown depth map as a Markov Random Field (MRF) with complex line process [7]. The model, formerly applied to natural images restoration [4, 5], is here tuned to the depth map interpolation problem. With respect to state-of-the-art depth interpolation techniques, the presented procedure has the featured novelty of being applicable without exploiting information from the high resolution luminance map. Therefore, it applies even in absence of a luminance/depth registration stage as well as in stand-alone depth estimation systems.

The structure of the chapter is as follows. After motivating the need for depth information in a number of future video services in Sect. 2, we recall state-of-the-art depth map interpolation in Sect. 3. We briefly recall the MRF model underlying the depth map interpolation procedure in Sect. 4. We describe the markovian interpolation procedure in Sect. 5. In Sect. 6 we report a few experimental results and Sect. 7 concludes the chapter.

2 Depth Map Enabled Innovative Video Services

Depth information enables various advanced video services, ranging from free view point television and 3D video, to advanced video surveillance, biometrics and virtual reality, to cite a few. Depth maps are exploited to render virtual view 3-D images from a given 2-D color image by means of depth image-based rendering techniques. Thus, autostereoscopic multiview displays for 3D home entertainment can exploit the depth information to synthesize numerous viewing angles from only a small set of given input views. Depth map estimation is also addressed by 2D to 3D conversion techniques, which allow to exploit rich encoded 2D video databases for enhanced user experience. Techniques for 2D to 3D video conversion usually generate the depth video from the original 2D video first as an intermediate step towards synthesizing the desired 3d video. Therefore, depth maps acquisition and compression are expected to be key technologies for future innovative video services [34].

The issue of depth map compression is addressed by the Multiview Video plus Depth coding techniques. The authors [30] present a 3D video coding scheme using multiview video plus depth format, which extends MVC using both disparity compensation and suitable representation of depth blocks. In Wildeboer [39] the authors show how depth up-sampling can be employed in depth compression method.

Coding efficiency and rendering quality depend on the tightness of the depth maps edges. Depth map coding is addressed in [20].

All the mentioned applications benefit of the availability of high quality depth maps, with temporally stable, sharp edges and smooth objects interior's regions. Thereby, all these applications rely on the availability of robust depth estimation and post-processing techniques, among which upsampling is of paramount importance.

3 Current Research Issues on Depth Map Interpolation and Processing

The problem of depth map upsampling arises mainly from technological limits of the range acquisition devices; in fact, due to the high cost of the range map acquisition technology, accurate and robust techniques for improving the resolution of measured depth maps are required. While high definition video and photo cameras are available on the market (e.g. 1920×1240 or larger), the on-the-shelf depth acquisition devices typically provide lower resolution (e.g. 176×144) maps. Moreover, in order to reduce the bandwidth occupancy of 3D or multi-view video systems, depth maps are usually downsampled before compression, so that a suitable upsampling stage is needed at receiver side.

Depth maps upsampling techniques recently debated in technical literature involve statistical, possibly Markovian, priors [24, 25], as well as video sequence analysis [37, 38]. In Wang et al. [37, 38], the depth map interpolation method exploits the existing pairs of key frames and their corresponding depth maps. The method requires frame selection, motion alignment, and updating and adjusting of the map. In Lee and Ho [21] the authors generate multi-view video sequences and their corresponding depth maps by making use of a multi-camera system enriched by one time-of-flight depth camera. An initial virtual depth map is generated at each viewpoint, and then the depth map edges are adapted to the estimated moving object edges. The work in [22, 23] deals with adaptive edge-preserving depth map smoothing, which counteracts typical depth based image rendering artifacts, ie holes on the generated virtual view images. In Zhu [42],method for combining the results from both active and passive techniques is built on the base of a pixel-wise reliability function computed for each acquisition method. In Jaesik et al. [19] high quality upsampling uses an additional edge-weighted nonlocal means filtering to regularize depth maps in order to maintain fine detail and structure. The depth image upsampling method in [16] exploits a novel edge layer concept and encompasses it in the design of a non-linear interpolation filter for depth map up-sampling. Edge preserving upsampling for depth map coding purposes appears in [26]. In Tseng and Lai [35], the depth map for all pixels at each frame is estimated by first applying correspondence search, computing the optical flow between selected scenes, and then refining the results by MRF. A depth map post processing scheme for FVT applications appears in [3]. In Xu et al. [40] the depth map preprocessing method using texture edge information to refine depth pixels around the large depth discontinuities. The method in [31] uses edge information from the video frame in the upscaling process and allows the use of sparse, non-uniformly distributed depth values. The method in Rong et al. [28] addresses sharpening edges of the depth maps possibliy degraded by coding. In Vijayanagar et al. [36] a post-processing technique corrects and sharpens the boundaries of the objects of the depth map and ensures local depth smoothness within the objects. The work in De Silva et al. [11] exploits the depth perception sensitivity of humans in suppressing the unnecessary spatial depth details, hence reducing the transmission overhead allocated to depth maps. In Ekmekcioglu [12] an edge adaptive depth map upsampling procedure stemming from an edge map of the original natural image has been proposed. The resulting upsampled depth maps exhibit an increased sharpness in edge regions with respect to classical upsampling such as bilinear interpolation and linear spatial scalable filters [33]. Since no information about the orientation of the edges is considered, some edges still exhibits visual artifacts which, in turn, may severely affect all of the stages where a correct high resolution depth map is required, such as, for instance, the rendering of free viewpoint images. Moreover, the work in Ekmekcioglu [12] estimates the edge map from the high resolution luminance map, thus needing the samples of the low resolution depth map to be correctly registered with the sample of the high resolution luminance map. This latter operation is computationally onerous; besides, it may affect the upsampling procedure when not perfectly performed (Table 1).

4 On the Adoption of MRF Model for Depth Map Interpolation

Depth maps are made up by homogeneous regions separated by abrupt boundaries. In this respect, MRFs, aiming to assign higher probabilities to configurations in which small differences between the pixel values occur in large regions, are well suited to be used as a statistical prior for depth maps. We model the unknown high resolution depth image as a realization of a bidimensional MRF$\mathbf{d}_{\mathscr{L}}$ defined on a rectangular lattice $\mathscr{L}$.

Such model has been successfully applied to natural image upsampling [7], where the model proved to be attractive under different points of view, namely (i) tightness, (ii) availability of low computational cost procedures, (iii) straightforward parameter tuning.

Let us then assume that the depth values are observed on a sub-lattice $\mathscr{L}' \in \mathscr{L}$: the observations' set is then given by $\mathbf{d}_{\mathscr{L}'}$. Here, we address the problem of interpolating the HR depth map $\mathbf{d}_{\mathscr{L}\setminus\mathscr{L}'}$ from the observed LR samples, namely $\mathbf{d}_{\mathscr{L}'}$, and we resort to the Maximum a Posteriori (MAP) estimation of the high-resolution samples $\mathbf{d}_{\mathscr{L}\setminus\mathscr{L}'}$ given the observations $\mathbf{d}_{\mathscr{L}'}$. The analytical expression of the estimator is a particular form of the estimators derived in [7] and it is inherently related to the depth map Markovian prior.

Table 1 Summary of state-of-the-art interpolation techniques

Reference	Principle
[35, 37, 38]	Video analysis
[24, 25]	Markovian priors
[3, 21, 42]	Measurements fusion
[11, 16, 26, 28, 31, 36]	Edge sharpening
[11, 19, 22, 23]	Interior smoothing

Let d_{mn} be the value of the random field $\mathbf{d}_{\mathscr{L}}$ at the pixel (m, n) and let $p\left(d_{mn}|\mathbf{d}_{\mathscr{L}\setminus(m,n)}\right)$ denote the probability density function (pdf) of d_{mn} conditioned to the values $\mathbf{d}_{\mathscr{L}\setminus(m,n)}$. The random field $\mathbf{d}_{\mathscr{L}}$ is said to be a MRF if, for every pixel (m, n), a neighborhood η_{mn} is found such that:

$$p\left(d_{mn}|\mathbf{d}_{\mathscr{L}\setminus(m,n)}\right) = p\left(d_{mn}|\mathbf{d}_{\eta_{mn}}\right) \tag{1}$$

A set of pixels such that all the pixels belonging to the set are neighbors of each other is called a clique. The joint pdf of a random field satisfying (1) takes the form of a Gibbs distribution [15], given by:

$$p\left(\mathbf{d}_{\mathscr{L}}\right) \stackrel{\text{def}}{=} \frac{1}{Z}\exp\left(-\frac{1}{T}\sum_c V_c\left(\mathbf{d}_c\right)\right) \tag{2}$$

where the functions $V_c\left(\mathbf{d}_c\right)$ operate on subsets of pixels $\mathbf{d}_c$ belonging to the same clique c, and the sum is carried out on all the cliques in the field. In this work we will consider cliques composed by two pixels, *i.e.* $\mathbf{d}_c = \{d_{mn} - d_c\}$. The functions $V_c\left(\mathbf{d}_c\right)$ are called *potential functions* and the parameter T driving the pdfcurvature is often referred to as the *temperature of the distribution*.

The MRF is characterized by the neighborhood system defined on $\mathscr{L}$ and by the form of the potential functions $V_c\left(\mathbf{d}_c\right)$, which ultimately determine the energy, and hence the probability, of the configuration $\mathbf{d}_{\mathscr{L}}$.

The neighborhood system η_{mn} and the potential functions $V_c\left(\mathbf{d}_c\right)$, representing the spatial continuity constraints, definetely identify the MRF. One of the most commonly adopted neighborhood system η_{mn} is depicted in Fig. 2. The system, formerly introduced in [15], encompasses only two pixels cliques $\mathbf{d}_c = \{d_{mn}, d_c\}$ oriented along different directions φ_c allowing the clique potential $V_c\left(\mathbf{d}_c\right)$ to adapt to up to 8 different edge directions. A commonly assumed form for the potential function $V_c\left(\mathbf{d}_c\right)$ is the parabolyc form:

$$V_c\left(\mathbf{d}_c\right) \stackrel{\text{def}}{=} k_c(d_{mn} - d_c)^2 \tag{3}$$

The quadratic term in (3) measures the contribution to the overall configuration energy related to the variations between the pixels d_{mn}, d_c. The term is to be interpreted as follows: high values of $k_c$lead to low values of the mass probability for the field configurations presenting abrupt variations along the direction φ_c of the clique c. Meanwhile, small values of k_c make the overall configuration probability independent on the same variations, and result in looser spatial continuity constraints. Thereby, the weights k_c definitely associate higher probabilities to configurations in which small differences between the pixel values occur in large regions.

On regions boundaries, discontinuities are allowed through the use of suitably defined line process, across which the spatial continuity constraints are relaxed. Uniform region boundaries have been modeled by means of suitable binary [15] or real valued [2] line processes. Recently, these models have been generalized by resorting to a complex valued line process [7], which formally takes into account visually relevant characteristics such as the edge intensity and orientation. In Colonnese et al. [7], the authors exploit the complex edge process e_{mn}, whose magnitude is proportional to the image edge intensity, and whose orientation is parallel to the edge orientation.

Therein, the weight k_c varies as a function of the angular distance between the clique direction φ_c and the local edge direction; the achieved maximum value depends on the edge intensity in (m, n). Let us then consider a generic site (m, n) and let us associate a clique direction φ_c to every clique $c \in \eta_{mn}$. The weight k_c is defined as the scalar product between the edge process e_{mn} and the versor $e^{j\varphi_c}$ of the clique direction.

The feasibility of the MRF model strictly depends on the availability of a procedure for estimation of the edge process e_{mn}. Parameter estimation is straightforwardly carried out by edge estimation, possibly carried out by a suitable computationally efficient band-pass filter [6].

The Circular Harmonic Functions (CHFs) provide an efficacious mean for estimation of visually relevant parameters. The functions, formerly defined in [18], have found applications in several image processing issues, mainly related to visual features extraction [9, 14]. The first order CHF $h^{(1)}_{mn}$ is a bandpass filter, defined by the following impulse response:

$$h^{(1)}_{mn} \propto \left(m^2 + n^2\right)^{1/2} e^{-(m^2+n^2)/\alpha^2} e^{-j \arctan n/m} \tag{4}$$

Filtering a bidimensional sequence with the first order CHF $h^{(1)}_{mn}$ leads to a complex image [6], whose magnitude is related to the local edge intensity and whose phase is orthogonal to the edge orientation.

In Fig. 1, we report a detail of a depth map of the video sequence Cones, adopted for performance evaluation in Scharstein [29] and publicly available at [17], and the estimated complex line process, represented by a field of vectors whose magnitude

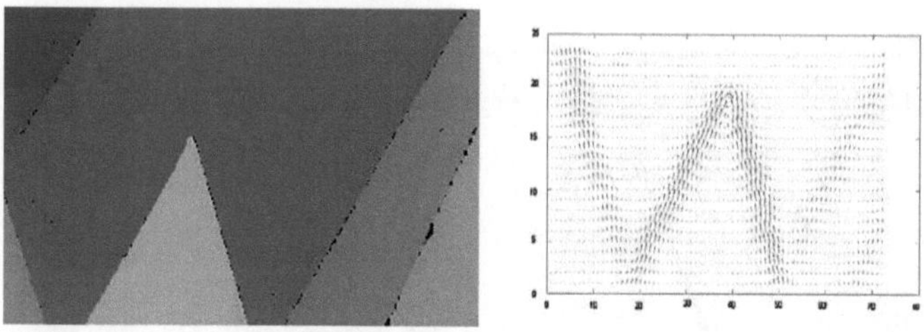

Fig. 1 Example of a detail of the depth map of the video sequence Cones [17] (*left*) and the estimated complex line process (*right*)

is proportional to $|e_{mn}|$ and whose phase equal to $\arg(e_{mn})$. Then, first-order CHF filtering, measures the edge strength and orientation and provides an estimate of the complex edge process e_{mn}.

5 MRF Based Depth Map Interpolation Algorithm

Herein, we adopt a closed form local Bayesian interpolator of the unknown high resolution depth map value d_{mn} given a set of measured values $d_c^{(LR)}$ extracted from the low-resolution depth map. Specifically, we estimate d_{mn} by interpolating $d_c^{(LR)}$ by suitable weights as follows:

$$\hat{d}_{mn} = \sum_{c \in \mathscr{C}_{\eta_{mn}}} \kappa_c d_c^{(LR)} \tag{5}$$

being $\kappa_c = k_c \cdot \left(\sum_{c \in \mathscr{C}_{\eta_{mn}}} k_c\right)^{-1}$. In Colonnese [7], interpolator (5) is proved to be the Maximum A Posteriori estimate of the unknown pixel d_{mn}. The interpolator weights the neighboring pixels by taking into account the normalized weights κ_c's. Since the effectively available set of neighboring pixels varies for each and every interpolated pixels, the weighted average involves differently selected neighbors at each pixel site. For non edge pixels, no favorite direction is taken into account and we refer to a reduced first-order neighboring set with uniform weights.

The MRF based interpolation procedure reads as follows.

1. The first stage of the interpolation algorithm is the estimation of the complex line process by means of the first order CHF. This task can be accomplished by performing a bilinear interpolation of the low-resolution depth map so as to provide a coarse estimate of the high resolution depth map over which the CHF filtering is performed. Remarkably, no registration is needed between the pixels of the high resolution natural image and those of the low-resolution depth map.

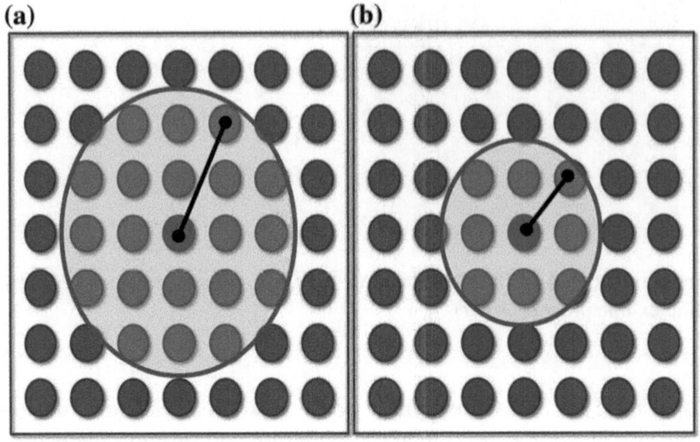

Fig. 2 Maximum extent of the cliques belonging to the neighborhood system for edge pixel interpolation (**a**) and for non edge pixels (**b**); the actual neighborhood system η_{mn} depends on the pixels available from the low-resolution depth map

2. For each clique, the weight is evaluated as the scalar product between the estimated complex edge process and the clique direction versor.
3. For each and every unknown pixel of the high resolution depth map, the edge magnitude is compared to a predefined threshold in order to detect the edge pixels;
   - on the so detected edge pixels, we evaluate the Markovian interpolator (5) by considering all the low-resolution depth map available values $d_c^{(LR)}$ within a circle of radius of $\sqrt{5}$ centered on the site (m, n) corresponding to the unknown high resolution depth map value d_{mn}; this geometry is exemplified in Fig. 2a;
   - on the remaining non edge pixels, we consider all the low-resolution depth map available values $d_c^{(LR)}$ within a circle of radius of $\sqrt{3}$ centered on the site (m, n), as shown in Fig. 2b.
4. Interpolation can be performed by cascading consecutive 2× interpolation stages; in this case, at each stage the available pixels may or not contain previously interpolated pixels (Fig. 3).

6 Experimental Results

We present here a few experimental results obtained on the video sequence Cones and Teddy, available [17]; two samples frames are reported in Figs. 3, 6, respectively. We have considered different resolutions, namely SQ (225 × 187), Q (450 × 375), H (900 × 750), F (1800 × 1500). The SQ map is obtained by decimation of the Q map without anti-aliasing filtering; the other resolutions are available at [17].

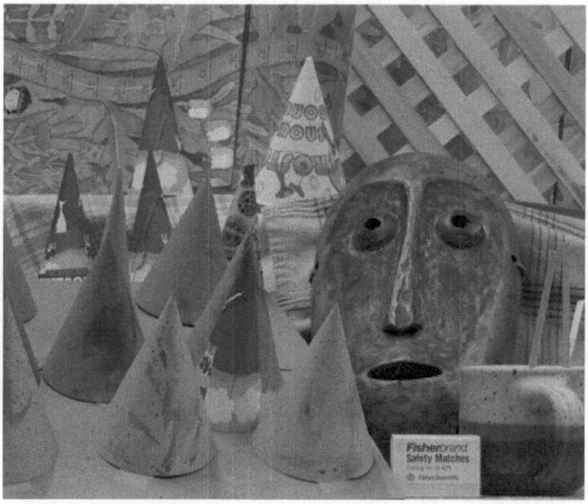

Fig. 3 Video sequence Cones: image [17]

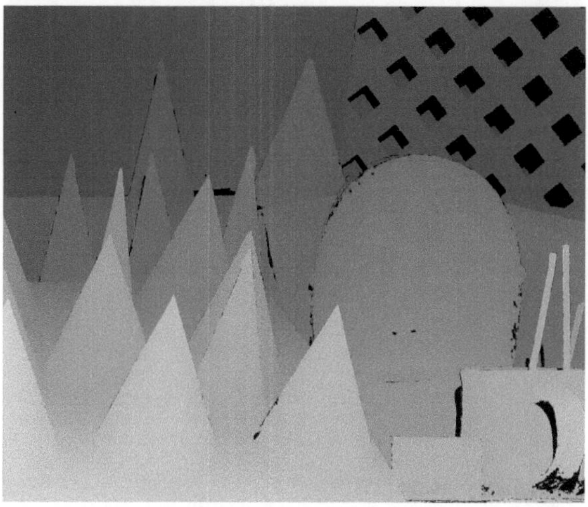

Fig. 4 Video sequence Cones: depth map [17]

In Table 2 we present results on the sequence Cones. Specifically, we report the PSNR observed adopting the herein presented MRF-based interpolation technique (BAY), the upsampling procedure presented in [12] (EKME), starting from the SQ resolution to Q (2× interpolation), H (4× interpolation) and F (8× interpolation).

In Fig. 5, we show the depth map estimated using the MRF based interpolation from the Q depth map (4× interpolation); for comparison sake, the Figure also shows

Table 2 PSNR achieved for different magnification factors: Cones

PSNR	2× (SQ → Q)	4× (SQ → H)	8× (SQ → F)
BAY	30.81	28.31	26.58
EKME	28.39	27.02	25.75

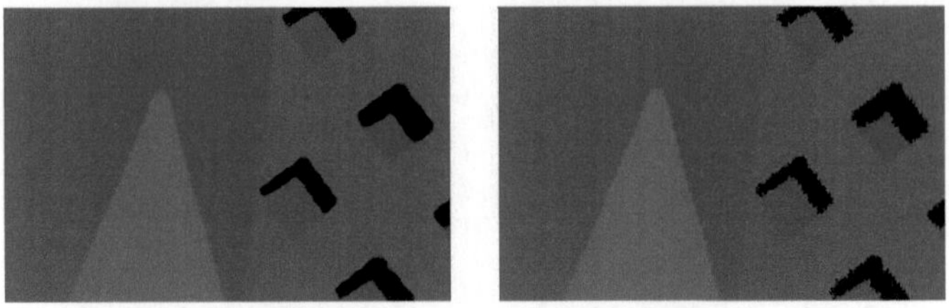

Fig. 5 Example of MRF based interpolation results: BAY 4× interpolated depth map (*left*), EKME 4× interpolated depth map (*right*)

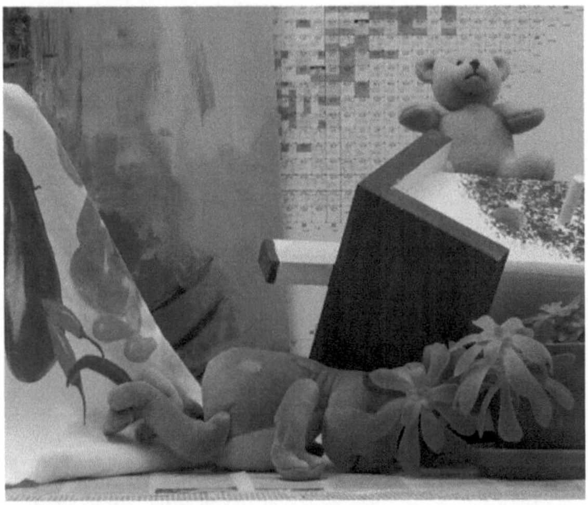

Fig. 6 Video sequence Teddy: image [17]

Table 3 PSNR achieved for different magnification factors: Cones

PSNR	2× (SQ → Q)	4× (SQ → H)	8× (SQ → F)
BAY	29.66	27.56	25.90
EKME	28.83	26.32	24.42

the result obtained by the edge adaptive upsampling technique in [12]. The MRF based interpolation favorably compares with the EKME interpolation.

Similar results have been obtained on the sequence Teddy. In Table 3 we report the PSNR results and in Fig. 8 we provide an example of the interpolation results.

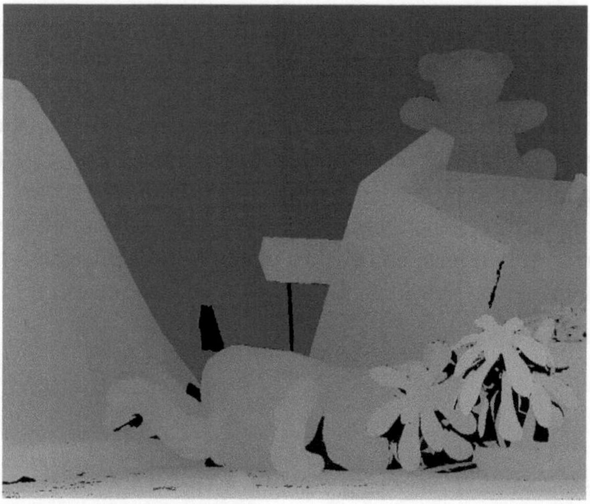

Fig. 7 Video sequence Teddy: depth map [17]

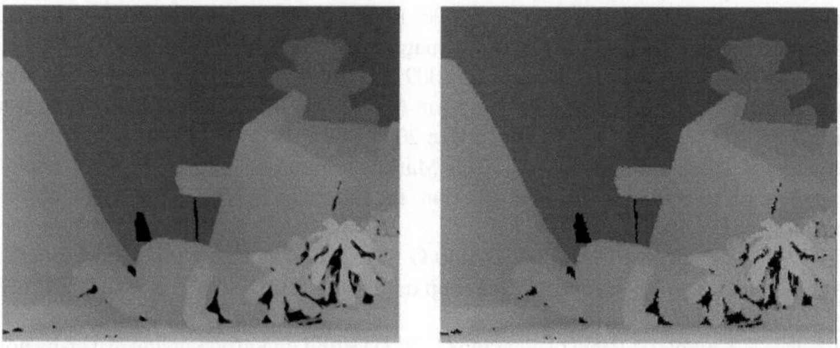

Fig. 8 Example of MRF based interpolation results: BAY 4× interpolated depth map (*left*), EKME 4× interpolated depth map (*right*)

To sum up, the markovian model proves to be very accurate in modeling depth map sequences, so as (i) to jointly enforce smoothness of interior regions and sharp regions' boundaries, and (ii) to account in a flexible ways for different interpolation geometries .

7 Conclusion and Further Work

In this chapter, we have summarized recent research results on depth map interpolation and we have described a fast procedure for MRF based interpolation of depth images. Markovian interpolation proved to be viable without side information on the reference high resolution luminance map. This allows application of the presented depth map interpolation technique independently by a luminance-depth registration stage and even in absence of a co-located luminance map. Besides, the procedure is applicable all over the map, without need of performing an initial segmentation over the edge map in order to identify textured and edge areas. As a matter of fact, this classification task is implicitly accomplished by a suitable band-pass filtering stage. Further investigation is to be carried out (i) on depth map boundary noise removal at large upscaling factors, which remain a critical task for both efficient coding and accurate rendering techniques, and (ii) on integration of differently reliable depth data obtained by means of hybrid active and passive techniques.

References

1. Ben Hadj S, Blanc-FTraud L, Maalouf E, Colicchio B, Dieterlen A (2012) Depth-variant image restoration in 3D fluorescence microscopy: two approaches under Gaussian and Poissonian noise conditions. In: IEEE International Symposium on Biomedical Imaging (ISBI), pp 1671–1674, 2–5 May 2012
2. Chantas GK, Galatsanos NP, Likas AC (2006) Bayesian resroration using a new nonstationary edge-preserving image prior. IEEE Trans Image Process 15(10):2987–2997
3. Chen CC, Chen YW, Yang FY, Peng WH (2009) A synthesis-quality-oriented depth refinement scheme for MPEG free viewpoint television (FTV). In: IEEE International Symposium on Multimedia, (ISM), pp 171–178, 14–16 Dec 2009
4. Colonnese S, Rinauro S, Scarano G (2011) Markov random fields using complex line process: an application to Bayesian image restoration. In: European Workshop on Visual Information Processing (EUVIP), 2–4 July 2011
5. Colonnese S, Randi R, Rinauro S, Scarano G (2010) Fast image interpolation using circular harmonic functions. In: European Workshop on Visual Information Processing (EUVIP), 5–7 July 2010
6. Colonnese S, Campisi P, Panci G, Scarano G (2004) Blind image deblurring driven by nonlinear processing in the edge domain. EURASIP J Appl Signal Process 16:2462–2475
7. Colonnese S, Rinauro S, Scarano G (2012) Bayesian image interpolation using Markov random fields driven by visually relevant image features. Signal Process: Image Commun 28(8):967–983
8. Colonnese S, Rinauro S, Scarano G (2012) Bayesian depth map interpolation using edge driven Markov Random fields. In: Computational Modeling of Objects Presented in Images: Fundamentals, Methods and Applications (COMPIMAGE), 5–7 Sept 2012
9. Colonnese S, Rinauro S, Rossi L, Scarano G (2009) Visual relevance evaluation using Rate Distortion analysis in the circular harmonic functions domain. In: IEEE International Conference Image Processing (ICIP)
10. Deng H, Yu L, Qiu J, Zhang J (2012) A joint texture/depth edge-directed up-sampling algorithm for depth map coding. In: IEEE International Conference on Multimedia and Expo (ICME), 9–13 July 2012
11. De Silva DVSX, Ekmekcioglu E, Fernando WAC, Worrall ST (2011) Display dependent preprocessing of depth maps based on just noticeable depth difference modeling. IEEE J Sel Topics Signal Process 5(2):335–351
12. Ekmekcioglu E, Mrak M, Worrall ST, Kondoz AM (2009) Edge adaptive upsampling of depth map videos for enhanced free-viewpoint video quality. IET Electron Lett 45(7):353–354
13. Garro V, dal Mutto C, Zanuttigh P, Cortelazzo GM (2009) A novel interpolation scheme for range data with side information. In: European Conference Visual Media Production (CVMP) , 12–13 Nov 2009

14. Goffredo M, Schmid M, Conforto S, Carli M, Neri A, D”Alessio T (2009) Markerless human motion analysis in Gauss-Laguerre transform domain: an application to sit-to-stand in young and elderly people. IEEE Trans Inf Technol Biomed 13(2):207–216
15. Geman S, Geman D (1984) Stochastic relaxation, Gibbs distribution, and the Bayesian restoration of images. IEEE Trans Pattern Anal Mach Intell PAMI-6(6):721–741
16. Graziosi DB, Dong T, Vetro A (2012) Depth map up-sampling based on edge layers. In: Asia-Pacific Signal & Information Processing Association Annual Summit and Conference (APSIPA ASC), 1–4, 3–6 Dec 2012
17. http://vision.middlebury.edu/stereo/
18. Jacovitti G, Neri A (2000) Multiresolution circular harmonic decomposition. IEEE Trans Signal Process 48(11):3242–3247
19. Jaesik P, Hyeongwoo K, Tai YW, Brown MS, Kweon I (2011) High quality depth map upsampling for 3D-TOF cameras. In: IEEE International Conference on Computer Vision (ICCV), pp 1623–1630, 6–13 Nov 2011
20. JSger F, Wien M, Kosse P (2012) Model-based intra coding for depth maps in 3D video using a depth lookup table. In: 3DTV-Conference: The True Vision—Capture, Transmission and Display of 3D Video (3DTV-CON), pp 1–4, 15–17 Oct 2012
21. Lee EK, Ho YS (2011) Generation of high-quality depth maps using hybrid camera system for 3-D video. J Vis Commun Image Represent 22(1):73–84
22. Lee PJ (2011) Nongeometric distortion smoothing approach for depth map preprocessing. IEEE Trans Multimedia 13(2):246–254
23. Lee PJ (2010) Adaptive edge-oriented depth image smoothing approach for depth image based rendering. In: IEEE International Symposium on Broadband Multimedia Systems and Broadcasting (BMSB), pp 1–5, 24–26 March 2010
24. Lee G, Ho Y (2011) Depth map up-sampling using random walk. In: Pacific Rim Symposiumv (PSIVT), 20–23 Nov 2011
25. Lu J, Min D, Singh Pahwa R, Do MN (2011) A revisit to MRF-based depth map super resolution and enhancement. In: IEEE International Conference on Acoustics, Speech and Signal Processing (ICASSP), 22–27 May 2011
26. Nguyen VA, Min D, Do MN (2012) Efficient edge-preserving interpolation and in-loop filters for depth map compression. IEEE International Conference on Image Processing (ICIP), pp 1293–1296 Sept 30–Oct. 3 2012
27. Palma V, Cancellaro M, Neri A (2011) Joint distributed source-channel coding for 3D videos. Image processing: algorithms and systems IX. In: Proceedings of the SPIE. doi:DOIurl10(1117/12):872878
28. Rong Z, Ying C, Karczewicz M (2012) Adaptive depth edge sharpening for 3D video depth coding. In: IEEE Visual Communications and Image Processing (VCIP), pp 1–6, 27–30 Nov 2012
29. Scharstein D, Szeliski R (2002) A taxonomy and evaluation of dense two-frame stereo correspondence algorithms. Int J Comput Vis 47(1–3):7–42
30. Schwarz H, Bartnik C, Bosse S, Brust H, Hinz T, Lakshman H, Marpe D, Merkle P, Mnller K, Rhee H, Tech G, Winken M, Wiegand T (2012) 3D video coding using advanced prediction, depth modeling, and encoder control methods. In: Picture Coding Symposium (PCS), pp 1–4, 7–9 May 2012
31. Schwarz S, Olsson R, Sjöström M, Tourancheau S (2012) Adaptive depth filtering for HEVC 3D video coding. In: Picture Coding Symposium (PCS), pp 49–52, 7–9 May 2012
32. Smisek J, Jancosek M, Pajdla T (2011) 3D with Kinect. In: IEEE International Conference on Computer Vision Workshops (ICCV Workshops), pp 1154–1160, 6–13 Nov 2011
33. Spatial Scalability Filters, ISO/IEC JTC1/SC29/WG11 and ITU-T SG16 Q.6 (2005) Doc. JVT-P007, Ponzan, Poland
34. Timmerer C, Mnller K (2010) Immersive future media technologies: from 3D video to sensory experiences. ACM Multimedia (Tutorial), 25–29 Oct 2010
35. Tseng SP, Lai SH (2011) Accurate depth map estimation from video via MRF optimization. In: IEEE Visual Communications and Image Processing (VCIP), pp 1–4, 6–9 Nov 2011

36. Vijayanagar KR, Loghman M, Joohee K (2012) Refinement of depth maps generated by low-cost depth sensors. In: International SoC Design Conference (ISOCC), pp 355–358, 4–7 Nov 2012
37. Wang HM, Huang CH, Yang JF (2011) Block-based depth maps interpolation for efficient multiview content generation. IEEE Trans Circuits Syst Video Technol 21(12):1847–1858
38. Wang HM, Huang CH, Yang JF (2010) Depth maps interpolation from existing pairs of keyframes and depth maps for 3D video generation. In: IEEE International Symposium on Circuits and Systems (ISCAS), pp 3248–3251, May 30 - June 2 2010
39. Wildeboer MO, Yendo T, Tehrani MP, Fujii T, Tanimoto M (2010) Color based depth up-sampling for depth compression. In: Picture Coding Symposium (PCS), pp 170–173, 8–10 Dec 2010
40. Xu X, Po LM, Cheung, KW, Ng KH, Wong KM, Ting CW (2012) A foreground biased depth map refinement method for DIBR view synthesis. In: IEEE International Conference on Acoustics, Speech and Signal Processing (ICASSP), pp 805–808, 25–30 March 2012
41. Zhang G, Jia J, Wong TT, Bao H (2009) Consistent depth maps recovery from a video sequence. IEEE Trans Pattern Anal Mach Intell 31(6):974–988
42. Zhu J (2011) Reliability fusion of time-of-flight depth and stereo geometry for high quality depth maps. IEEE Trans Pattern Anal Mach Intell 33(7):1400–1414

Iris Image Correction Method from Unconstrained Images

Eliana Frigerio and Marco Marcon

Abstract The use of iris as biometric trait has emerged as one of the most preferred method because of its uniqueness, lifetime stability and regular shape. Moreover it shows public acceptance and new user-friendly capture devices are developed and used in a broadened range of applications. Currently, iris recognition systems work well with frontal iris images from cooperative users. Nonideal iris images are still a challenge for iris recognition and can significantly affect the accuracy of iris recognition systems. Moreover, accurate localization of different eye's parts from videos or still images is a crucial step in many image processing applications that range from iris recognition in Biometrics to gaze estimation for Human Computer Interaction (HCI), impaired people aid or, even, marketing analysis for products attractiveness. Notwithstanding this, actually, most of available implementations for eye's parts segmentation are quite invasive, imposing a set of constraints both on the environment and on the user itself limiting their applicability to high security Biometrics or to cumbersome interfaces. In the first part of this Chapter, we propose a novel approach to segment the *sclera*, the white part of the eye. We concentrate on this area since, thanks to the dissimilarity with other eye's parts, its identification can be performed in a robust way against light variations, reflections and glasses lens flare. An accurate sclera segmentation is a fundamental step in iris and pupil localization, even in non-frontal noisy images. Furthermore its particular geometry can be fruitfully used for accurate eyeball rotation estimation. The proposed technique is based on a statistical approach (supported by some heuristic assumptions) to extract discriminating descriptors for sclera and non-sclera pixels. A Support Vector Machine (SVM) is then used as a final supervised classifier. Once the eyeball rotation angle respect to the camera optical axis is estimated and the *limbus* (the boundary between the iris and the sclera) is extracted, we propose a method to correct off-angle

F. Eliana (✉) · M. Marco (✉)
ISPG, DEIB, Politecnico di Milano, P.zza Leonardo Da Vinci, 32, 20133 Milano, Italy
e-mail: efrigerio@elet.polimi.it

M. Marco
e-mail: marcon@elet.polimi.it

P. Di Giamberardino et al. (eds.), *Computational Modeling of Objects Presented in Images*, Lecture Notes in Computational Vision and Biomechanics 15,
DOI: 10.1007/978-3-319-04039-4_12,

iris image. Taking into account the eye morphology and the reflectance properties of the external transparent layers, we can evaluate the distorting effects that are present in the acquired image. The correction algorithm proposed includes a first modeling phase of the human eye and a simulation phase where the acquisition geometry is reproduced and the distortions are evaluated. Finally we obtain an image which does not contain the distorting effects due to jumps in the refractive index. We show how this correction process reduces the intra-class variations for off-angle iris images.

Keywords Sclera segmentation · Iris correction · 3D eye model · Gaze estimation · Eikonal equation

1 Introduction

Biometrics uses physical, biological and behavioral traits to automatically identify and verify a person. The human iris, an annular portion between the pupil and the white sclera, has an extraordinary structure and provides many minute interlacing characteristics such as freckles, coronas, stripes and the collarette area, which are unique to each subject [4]. The unique structure of iris, the stability of iris pattern throughout the person's lifetime, the non invasiveness of the system (iris is an internal as well as an externally visible organ), the public acceptance, and a wide range of applications influence the increased interest in the iris as one of the most reliable biometric technologies in recent years. Most of the literature is focused on processing of ideal iris images, acquired in typical quite constrained scenarios: subjects stop and stare relatively close to the acquisition device while their eyes are illuminated by a near-infrared light source, enabling the acquisition of high-quality data. Starting from the pioneer work of Daugman [5], which is still the reference processing approach, many other approaches were proposed during years [16, 21, 22, 25, 30, 39, 45].

Several researchers are currently working on lowering these constraints without significantly impacting performance while increasing system usability. These include processing and encoding of a "nonideal iris" that is defined as accounting for the off-angle, occluded, blurred and noisy images, and "iris at a distance" that is defined as a snapshot of an iris captured from a moving individual at a large distance (more than a meter) [32]. Under a nonideal situation, traditional iris recognition systems would not work well. We focalize our attention on compensating off-angle iris images. It is not practical to assume that a user always aligns his/her optical axis with the camera's optical axis. Previous techniques for nonideal iris recognition do not specifically adjust for iris images captured off-angle. Exceptions are the early work of Sung et al. [35], where they apply an inner eye corner detector in combination with a Sobel edge detector and a least square elliptical fit, and the work of Takano et al. [36], that uses a rotation-spreading neural network. Santos et al. propose a novel fusion of different recognition approaches [31] and describe how they can contribute to more reliable noncooperative iris recognition. The limitation of these papers is that the datasets used for testing do not specifically include the off-angle images. Li [19], Dorairaj et al. [8] and Schuckers et al. [32] use the West Virginia University database, specifically developed to address this issue. In particular, Dorairaj et al. [8] design a system to process non-ideal iris images in two steps: (i) estimation of the gaze direction and (ii) processing and encoding of the rotated iris image. The limitation of all these papers is that homographic transformations are applied to the distorted images in order to obtain a synthetic frontal view with iris having circular boundaries. Our approach uses a 3D iris model and a ray-tracing algorithm in order to compensate also the distortions introduced by transparent surface layers and to obtain a more reasonable iris frontal view. Moreover we propose a method that does not change the core parts of the traditional systems but adds additional software modules in order to compensate geometric distortions due to jumps in the refractive index of the external transparent layers.

Before compensating the distortions introduced by transparent surface layers, it is necessary to estimate the gaze direction. *Gaze direction* is either modeled, in the literature, as the optical axis (Line of Gaze LoG) or as the visual axis (Line of Sight LoS). The optical axis is the line connecting the pupil center, cornea center and eyeball center. The visual axis is the line connecting the fovea (small region in the center of the retina) and the cornea center. The *point of regard* (PoR) is often used too. It is computed as the intersection of the gaze direction vector with the nearest object of the scene [13]. In the following we are interested in estimating the gaze direction respect to the camera optical axis, that is the LoG in the camera reference system. A person can change gaze direction by rotating the eyeball while keeping the head stationary, or by moving the head while keeping the eye stationary respect to the head. Considering a user looking at the camera optical center, the image of his eye will be different for different head positions. Head pose, therefore, determines the coarse-scale gaze direction, while the eyeball orientation determines the local and detailed gaze direction. In general, the non-intrusive vision-based gaze estimation techniques can be classified into two groups [47]: 2D mapping-based gaze estimation methods (regression-based) [26] and direct 3D gaze estimation methods [24, 34, 40]. They are both called feature-based methods [13]. Instead of using explicit geometric features like contours and corners, an alternative approach to gaze estimation is to implement an appearance-based algorithm [37]. An image is treated as a point in a high-dimensional space and the PoR is estimated comparing the whole image with a database of hand labeled images. The main drawbacks of this class of methods are the necessity of a large database of eye images in order to estimate the prototypes and the inability to estimate the 3D LoS. Only the PoR, usually respect to a monitor placed in the scene and used for the database acquisition, can be estimated. In the regression-based methods, the eye gaze is estimated from 2D eye movement features extracted from the images. The 2D features change with the gaze and the relationship between them can be encoded by a calibrated gaze mapping function. The gaze mapping function varies significantly with the user (a calibration for each user is needed) and, moreover, with the head position [47]. These are the main problems of 2D mapping-based methods. Wang et al. [42–44] show the possibility to allow more freedom of head movements using a couple of cameras: a fixed camera to estimate the head pose, and a pan/tilt camera that zooms to the user eye to acquire the eye image.

However, the system still requires a user calibration in order to estimate the gaze. 3D model-based approaches model the physical structure of the human eye in order to calculate the gaze direction vector. They are not constrained by the head position and the PoR can be obtained simply intersecting the estimated 3D gaze line with any object in the scene. The system independence from a user calibration depends on the number of lights and/or cameras used. Shih et al. [34] demonstrate that at least two cameras and at least two point light sources are needed to recover the LoG without any head-position constraint or user calibration. Considering the proposed algorithm to compensate the distortions on the iris image introduced by transparent surface layers, we focalize our attention on the latter class of methods because we are interested on estimating the 3D LoG without any head-position constraint.

Due to the importance for the gaze estimation and for the iris correction algorithm, an accurate eye parts segmentation is the first requirement for any successive processing. At the beginning of this Chapter we focus on this topic, in particular we tackle sclera localization. The sclera is the white part of the eye and its accurate segmentation can offer considerable advantages in localizing the iris, possible eyelids occlusions, and accurate estimation of eyeball rotation with respect to the facial pose.

The rest of the contribution is organized as follows. In Sect. 2, we introduce the two databases used for sclera segmentation, gaze estimation and iris correction, highlighting the strengths of both. Section 3 describes the algorithm developed for sclera segmentation together with some experimental results. Section 4, after a brief review of the state of the art methods that are well suited to our acquisition configuration, proposes a gaze-estimation technique. Section 5 explains the iris correction process (Sect. 5.1 illustrates the 3D eye model used). Conclusions (Sect. 6) end the paper.

2 Database Definition

The database used for sclera segmentation algorithm tuning and test evaluation is the UBIRIS v.2 database [27]. This database differs from other iris databases, like CASIA [38] or UPOL [7], since in UBIRIS the acquired iris images are far from those relative to perfect acquisition conditions and are very similar to those that could be acquired by a non-invasive and passive system. In particular UBIRIS is composed by 11102 images collected from 261 persons. Images were actually captured on non-constrained conditions (at-a-distance, on-the-move and on the visible wavelength), with corresponding more realistic noise factors. The acquisition setup is shown in Fig. 1a [27]. The images present the following types of "imperfections" with respect to optimal acquisitions (shown in Fig. 2):

- *Images acquired at different distances* from 3 to 7 m with different eye's size in pixel (e.g. Fig. 2a, b);
- *Rotated images* when the subject's head is not upright (e.g. Fig. 2c;

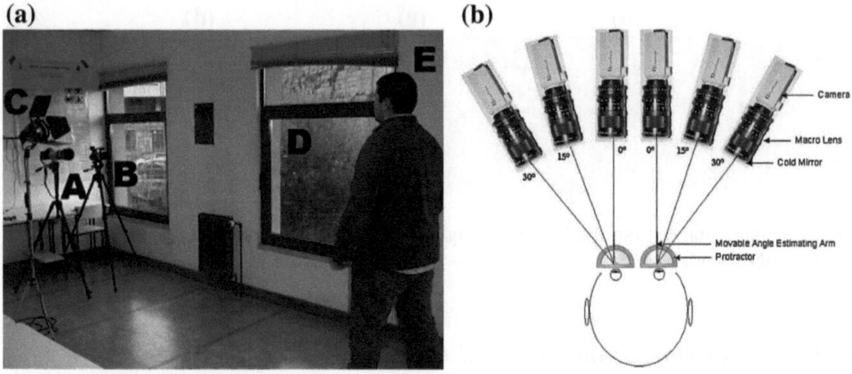

Fig. 1 **a** Overview of the used image acquisition framework (*A*, *B*), light sources (*C*, *D*) and subjects location (*E*) for the UBIRIS v.2 database (courtesy of Proença and Alexandre [27]). **b** Schematic data collection setup for the off-angle iris images of the WVU database. The subjects head is positioned on a chin/head rest and he is asked to focus straight ahead on a LED. The camera is rotated 15° and 30° as measured by a protractor on a movable arm positioned under the eye (courtesy of Schuckers et al. [32])

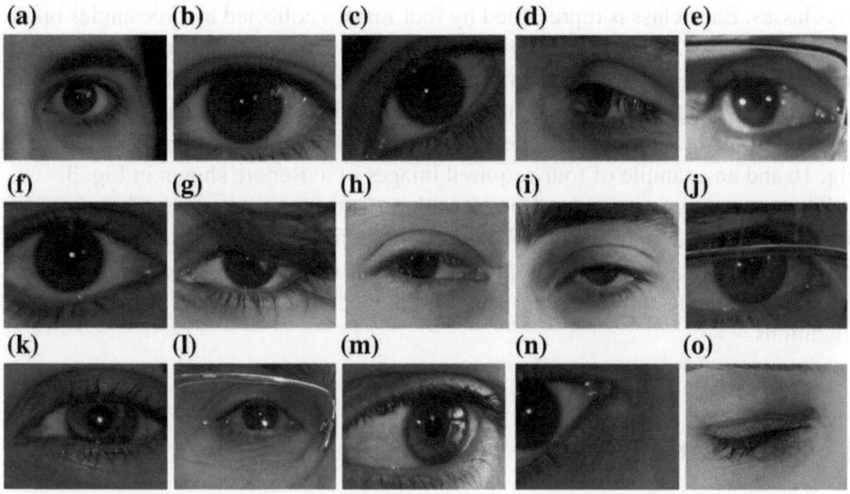

Fig. 2 Examples of UBIRIS v.2 images presenting different noise sources. See text above for a description of the "imperfections" with respect to optimal acquisitions

- *Iris images off-axis* when the iris is not frontal to the acquisition system (e.g. Fig. 2d, e);
- *Fuzzy and blurred images* due to subject motion during acquisition, eyelashes motion or out-of-focus images (e.g. Fig. 2e, f);
- *Eyes clogged by hair* Hair can hide portions of the iris (e.g. Fig. 2g);
- *Iris and sclera parts obstructed by eyelashes or eyelids* (e.g. Fig. 2h, i);

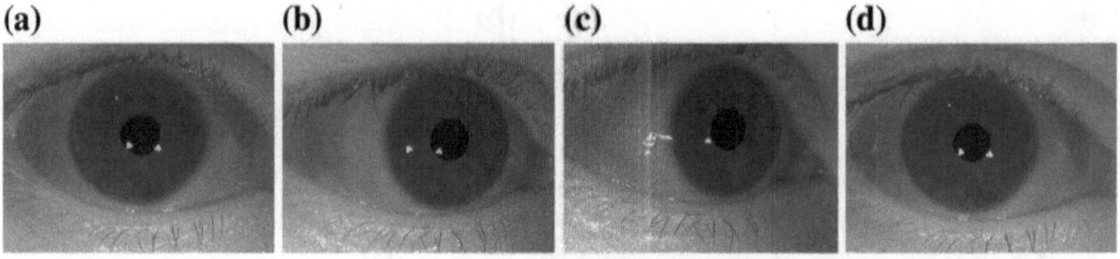

Fig. 3 Sample images from the WVU off-angle iris database. **a** 0° angle; **b** 15° off-angle; **c** 30° off-angle; **d** 0° angle

- *Eyes images clogged and distorted by glasses or contact lenses* (e.g. Fig. 2j, k and l);
- *Images with specular or diffuse reflections* Specular reflections give rise to bright points that could be confused with sclera regions (e.g. Fig. 2l, m);
- *Images with closed eyes or truncated parts* (e.g. Fig. 2n, o).

To verify the proposed correction method for nonideal iris recognition, we use part of the West Virginia University off-angle iris database. The dataset consists of 200 iris classes. Each class is represented by four images collected at three angles on the order of 0°, 15°, 30°, and again 0° [32]. The acquisition setup is more-constrained respect to the UBIRIS v.2 acquisition conditions: the images collected are in the near infrared range (above 700 nm) and the illumination is performed by six LEDs attached at the bottom of the camera. The schematic acquisition setup is showed in Fig. 1b and an example of four acquired images of a user are shown in Fig. 3.

There are no eye gaze estimation algorithms working well in natural light acquisition setup [13] and moreover the WVU off-angle iris database provides a rough LoG estimation, useful to verify the proposed algorithm. On the other hand the UBIRIS v.2 database is more useful to test the sclera segmentation algorithm in non-constrained conditions.

3 Sclera Segmentation

The term sclera refers to the white part of the eye that is about 5/6 of the outer casing of the eyeball. It is an opaque and fibrous membrane that has a thickness between 0.3 and 1 mm, with both structural and protective function. Its accurate segmentation is particularly important for gaze tracking to estimate eyeball rotation with respect to head pose and camera position but it is also relevant in Iris Recognition systems: since the limbus is the boundary between the iris and the sclera, an accurate segmentation of the sclera is helpful to estimate the external edge of the iris.

3.1 Coarse Sclera Segmentation

The first step in the proposed Sclera segmentation approach is based on a dynamic enhancement of the Red, Green, Blue channel histograms. Being the sclera a white area, this will encourage the emergence of the region of interest. Calling x_{min} and x_{max} the lower and the upper limit of the histogram of the considered channel, assuming that the intensities range from 0 to 1, we apply, independently on each channel, a non-linear transform based on a sigmoid curve where the output intensity y is given by:

$$y = \frac{1}{1 + exp\left(-\alpha\frac{x-\bar{x}}{\sigma}\right)}, \tag{1}$$

where $\bar{x}$ is the mean value of x , σ is the standard deviation and we assume $\alpha = 10$. The latest value is chosen making various tests trying to obtain a good contrast between sclera and non-sclera pixels.

We manually segment 100 randomly-chosen images from the whole preprocessed database, dividing pixels into Sclera (ω_S) and Non-Sclera (ω_N) classes. Each pixel can be considered as a vector in the three dimensions (Red, Green and Blue) color space $\Re^3$. These vectors are then used in minimum Mahalanobis distance classifier with the two aforementioned classes, combined with Linear Discriminant Analysis (LDA) [9]. LDA projects data through a linear mapping that maximizes the between-class variance while minimizes the within-class variance [23]. Calling $\mathbf{x}$ the projected vector, corresponding to a pixel to be classified, accordingly to a minimum Mahalanobis distance criterium we define a Sclera pixel as:

$$M_S = \begin{cases} 1 \texttt{ if } & D_S(\mathbf{x}) \leq D_N(\mathbf{x}) \\ 0 \texttt{ if } & D_S(\mathbf{x}) > D_N(\mathbf{x}) \end{cases}, \tag{2}$$

where $D_S(\mathbf{x})$ and $D_N(\mathbf{x})$ are the distances respectively from ω_S and ω_N. We recall that:

$$D_i(\mathbf{x}) = \sqrt{(\mathbf{x} - \mu_i)^T\, \Sigma_i^{-1}\, (\mathbf{x} - \mu_i)}, \tag{3}$$

where μ_i is the average vector and Σ_i is the Covariance Matrix [9]. Therefore, using this simple linear classifier we can obtain a coarse mask for Sclera and Non-Sclera pixels using the Mahalanobis distances.

3.2 Dealing with Reflections

Specular reflections are always a noise factor in images with non-metallic reflective surfaces such as cornea or sclera. Since sclera is not a reflective metallic surface, the presence of glare spots is due to incoherent reflection of light incident on the cornea. Typically, the pixels representing reflections have a very high intensity, close to pure white. Near to their boundaries, there are sharp discontinuities due to strong variations in brightness. The presented algorithm for the reflexes identification consists mainly of two steps:

- Identification of possible reflection areas by the identification of their edges through the use of a Sobel operator;
- Intensity analysis within the selected regions.

The first step, using a gray-scaled version of the image, is based on an approximation of the modulus of the image gradient, $\nabla I(x, y)$, by the Sobel 3×3 operator:

$$G_x = \begin{bmatrix} -1\,0\,1 \\ -2\,0\,2 \\ -1\,0\,1 \end{bmatrix}. \tag{4}$$

So $|\nabla I(x, y)| = \sqrt{G_x^2 + G_y^2}$, where $G_y = G_x^T$. Due to the sharp edges present on reflexes we adopt a threshold of 0.1 to define reflex edges; the threshold value is chosen as the best for the 100 images used for training. For each candidate region we then check, through a morphological filling operation for 8-connected curves [11], if it is closed, and, if this is the case, we assume it as a reflex if all pixels inside have an intensity above the 95 % of the maximum intensity present in the whole image (regions with high intensity pixels). These steps are shown in Fig. 4 where reflexes are insulated.

The location of the estimated reflections defines a "region of interest" in which the pixels are classified as Sclera or Non-Sclera following the aforementioned process. Avoiding all the pixels that are outside the "reflex regions" from the previously defined candidates for the Sclera regions provides us with the first rough estimation of Sclera Regions. Some rough results are shown in Fig. 5.

3.3 Results Refinement

A first improvement with respect to the aforementioned problems is obtained using morphological operators. They allow small noise removal, holes filling and image regions clustering. We apply the following sequence of operators:

- Opening with a circular element of radius 3. It allows to separate elements weakly connected and to remove small regions.
- Erosion with a circular element of radius 4. It can help to eliminate noise still present after the opening and insulate objects connected by thin links.
- Removal of elements with area of less than 4 pixels.
- Dilation with a circular element of radius 7 to fill holes or other imperfections and to join neighbor regions.

Radii of structuring elements to perform aforementioned tasks are heuristically found. They perform well on UBIRIS v.2 images, but different acquisition setups

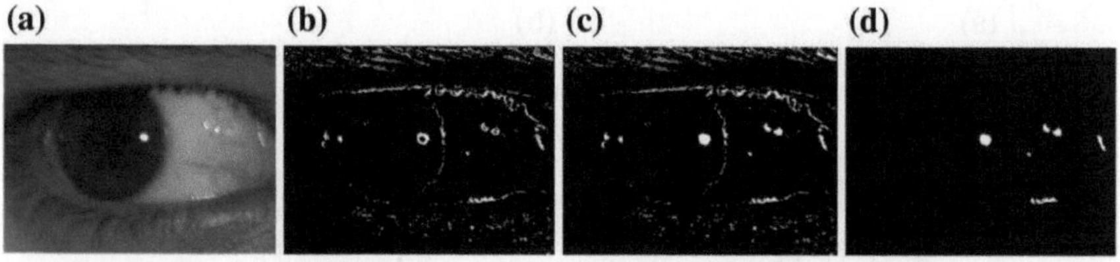

Fig. 4 **a** Original, normalized image, **b** binary mask where '1' represents pixels whose gradient modulus ($|\nabla I(x, y)|$) is above 0.1, **c** binary mask with filled regions, and **d** binary mask only with regions of high intensity pixels

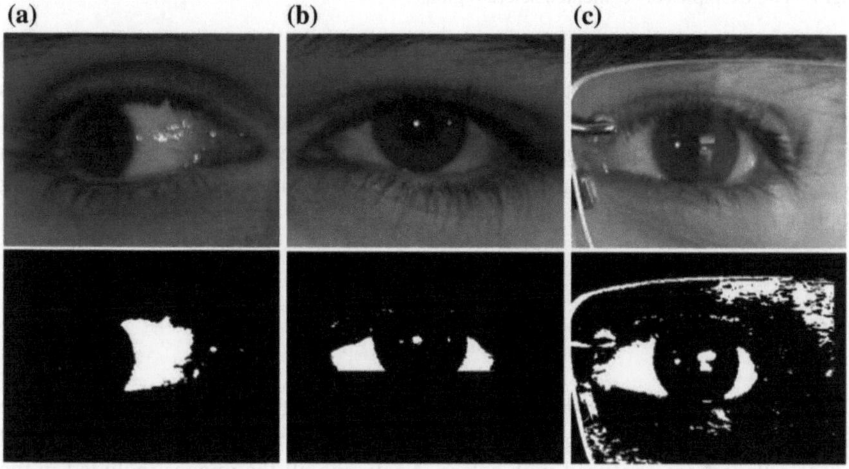

Fig. 5 Preliminary results identifying the "reflex region": (*top row*) original images and (*bottom row*) binary Sclera masks. In (**c**) many classification errors are still present due to glasses lens and frame

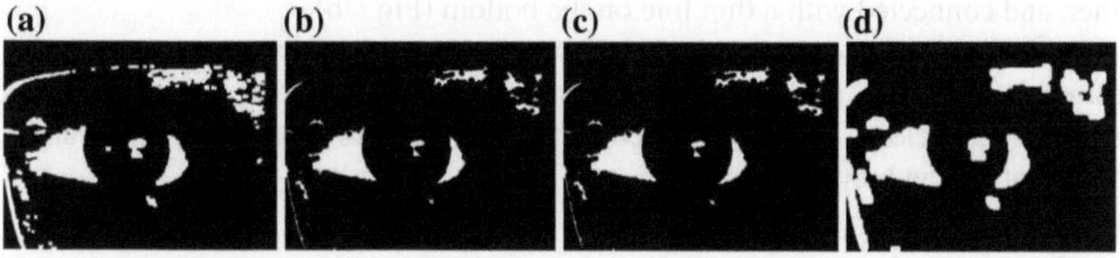

Fig. 6 Results of the application of the 4 morphological operators described in Sect. 3.3 on the binary mask shown in Fig. 5c. **a** Opening with a circular element of radius 3. **b** Erosion with a circular element of radius 4. **c** Removal of elements with area of less than 4 pixels. **d** Dilation with a circular element of radius 7

may require a different tuning. Intensity analysis within the selected regions fits well with the UBIRIS database, but, in case of different resolution images should scale accordingly to the eye size. An example of the results obtained following the aforementioned steps is shown in Fig. 6.

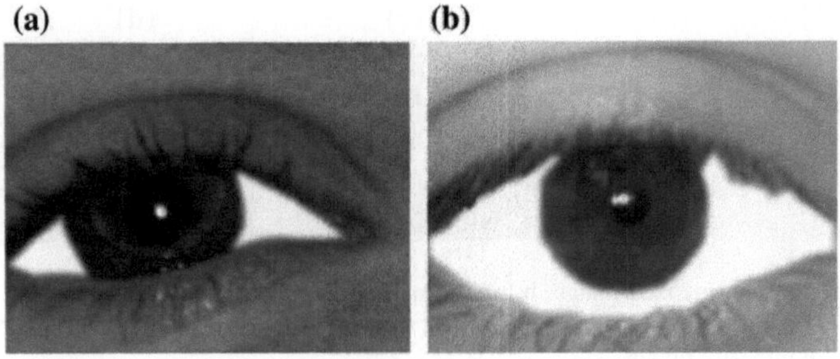

Fig. 7 Two examples of segmented sclera regions

The center of the different regions are then used as seeds for a Watershed analysis [41] that allows us to obtain accurate edges for each region in the image. Different regions, accordingly to the gradient formulation, are then defined whenever a basin area is not significantly changing for consistent intensities variation (water filling approach [2, 46]).

3.4 Final Classification Step

The aforementioned algorithm provides no false negative regions but many false positives are present in images where ambiguous regions, due to glasses or contact lenses reflexes, are confused with sclera. Analyzing all the images included in the considered database, we observe that the true sclera region have only two possible configurations: (1) like a triangle with two extruded sides and one intruded (Fig. 7a) or, when the subject is looking up, (2) like two of the previous triangles, facing each other, and connected with a thin line on the bottom (Fig. 7b).

On the basis of these considerations, we decide to define a set of shape-based features that can be used to separate, among all the selected regions, those that represent real scleras. The vector is composed by the following elements (invariant to translations and rotations):

- Region area in pixels;
- Ratio between region area and its perimeter;
- 7 Hu invariant moments [15]. Concerning the seventh moment I_7 [15], we use its module since we do not want to distinguish mirror images.

The final region classifier is then based on a Support Vector Machine accordingly to the Cortes-Vapnik formulation [3]. Sclera and Non-Sclera regions are classified accordingly to:

$$\hat{y} = sign\,(f(\mathbf{x}))\,, \tag{5}$$

where

$$f(\mathbf{x}) = \sum_{i \in S} \alpha_i y_i \Phi(\mathbf{x}_i) \cdot \Phi(\mathbf{x}) + b = \sum_{i \in S} \alpha_i y_i \mathcal{K}(\mathbf{x}_i, \mathbf{x}) + b. \quad (6)$$

α_i are Lagrange multipliers, b is a constant, S are elements for which the relative multiplier α_i is non-null after optimization process and $\mathcal{K}$ is the non-linear kernel. In this case $\mathcal{K}$ is:

$$\mathcal{K}(\mathbf{a}, \mathbf{b}) = (\mathbf{a} \cdot \mathbf{b} + 1)^2 . \quad (7)$$

This is a Quadratic Programming Problem that can be solved using optimization algorithms [14].

3.5 Results

Evaluating the segmentation results achieved over all the 250 chosen images (100 of them are also used for training) of the UBIRIS v.2 database, we obtain a 100 % recognition of closed eyes (no sclera pixels at all), 2 % false negative (with respect to the handmade segmented region) in the rare cases of very different brightness from left to right eye parts (due to a side illumination), and we also report a 1 % of false positive (with respect to the handmade segmented region) for particular glass-frames that locally resemble sclera regions.

4 Gaze Estimation

This Section, after a brief review of the state of the art methods that are well suited to our acquisition configuration, proposes a gaze-estimation technique. Normally, infrared (IR) light-emitting diodes (LEDs) are used in gaze estimation systems, as this light is not visible to humans and produces reflections on the cornea that are visible on the acquired images, called glints (see Fig. 8). When a beam light enters the cornea surface of a human eye, part of the light is reflected by the surface and part is refracted after traveling through the surface. The light which is reflected by the exterior cornea surface is called the first Purkinje image (see Fig. 8). Since the first Purkinje image is a result of specular reflection, observations at different directions will observe different images. Corneal reflections, together with the pupil center or the pupil contour or the limbus, are the eye features commonly used for gaze estimation. In particular, considering the WVU iris database acquisition setup, we estimate the gaze using corneal reflections (at least 2 are present in each image) and the pupil center (highlighted in Fig. 9b).

Most of the 3D model-based approaches employ 3D eye models and calibrated scenarios (calibrated cameras, light sources, and camera positions). Shih et al. [34] use the eye model proposed by Le Grand [17], where the shape of the cornea is assumed to be a portion of an imaginary sphere with center at $\mathbf{c}$ and radius R =

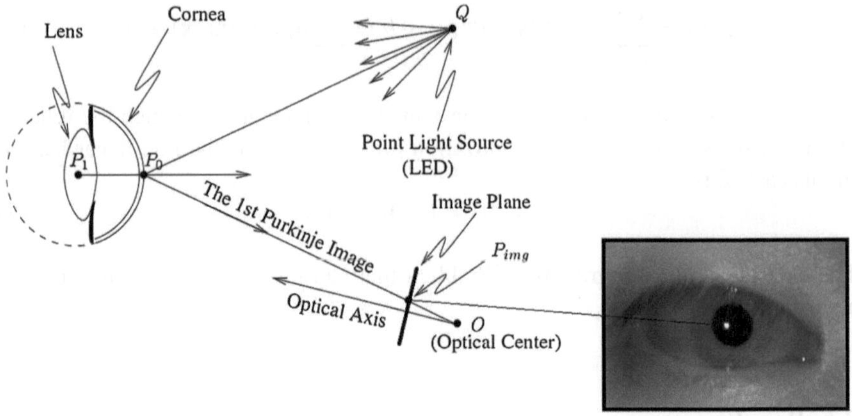

Fig. 8 Schematic diagram illustrating the geometry relationship between the point light source, the cornea, the first Purkinje image, and the camera. The bright spot in the image is the recorded first Purkinje image of an infrared LED (courtesy of Shih and Liu [33])

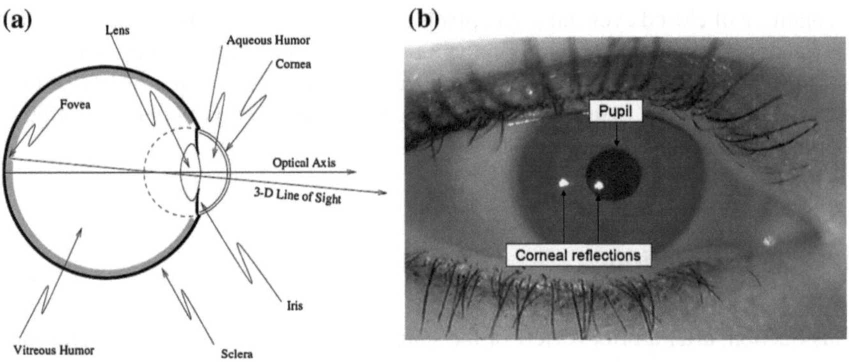

Fig. 9 **a** Structure of Le Grand's simplified eye [17]. **b** Example of image of the WVU iris database, highlighting the features used for gaze estimation

7.8 mm. The pupil is a circle on a plane distant h = 4.2 mm respect to the cornea center. The pupil and cornea centers define the optical axis (LoG). The cornea and the aqueous humor can be modeled as a convex spherical lens having uniform refraction index (as shown in Fig. 9a).

The reflective properties of the cornea influence the position of the glint(s) in the image, while its refractive properties modify the pupil image. The pupil image is not the projection of the pupil, but the projection of the refracted pupil and this concept is fundamental also in the proposed iris correction method [40]. Figure 10 shows the 3D pupil inside the cornea and the pupil shape after refraction. The methods proposed by Villanueva et al. [40], Shih et al. [34] and Guestrin and Eizenman [12] are all based on the use of multiple light sources and one or more cameras for estimating the optical axis using pupil center and corneal reflections. In particular, we

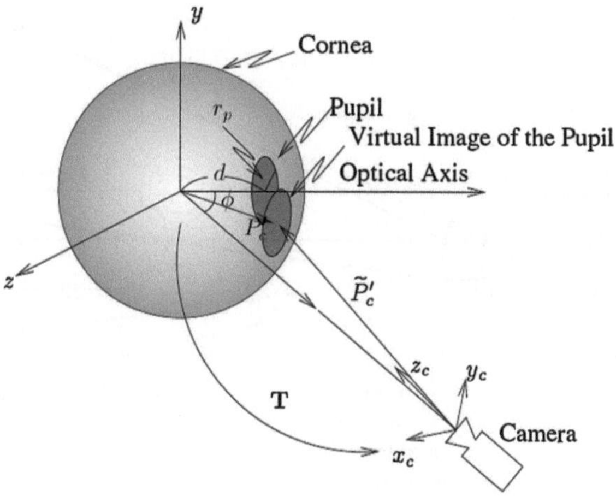

Fig. 10 3D model representing the real pupil and the virtual image of the pupil due to the refractive properties of the cornea (courtesy of Shih and Liu [33])

follow the latter method, even if the algorithms and the results of the aforementioned estimation processes are absolutely comparable. We work in the assumption that the light sources are modeled as point sources and the camera as a pin-hole camera [12]. Figure 11 presents a ray tracing diagram of the system and the eye for a single light and a single camera. We assume that the whole system is calibrated: the intrinsic camera parameters are known together with the positions of the LEDs respect to the camera (a plane mirror can be used to estimate each LED position as suggested by Shih and Liu [33]). All points are represented in a right-handed Cartesian world coordinate system aligned with the canonical camera reference system.

4.1 Mathematical Model

Consider a ray that comes from light source i, placed at $\mathbf{l}_i$, and reflects at a point $\mathbf{q}_{ij}$ on the corneal surface such that the reflected ray passes through the j-camera optical center, $\mathbf{o}_j$, and intersects the camera image plane at a point $\mathbf{u}_{ij}$.

The condition that the ray coming from the point of reflection $\mathbf{q}_{ij}$ and, passing camera optical center $\mathbf{o}_j$, intersects the camera image plane at point $\mathbf{u}_{ij}$, can be expressed in parametric form as:

$$\mathbf{q}_{ij} = \mathbf{o}_j + k_{q,ij}(\mathbf{o}_j - \mathbf{u}_{ij}) \tag{8}$$

for a scaling factor $k_{q,ij}$.

The condition that the point of reflection is on the corneal surface can be written as:

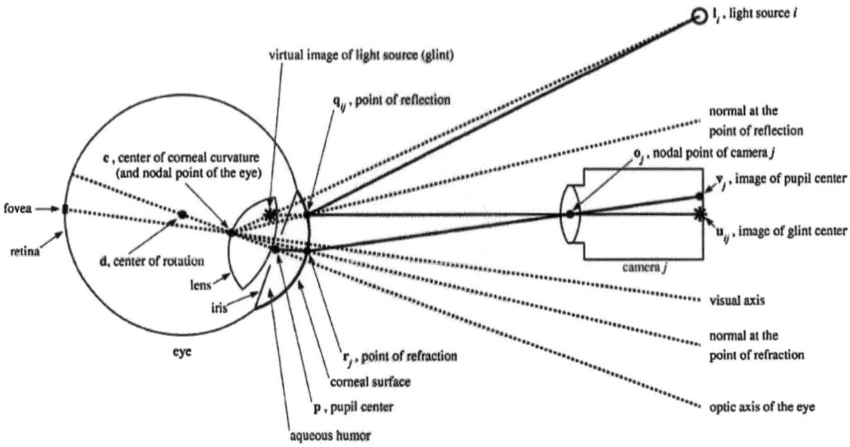

Fig. 11 Schematic representation of the eye, a camera, a light source, the 3D point of refection, the 3D refracted pupil center and their image on the camera image plane (courtesy of Guestrin and Eizenman [12])

$$\|\mathbf{q}_{ij} - \mathbf{c}\| = R, \tag{9}$$

where **c** is the unknown center of corneal curvature and R is the radius of the corneal surface.

The law of reflection states two conditions:

(1) the incident ray $(\mathbf{q}_{ij} - \mathbf{l}_j)$, the reflected ray $(\mathbf{o}_j - \mathbf{q}_{ij})$, and the normal at the point of reflection are coplanar. Since vector $(\mathbf{q}_{ij} - \mathbf{c})$ is normal to the spherical surface at the point of reflection $\mathbf{q}_{ij}$, this condition implies that points $\mathbf{l}_i$, $\mathbf{q}_{ij}$, $\mathbf{c}$, and $\mathbf{o}_j$ are coplanar. Therefore this condition can be formalized as:

$$(\mathbf{l}_i - \mathbf{o}_j) \times (\mathbf{q}_{ij} - \mathbf{o}_j) \cdot (\mathbf{c} - \mathbf{o}_j) = 0, \tag{10}$$

considering that three coplanar vectors $\mathbf{a}_1$, $\mathbf{a}_2$, and $\mathbf{a}_3$ satisfy $\mathbf{a}_1 \times \mathbf{a}_2 \cdot \mathbf{a}_3 = 0$.

(2) the angles of incidence and reflection are equal. Since the angle θ between two vectors $\mathbf{a}_1$ and $\mathbf{a}_2$ can be obtained from the scalar product $\mathbf{a}_1 \cdot \mathbf{a}_2 = \|\mathbf{a}_1\|\|\mathbf{a}_2\|cos(\theta)$, this condition can be expressed as:

$$(\mathbf{l}_i - \mathbf{q}_{ij}) \cdot (\mathbf{q}_{ij} - \mathbf{c})\|\mathbf{o}_j - \mathbf{q}_{ij}\| = (\mathbf{o}_j - \mathbf{q}_{ij}) \cdot (\mathbf{q}_{ij} - \mathbf{c})\|\mathbf{l}_i - \mathbf{q}_{ij}\|. \tag{11}$$

Next, consider a ray that comes from the unknown pupil center, **p**, and refracts at point $\mathbf{r}_j$ on the corneal surface such that the refracted ray passes through the camera j optical center $\mathbf{o}_j$ and intersects the camera image plane at a point $\mathbf{v}_j$. The condition that the ray coming from the point of refraction $\mathbf{r}_j$, passing through $\mathbf{o}_j$, intersects the camera image plane at point $\mathbf{v}_j$, can be expressed in parametric form as:

$$\mathbf{r}_j = \mathbf{o}_j + k_{r,j}(\mathbf{o}_j - \mathbf{v}_j) \tag{12}$$

for a scaling factor $k_{r,j}$.

The condition that $\mathbf{r}_j$ is on the corneal surface can be written as:

$$\|\mathbf{r}_j - \mathbf{c}\| = R. \tag{13}$$

The law of refraction states two conditions:

(1) the incident ray $(\mathbf{r}_j - \mathbf{p})$, the refracted ray $(\mathbf{r}_j - \mathbf{o}_j)$, and the normal at the point of refraction are coplanar. Since vector $(\mathbf{r}_j - \mathbf{c})$ is normal to the spherical surface at the point of refraction $\mathbf{r}_j$, this condition implies that points $\mathbf{p}$, $\mathbf{r}_j$, $\mathbf{c}$, and $\mathbf{o}_j$ are coplanar, which can be formalized as:

$$(\mathbf{r}_j - \mathbf{o}_j) \times (\mathbf{c} - \mathbf{o}_j) \cdot (\mathbf{p} - \mathbf{o}_j) = 0. \tag{14}$$

(2) the angle of incidence, θ_1, and the angle of refraction, θ_2, satisfy Snell's law ($n_1 sin(\theta_1) = n_2 sin(\theta_2)$, where n_1 and n_2 are the indices of refraction of mediums 1 and 2). Since the sine of the angle θ between two vectors $\mathbf{a}_1$ and $\mathbf{a}_2$ can be obtained from the modulus of the vector product $\|\mathbf{a}_1 \times \mathbf{a}_2\| = \|\mathbf{a}_1\| \|\mathbf{a}_2\| sin(\theta)$, this condition can be expressed as:

$$n_1 \|(\mathbf{r}_j - \mathbf{c}) \times (\mathbf{p} - \mathbf{r}_j)\| \|\mathbf{o}_j - \mathbf{r}_j\| = n_2 \|(\mathbf{r}_j - \mathbf{c}) \times (\mathbf{o}_j - \mathbf{r}_j)\| \|\mathbf{p} - \mathbf{r}_j\|, \tag{15}$$

where n_1 is the effective index of refraction of the aqueous humor and cornea combined and n_2 is the index of refraction of air ($\approx$1).

In this model, the refraction at the aqueous humor-cornea interface is neglected since the difference in their indices of refraction is small relative to that of the cornea-air interface. Only the refraction at the cornea-air interface is taken into account and the aqueous humor and cornea are considered as a homogenous medium.

Finally, considering the distance h between the pupil center and the center of corneal curvature leads to:

$$\|\mathbf{p} - \mathbf{c}\| = h. \tag{16}$$

Since the optic axis of the eye passes through the pupil center $\mathbf{p}$ and the center of corneal curvature $\mathbf{c}$, if the above system of equations is solved for $\mathbf{c}$ and $\mathbf{p}$, the optic axis of the eye in space can be reconstructed as the line defined by these two points [12]. Notice that in order to solve the above system of equations, the eye parameters R, h and n_1 have to be known. These eye parameters are subject-specific and are not easily measured directly. If at least two light sources and at leas two cameras are used, their estimation is not necessary and the LoG can be estimated without any user calibration procedure [33]. Typical values of these eye parameters are: R = 7.8 mm, h = 4.2 mm, and n_1 = 1.3375 [10].

4.2 Proposed Approach

The use of two light sources $i = 1, 2$ (and $j = 1$) allows the solution of the system of Eqs. (8)–(16) if the eye parameters R, h n_1 are known. The center of corneal curvature $\mathbf{c}$ belongs to each plane defined by the camera optical center $\mathbf{o}_j$, light source $\mathbf{l}_i$, and its corresponding image point $\mathbf{u}_{ij}$:

$$(\mathbf{l}_i - \mathbf{o}_j) \times (\mathbf{u}_{ij} - \mathbf{o}_j) \cdot (\mathbf{c} - \mathbf{o}_j) = 0. \tag{17}$$

Since there is only one camera, the subscript that identifies the camera can be dropped for simplicity of notation and the two Eq. (17), for $j = 1, 2$, can be written in matrix form:

$$\begin{bmatrix} [(\mathbf{l}_1 - \mathbf{o}) \times (\mathbf{u}_1 - \mathbf{o})]^T \\ [(\mathbf{l}_2 - \mathbf{o}) \times (\mathbf{u}_2 - \mathbf{o})]^T \end{bmatrix} (\mathbf{c} - \mathbf{o}) = M(\mathbf{c} - \mathbf{o}) = 0. \tag{18}$$

Since Eq. (18) represents the intersection of two planes, it follows that matrix M has, at most, rank 2 [12]. If M has rank 2, the solution to Eq. (18) is given by an equation of the form:

$$(\mathbf{c} - \mathbf{o}) = k_{c,b}\mathbf{b}_{norm} \tag{19}$$

which defines the vector $(\mathbf{c} - \mathbf{o})$ up to a scale factor. In particular, $\mathbf{b}_{norm}$ is a unit vector in the direction of the line of intersection of the planes whose normals are given by $[(\mathbf{l}_1 - \mathbf{o}) \times (\mathbf{u}_1 - \mathbf{o})]$ and $[(\mathbf{l}_2 - \mathbf{o}) \times (\mathbf{u}_2 - \mathbf{o})]$, thus:

$$\mathbf{b}_{norm} = \frac{\mathbf{b}}{\|\mathbf{b}\|} \tag{20}$$

$$\mathbf{b} = [(\mathbf{l}_1 - \mathbf{o}) \times (\mathbf{u}_1 - \mathbf{o})] \times [(\mathbf{l}_2 - \mathbf{o}) \times (\mathbf{u}_2 - \mathbf{o})]. \tag{21}$$

Summarizing, in order to estimate the LoG, the image coordinates of the pupil center $\mathbf{v}$ and the glints $\mathbf{u}_1$, and $\mathbf{u}_2$ are first transformed into world coordinates. Next, the center of corneal curvature, $\mathbf{c}$, is calculated from Eqs. (8), (9), (11), (19), and (21). They are equivalent to 13 scalar equations with 12 scalar unknowns. Knowing $\mathbf{c}$, Eqs. (12) and (13) are used to compute the point of refraction $\mathbf{r}_j = \mathbf{r}$. Knowing $\mathbf{c}$ and $\mathbf{r}$, Eqs. (14), (15), and (16) are used to compute $\mathbf{p}$. Knowing $\mathbf{c}$ and $\mathbf{p}$, the optic axis of the eye in space is reconstructed as the line defined by these two points.

The only two aspects that still need to be clarified are the estimation of the pupil center $\mathbf{v}$ and the glints $\mathbf{u}_1$, and $\mathbf{u}_2$ on each image. For the glints estimation, we use the procedure already described in Sect. 3.2. The pupil center is estimated with sub-pixel accuracy as the center (intersection of the two axes) of the ellipse fitted on the limbus, procedure described in the next Sect. 4.3 (taking inspiration from the idea proposed by Zhu and Yang [24]).

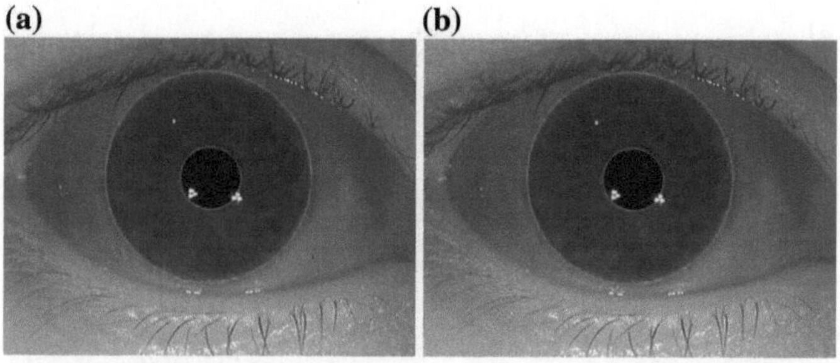

Fig. 12 Segmented iris images from the WVU off-angle iris database. **a** 0° angle; **b** 30° off-angle

4.3 Iris Segmentation

The proposed sclera segmentation algorithm performs well on the WVU non-frontal iris database and highlights the limbus in the image. The iris contour is extracted fitting an ellipse on the edge map empathized using the sclera boundaries (estimated using the previously described algorithm). There are several approaches focused on localization of non-circular iris boundaries [6, 18]. Daugman [6] reportes some advances in accurate iris boundaries localization with active contour, while Li et al. [18] use RANSAC-based algorithm for localizing iris outer boundaries with ellipses. Other approaches consider that, in the cases of non-ideal iris images, which are affected by gaze direction, motion blur, pupil dilation, nonlinear deformations, eyelids and eyelashes occlusions, reflections, etc, iris may appear as noncircular or nonelliptical [28, 29]. Roy et al, for example, to segment the inner boundary from a nonideal iris image, apply a level set based curve evolution approach using the edge stopping function, and to detect the outer boundary, they employ the curve evolution approach using the regularized Mumford-Shah segmentation model with an energy minimization approach [28, 29]. In our case we can take advantages considering only off-angle acquisitions, that means that the ellipses must have long and short axes parallel to vertical and horizontal directions.

The segmentation process results and the extracted iris regions are shown in Fig. 12 (for two examples of acquired images).

The described algorithm for gaze estimation allows to obtain an accurate estimation of the LoG of the acquired eye respect to the camera optical axis. This is a prerequisite information for the next phase of iris-image correction process, as described in detail in the following Section.

5 Iris correction Algorithm

Regarding the image acquisition for the iris correction algorithm, we consider two cases (see Fig. 3): frontal and off-angle acquisition. In the frontal acquisition case the camera optical axis is aligned with the user's optical axis. Iris and pupil boundaries are

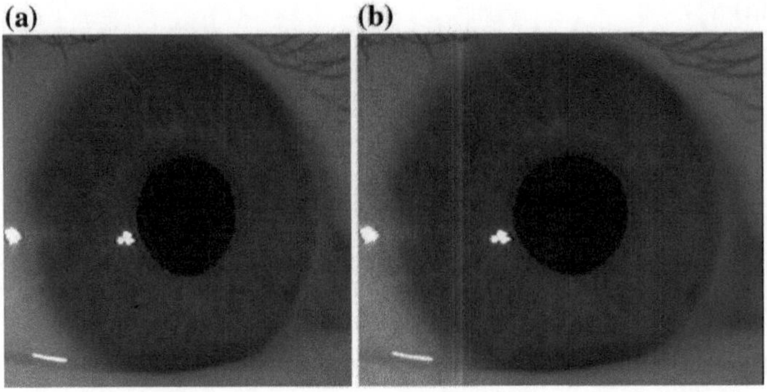

Fig. 13 **a** Example of WVU database image acquired with 30° off-angle. **b** Image obtained after rotation around the vertical axis

well approximated as having circular boundaries. In the off-angle acquisition case, the camera and the eyes are at the same height but the user is looking at a different horizontal direction respect to the camera optical axis. Iris and pupil boundaries could be approximated as ellipses, whose long and short axes are parallel to the vertical and the horizontal directions [19].

Considering the off-angle image, we can make a first correction compensating the distortions associated with the off-angle acquisition. We restore the circular shape of the iris and pupil acting directly on the image by changing the shape of the image content. This method does not consider how the distortions are effectively introduced on the image during its acquisition (see Fig. 13). We can observe a loss of horizontal resolution due to the interpolation of a greater number of pixels. Using a 3D model of the eye and considering the estimated gaze, a more reasonable correction method can be developed.

5.1 3D Eye Model

Taking into account the morphology and the properties that characterize the superficial layers that protect the iris, distortions that are present in the acquired image could be effectively corrected, both for frontal and for off-angle acquisitions. The transparent surface layers, cornea and aqueous humor, have different refractive indices and refract incident light, focusing it on the retina. The way in which a generic ray of light is refracted by an interface between two media depends on the incident angle and the interface properties. As a result of the refraction indexes jumps and of the cornea curvature, the iris in the image appears always distorted. The idea behind the implemented method is to determine and compensate the distortions introduced on the iris image, due to both the off-angle acquisition condition and the refraction generated by cornea and aqueous humor. We use a 3D model of the human eye, more detailed than the one used for gaze estimation, as shown in Fig. 14a. It takes inspiration from the model proposed by Liou et al. [20]:

- cornea is modeled by a meniscus with:
  - anterior radius $r_a = 7.2$ mm;
  - distance between sclera center and anterior corneal center of curvature $d_2 = 5.62$ mm;
  - posterior radius $r_p = 6.8$ mm;
  - distance between sclera center and posterior corneal center of curvature $d_1 = 5.54$ mm;
  - minimum corneal thickness $s_{min} = 0.5$ mm;
  - maximum corneal thickness $s_{max} = 0.65$ mm;
  - refraction index $n_c = 1.376$;
- iris is assumed to be planar and with constant thickness:
  - radius $r_i = 5.75$ mm;
  - distance between sclera center and iris $d_3 = 9.95$ mm;
- aqueous humor is the spherical cap between the iris and posterior part of the cornea. Its refraction index is $n_a = 1.336$;
- sclera, the white part of the eye, has radius $r_s = 11.5$ mm;
- pupil is assumed to be planar with mean radius $r_{pp} = 2.75$ mm.

In agreement with the geometry of the 3D model, a refractive map is created to define refraction index values for each point belonging to cornea and aqueous humor (Fig. 14b).

5.2 Eikonal Equation

The next step is the analysis of the introduced distortions: knowing the camera position and starting from the grid of equally spaced points on the iris image, the points of impact on the iris model are computed. The angle of each ray connecting the camera center and each point of impact on the model, in the absence of discontinuities, is estimated. At this point of the process, we assume that the off-angle is known.

We use the Eikonal equation in order to determine the trajectory of each ray that, starting from each pixel on the camera image plane, passes trough the optical center, is refracted by the cornea and then by aqueous humor before impact on iris. We find that this method is more useful than applying the Snell equation when we work with a trajectory meeting two interfaces: air versus cornea first and cornea versus aqueous humor after. Using the Eikonal equation, we are able to determine the trajectories of the rays that, emitted from a point source, propagate up to the discontinuities that characterize the surface layers of the eyeball, where are refracted, and then impact on the iris or pupil. The Eikonal equation can be written as:

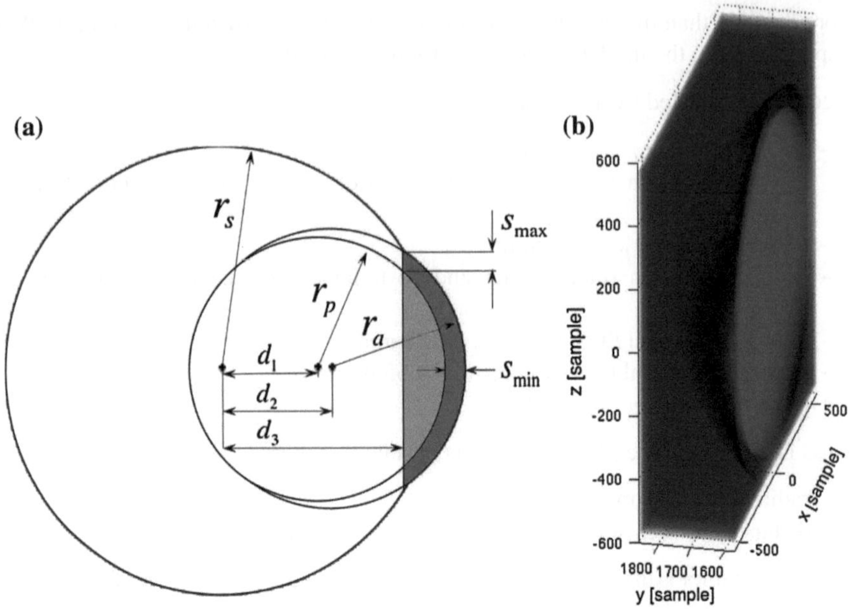

Fig. 14 **a** Geometry of the considered model. **b** Refraction index map

$$\frac{dT}{dl} = s(\mathbf{x}) \tag{22}$$

where $T(\mathbf{x})$ is the phase of the wave, l is the distance along the ray trajectory and $s(\mathbf{x}) = n(\mathbf{x})/c_0$ is the slowness of the medium. We indicate with c_0 the light speed in vacuum and with $n(\mathbf{x})$ the refraction indexes distribution in the model. The Eq. (22) states that, moving along the ray trajectory, the phase derivative varies according to the slowness of the medium at the point considered $\mathbf{x}$. We use the Runge-Kutta method [1] in order to estimate all the trajectories from the camera center to the iris.

5.3 *Interpolation*

Downstream the ray-tracing step, we obtain a new grid of points on the iris, non-linearly distorted due to the refraction introduced by the discontinuities that precede the iris from the outside toward the interior. The iris image is considered as a spatially uniform sampling of the distorted grid obtained with ray-tracing, as shown in Fig. 15 with points (representing the pixels centers) and arrows (representing the distorted grid) for images with 0° and 30° acquisition angles. It can be seen that in the frontal case the grid is compressed towards the pupil center symmetrically, while in the off-angle case the compression is symmetric only respect to the horizontal axis. In

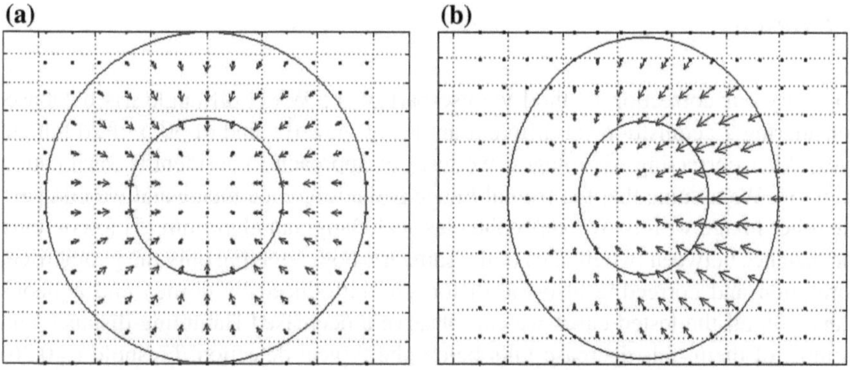

Fig. 15 Original and distorted grids for iris images acquired under **a** 0° angle; **b** 30° off-angle

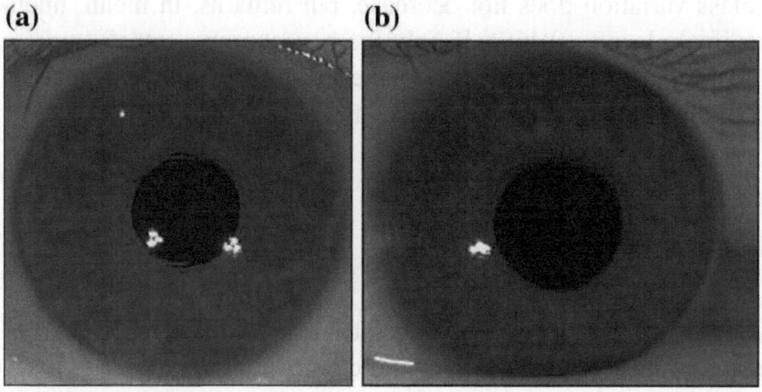

Fig. 16 Corrected iris images from the WVU off-angle iris database. **a** 0° angle; **b** 30° off-angle

both cases the distortion is bigger for points further away from pupil center that, because of cornea radius of curvature, undergoes refraction with a bigger angle. The intensity value of each point of the distorted grid is the corresponding intensity of the pixel originally considered. The intensity values of the corrected image are estimated interpolating the values of the 4 nearest "distorted" pixels on the acquired images:

$$\hat{I}_j = \frac{\sum_{i=1}^{4} \frac{1}{d_{i,j}^2} I_i}{\sum_{i=1}^{4} \frac{1}{d_{i,j}^2}} \tag{23}$$

where $I_i (i = 1, ...4)$ represents the intensity values of the 4 nearest pixels, $\hat{I}_j$ represents the interpolated intensity value on the regular corrected grid, and $d_{i,j}$ is the distance between the points in pixel unit. The corrected image is obtained by interpolating the values at the positions on the camera image plane obtained downstream the ray-tracing (performed independently from the cornea and aqueous humor). Two examples of corrected images are shown in Fig. 16.

5.4 Results

To verify our correction method we use part of the WVU off-angle iris database, considering 2 acquisitions at different angles of view (0° and of 30°) of 20 human eyes. After correcting iris images, we test our approach in an identity verification scenario. We assume that the frontal image is the reference image and we compare the other image with it. We apply the classical Daugman algorithm [5] to compute the distance between two images of the same iris both applying only the geometrical correction and correcting also the distortions introduced by cornea and aqueous humor. In all the tested cases we can observe a decreased Hamming-distance and in most of them, this decrease falls below the typical detection threshold (=0.36) experimentally founded by Daugman for frontal images from the CASIA databases. We obtain a reduction of the mean distance from 0.39075 till 0.3615. At the same time inter-class variation does not decrease, but remains, in mean, unchanged till the third decimal place (=0.460). If only the homographic transform is applied, as illustrated in Fig. 13, a less decrease of the mean intra-class distance is obtained (=0.3802), unable to reduce the false non-matching rate.

6 Conclusions

In this chapter we propose a novel approach to correct off-angle iris images. Starting from the acquired image of a human eye, the portion of the Sclera is first localized. This is useful both to estimate the gaze direction and to accurately localize the limbus. Once the eyeball rotation angle respect to the camera optical axis is estimated and the *limbus* (the boundary between the iris and the sclera) is extracted, we propose a method to correct off-angle iris image. In particular, through the study and modeling of human eye discontinuities, it is possible to introduce a correction method for iris acquired both frontal and off-angle. It can be seen from Fig. 16 how, after the correction process, the circular shape of iris and pupil is obtained also for images acquired with angle of view different from 0°. This correction method, added in a traditional iris recognition system, allows to obtain a reduction of the Hamming distance between templates belonging to the same subject but acquired with different angles of view. This effectively decreases the intra-class variation, fundamental for reducing false non-matching rate and that is shown to increase when working with off-angle iris [19]. At the same time inter-class variation does not decrease, maintaining a low false acceptance rate. The proposed algorithm works in theory for all the possible Line of Gaze, but deeper tests must be conducted to verify its effectiveness in more general acquisition setups.

References

1. Benamou J (1995) Big ray tracing: Multivalued travel time field computation using viscosity solutions of the eikonal equation. J Comput Phys 128(2):463–474
2. Colletto F, Marcon M, Sarti A, Tubaro S (2006) A robust method for the estimation of reliable wide baseline correspondences. Proc Int Conf Image Process 2006:1041–1044
3. Cortes C, Vapnik V (1995) Support-vector networks. Mach Learn 20:273–297
4. Daugman J (2003) The importance of being random: statistical principles of iris recognition. Pattern Recogn 36(2):279–291
5. Daugman J (2004) How iris recognition works. IEEE Trans Circuits Syst Video Technol 14(1):21–30
6. Daugman J (2007) New methods in iris recognition. IEEE Trans Syst Man Cybern Part B Cybern 37(5):1167–1175
7. Dobes M, Machala L (2004) Upol iris image database, link: http://phoenix.inf.upol.cz/iris/
8. Dorairaj V, Schmid N, Fahmy G (2005) Performance evaluation of non-ideal iris based recognition system implementing global ica encoding. In: ICIP 2005. IEEE international conference on image processing. IEEE , 2005, vol 3, pp III 285
9. Fukunaga K (1990) Introduction to statistical pattern recognition, 2nd edn. Wiley, New York
10. Gale A (1982) A note on the remote oculometer technique for recording eye movements. Vision Res 22(1):201–202
11. Gonzalez R, Woods R (1992) Digital image processing. Addison-Wesley Publishing Company, New York
12. Guestrin E, Eizenman M (2006) General theory of remote gaze estimation using the pupil center and corneal reflections. IEEE Trans Biomed Eng 53(6):1124–1133
13. Hansen D, Ji Q (2010) In the eye of the beholder: A survey of models for eyes and gaze. IEEE Trans Pattern Anal Mach Intell 32(3):478–500
14. Hiller F, Lieberman GJ (1995) Introduction to mathematical programming. McGraw-Hill, New York
15. Hu MK (1962) Visual pattern recognition by moment invariants. IRE Trans Inf Theory 8:179–187
16. Krichen E, Mellakh M, Garcia-Salicetti S, Dorizzi B (2004) Iris identification using wavelet packets. In: ICPR 2004. Proceedings of the 17th international conference on pattern recognition, 2004. IEEE, vol 4, pp 335–338
17. Le Grand Y, Hunt R, Walsh J (1957) Light, colour and vision. Chapman & Hall, London
18. Li P, Ma H (2011) Iris recognition in non-ideal imaging conditions. Pattern Recogn Lett 33(8):1012–1018
19. Li X (2005) Modeling intra-class variation for nonideal iris recognition. Advances in biometrics. Springer, Berlin, pp 419–427
20. Liou H, Brennan N (1997) Anatomically accurate, finite model eye for optical modeling. JOSA A 14(8):1684–1695
21. Ma L, Tan T, Wang Y, Zhang D (2003) Personal identification based on iris texture analysis. IEEE Trans Pattern Anal Mach Intell 25(12):1519–1533
22. Masek L et al (2003) Recognition of human iris patterns for biometric identification. Master's thesis, The University of Western Australia
23. Mika S, Ratsch G, Weston J, Scholkopf B, Mullers K (1999) Fisher discriminant analysis with kernels. In: Neural Networks for Signal Processing IX, 1999. Proceedings of the 1999 IEEE Signal Processing Society, Workshop, pp 41–48
24. Morimoto C, Mimica M (2005) Eye gaze tracking techniques for interactive applications. Comput Vis Image Underst 98(1):4–24
25. Park C, Lee J, Oh S, Song Y, Choi D, Park K (2003) Iris feature extraction and matching based on multiscale and directional image representation. In: Scale space methods in computer vision, Springer, pp 576–583.
26. Parker J, Duong A (2009) Gaze tracking: a sclera recognition approach. In: SMC 2009. IEEE international conference on systems, man and cybernetics, 2009. IEEE, pp. 3836–3841

27. Proença H, Alexandre LA (2004) Ubiris iris image database, link: http://iris.di.ubi.pt
28. Roy K, Bhattacharya P (2009) Nonideal iris recognition using level set approach and coalitional game theory. In: Computer vision systems: 7th international conference on computer vision systems, ICVS 2009, Lecture Notes in Computer Science, vol 5815, pp 394–402.
29. Roy K, Bhattacharya P, Suen C (2011) Towards nonideal iris recognition based on level set method, genetic algorithms and adaptive asymmetrical svms. Eng Appl Artif Intell 24(3):458–475
30. Sanchez-Avila C, Sanchez-Reillo R (2005) Two different approaches for iris recognition using gabor filters and multiscale zero-crossing representation. Pattern Recogn 38(2):231–240
31. Santos G, Hoyle E (2011) A fusion approach to unconstrained iris recognition. Pattern Recogn Lett 33(8):984–990
32. Schuckers S, Schmid N, Abhyankar A, Dorairaj V, Boyce C, Hornak L (2007) On techniques for angle compensation in nonideal iris recognition. IEEE Trans Syst Man Cybern Part B Cybern 37(5):1176–1190
33. Shih S, Liu J (2004) A novel approach to 3-d gaze tracking using stereo cameras. IEEE Trans Syst Man Cybern Part B Cybern 34(1):234–245
34. Shih S, Wu Y, Liu J (2000) A calibration-free gaze tracking technique. In: Proceedings of 15th international conference on pattern recognition, 2000. IEEE, vol 4, pp 201–204
35. Sung E, Chen X, Zhu J, Yang J (2002) Towards non-cooperative iris recognition systems. In: ICARCV 2002. 7th international conference on IEEE, vol 2, pp 990–995
36. Takano H, Kobayashi H, Nakamura K (2006) Iris recognition independent of rotation and ambient lighting variations. In: IJCNN'06. International joint conference on neural networks, 2006. IEEE, pp 4056–4062
37. Tan K, Kriegman D, Ahuja N (2002) Appearance-based eye gaze estimation. In: Proceedings of sixth IEEE workshop on applications of computer vision, 2002 (WACV 2002). IEEE, pp 191–195
38. Tan T (2010) Chinese accademy of science institute of automation casia iris database, link: http://biometrics.idealtest.org/
39. Vijaya Kumar B, Xie C, Thornton J (2003) Iris verification using correlation filters. In: Audio- and video-based biometric person authentication. Springer, pp 697–705
40. Villanueva A, Cabeza R (2008) A novel gaze estimation system with one calibration point. IEEE Trans Syst Man Cybern Part B Cybern 38(4):1123–1138
41. Vincent L, Soille P (1991) Watersheds in digital spaces: an efficient algorithm based on immersion simulations. IEEE Trans Pattern Anal Mach Intell 13(6):583–598
42. Wang J, Sung E (2002) Study on eye gaze estimation. IEEE Trans Syst Man Cybern Part B Cybern 32(3):332–350
43. Wang J, Sung E, Venkateswarlu R (2003) Eye gaze estimation from a single image of one eye. In: Proceedings of ninth IEEE international conference on computer vision, 2003. IEEE, pp 136–143
44. Wang J, Sung E, Venkateswarlu R (2005) Estimating the eye gaze from one eye. Comput Vis Image Underst 98(1):83–103
45. Yu L, Zhang D, Wang K (2007) The relative distance of key point based iris recognition. Pattern Recogn 40(2):423–430
46. Zhao Y, Liu J, Li H, Li G (2008) Improved watershed algorithm for dowels image segmentation. In: WCICA 2008. 7th world congress on intelligent control and automation, 2008, p 7644
47. Zhu Z, Ji Q (2007) Novel eye gaze tracking techniques under natural head movement. IEEE Trans Biomed Eng 54(12):2246–2260

Texture Image Segmentation by Weighted Image Gradient Norm Terms Based on Local Histogram and Active Contours

Juan C. Moreno

Abstract New variational image segmentation models for images with texture information are proposed in this chapter. This is accomplished by defining new fitting terms based on the original image, its local histogram information, and the image gradient norm, which are combined in two different ways. The first fitting term is the smoothed product of the image with the corresponding image gradient norm, and the second fitting term is the product of a smoothed version of the image gradient norm and a function depending on the image local histograms. A fast minimization algorithm for the models based on the dual formulation of the total variation (TV) term is proposed and experimented on real images.

Keywords Active contours · Image gradient norm · Texture segmentation

1 Introduction

Texture image segmentation plays an important role in computer vision based tasks such as object recognition and classification. The main idea in image segmentation is to obtain a partition of the input image into a finite number of disjoint homogeneous objects. Nevertheless, it is not always easy to get a good partition in regions with texture information, since it is difficult to differentiate the boundaries between two textures due to the lack of sharp differences between them. Therefore, it is necessary to introduce extra features to the usual segmentation algorithm. Different approaches deal with the extraction of homogeneous features from textures. Many of these texture descriptors go from statistical models to filtering methods, and to

J. C. Moreno (✉)
Department of Mathematics, University of Coimbra, 3001–501 Coimbra, Portugal
e-mail: jmoreno@mat.uc.pt; jmoreno@ubi.pt

IT—Instituto de Telecomunicações Department of Computer Science,
University of Beira Interior, 6201–001 Covilhã, Portugal

P. Di Giamberardino et al. (eds.), *Computational Modeling of Objects Presented in Images*, Lecture Notes in Computational Vision and Biomechanics 15,
DOI: 10.1007/978-3-319-04039-4_13,

geometric approaches [16]. Active contour based solutions for image segmentation have become very popular in image procession literature [3, 14]. One of the most important contributions is due to the Chan and Vese (CV) model for image segmentation trough level set methods [12, 13, 15, 28]. CV segmentation model is based on the Mumford and Shah functional for segmentation [31] an it is an improvement of the classical geodesic active contour model proposed by Caselles et al. [9] whose main idea is based on curve evolution of an edge-detector function. However, the CV model does not consider local region properties and hence can not handle texture images. Then the minimization of CV energy can often be trapped in the local solution leading to wrong segmentation results.

An extension of the CV model to manage images with texture information is proposed by considering the image gradient norm information [18, 19, 29, 30, 34]. To capture texture objects new hybrid input channels for the energy minimization based on weighted versions of the image gradient norm are utilized. The new weighted functions for the proposed input channels make use of the original image, as well as local intensity information in neighbors around image-pixels via local histograms. All these features are combined by means of the product which makes possible to distinguish different texture information from images. Color extension of the studied segmentation models based on the traditional multichannel CV model [13] are also proposed in this chapter.

The performance of the proposed models are compared with some recent different approaches involving extended structure tensor and histograms information via the segmentation of real images carrying different texture segmentation [5, 32, 37]. For the numerical implementation of the proposed segmentation models it is implemented the dual minimization approach of the TV-norm [6, 10]. As an application of the weighted input segmentation models, the segmentation of polyps in wireless capsule endoscopy images is considered [20].

2 Description of the Model

Let Ω be an open and bounded set in $\mathbb{R}^2$, and $I : \overline{\Omega} \longrightarrow [0, L]$ a scalar function, representing the observed grayscale input image. Based on the CV model [12, 15], the minimization problem to consider is

$$\min_{\substack{u\in\{0,1\}\\ \mathbf{c}}} \left\{ G(\mathbf{c}, u) = \int_\Omega |\nabla u| \, \mathrm{d}\mathbf{x} + \sum_{i=1}^{n} \lambda_i^{in} \int_\Omega r_i\big(c_i^{in}, f_i(I)\big) u \, \mathrm{d}\mathbf{x} \right.$$
$$\left. + \sum_{i=1}^{n} \lambda_i^{out} \int_\Omega r_i\big(c_i^{out}, f_i(I)\big)(1-u) \, \mathrm{d}\mathbf{x} \right\}, \tag{1}$$

where for each i, $f_i(I)$ is some feature input channel depending on the image, the vector $\mathbf{c} = (\mathbf{c}^{in}, \mathbf{c}^{out})$ with $\mathbf{c}^{in} = (c_i^{in})$ and $\mathbf{c}^{out} = (c_i^{out})$ are inside and outside unknown averages of $f_i(I)$, respectively. There are also $r_i(c_i^{in}, f_i(I)) = (f_i(I) -$

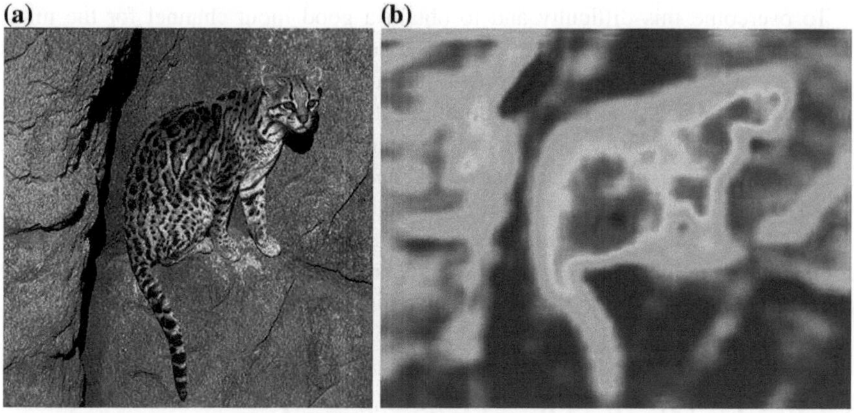

Fig. 1 **a** Image with texture information, **b** input feature $f_1(I)$ computed from (**a**) with $\sigma = 10$, see (2)

$c_i^{in})^2$ and $r_i(c_i^{out}, f_i(I)) = (f_i(I) - c_i^{out})^2$. Vector $\lambda = (\lambda_i^{in}, \lambda_i^{out})$ has constant components that weight fitting terms.

2.1 The Proposed Feature Input Channels

Derivatives are a powerful tool for the extraction of features in images with texture (see e.g. [23]). Given a grayscale texture image displaying two different texture information, it is possible to discriminate between textures using the gradient vector and its norm [19].

Indeed, given a scalar image $I : \Omega \subset \mathbb{R}^2 \to \mathbb{R}$, the new input channel is

$$f_1(I) = (|\nabla I|)_\sigma, \tag{2}$$

where the lower subscript σ in (2) means a smoothed version of the corresponding indexed function. Smoothing is done using a Gaussian function

$$G_\sigma(\mathbf{x}) = (2\pi\sigma)^{-1} e^{-\frac{|\mathbf{x}|^2}{2\sigma}}. \tag{3}$$

This new input channel $f_1(I)$ embodies different texture information. Nevertheless, it is not able to differentiate between similar scale textures in natural images, as can be seen in Fig. 1b. The input *Leopard* image, Fig. 1a, is an example of a natural image containing a texture object. In the image with comparable texture information both inside and outside the object of interest, the corresponding feature channel $f_1(I)$ can not adequately distinguish the object itself, potentially leading to poor segmentation.

To overcome this difficulty and to obtain a good input channel for the minimization approach (1), an image feature data descriptor is proposed using functions ($\Psi : \Omega \to \mathbb{R}$) which contain information about image intensity. This will be combined with channel $|\nabla I|$ using the multiplication operation. The main idea about using Ψ is to help identify the edges between the texture object and the background. In this chapter, two different choices of the function Ψ are proposed.

- The first natural choice is $\Psi_1 = I$ (global information).
- Another choice for Ψ, called Ψ_2, is selected based on local cumulative distribution around a neighborhood of a given pixel, and then computing the total intensity given by the area under the local cumulative distribution curve (local information).

2.2 *Weighted Gradient Based Fitting Terms I*

Given a grayscale image $I : \Omega \to [0, L]$, using the Gaussian function (3) the following smoothed input channel is obtained:

$$f_2(I) = (|\nabla I|\Psi_1)_\sigma = (|\nabla I|I)_\sigma. \tag{4}$$

Then, the new fitting term is

$$\lambda \int_\Omega r_2\big(c_2^{in}, f_2(I)\big)u \, d\mathbf{x} + \lambda \int_\Omega r_2\big(c_2^{out}, f_2(I)\big)(1-u) \, d\mathbf{x}. \tag{5}$$

It should be noticed that $f_2(I)$ involves computing three feature channels for each scale, $I_x I_y$ and $|\nabla I|$, differentiating the proposed model from the Gabor filters [33, 36] for texture image segmentation. Gabor filters have the drawback of inducing a lot of redundancy feature channels. Other texture features involving image gradient were also considered by Brox et al. [7, 35]. They used the structure tensor notion defined by the matrix

$$\begin{pmatrix} I_x^2 & I_x I_y \\ I_y I_x & I_y^2 \end{pmatrix}. \tag{6}$$

2.2.1 Color Extension

The proposed model can be extended to color images using the vector-value CV model extension [13]. For a color image $\mathbf{I} = (I_1, I_2, I_3)$, where I_1, I_2 and I_3 represent red, green and blue input channels, respectively, the new fitting terms are

$$\lambda \sum_{j=1}^{3} \int_\Omega r_{2_j}\big(c_{2_j}^{in}, f_2(I_j)\big) \, u \, d\mathbf{x} + \lambda \sum_{j=1}^{3} \int_\Omega r_{2_j}\big(c_{2_j}^{out}, f_2(I_j)\big) \, (1-u) \, d\mathbf{x}. \tag{7}$$

2.3 Weighted Gradient Based Fitting Terms II

Another weighted gradient based fitting term is proposed herein using local histograms. Local histograms give a complete description of image intensity around each pixel and do not depend on regions [2, 11, 32]. For a given grayscale image $I : \overline{\Omega} \longrightarrow [0, L]$, let $\mathcal{N}_{\mathbf{x},r}$ be the local region centered at a pixel $\mathbf{x}$ with radius r. The local histogram of a pixel $\mathbf{x} \in \Omega$ and its corresponding cumulative distribution function for input channel I are defined, respectively, by

$$P_{\mathbf{x}}(I, \mathsf{y}) = \frac{|\{\mathbf{z} \in \mathcal{N}_{\mathbf{x},r} \cap \Omega \mid I(\mathbf{z}) = \mathsf{y}\}|}{\mathcal{N}_{\mathbf{x},r} \cap \Omega},$$

and

$$F_{\mathbf{x}}(I, \mathsf{y}) = \frac{|\{\mathbf{z} \in \mathcal{N}_{\mathbf{x},r} \cap \Omega \mid I(\mathbf{z}) \leq \mathsf{y}\}|}{\mathcal{N}_{\mathbf{x},r} \cap \Omega},$$

for $0 \leq \mathsf{y} \leq L$. Then, $\Psi_{2,I} : \Omega \rightarrow \mathbb{R}$ is defined

$$\Psi_{2,I}(\mathbf{x}) = \int_0^L F_{\mathbf{x}}(I, \mathsf{y})\, d\mathsf{y}.$$

With $\Psi_{2,I}(\mathbf{x})$ the total intensity weight within the neighborhood $\mathcal{N}_{\mathbf{x},r}$ of $\mathbf{x}$ is obtained, in contrast with $\Psi_1(\mathbf{x}) = I(\mathbf{x})$, which only gives the intensity value in $\mathbf{x}$. Together with the image gradient norm, the following input channel is considered:

$$f_3(I)(\mathbf{x}) = \Psi_{2,I}(\mathbf{x}) f_1(I)(\mathbf{x}) = \Psi_{2,I}(\mathbf{x}) |\nabla I(\mathbf{x})|_\sigma, \tag{8}$$

with an associated fitting term

$$\lambda \int_\Omega r_3(c_3^{in}, f_3(I))\, u\, d\mathbf{x} + \lambda \int_\Omega r_3(c_3^{out}, f_3(I))\, (1 - u)\, d\mathbf{x}.$$

The notion of local histogram for texture image segmentation has also been taken into account by Ni et al. [22, 32]. The current approach differs from previous work mainly because it does not use the Wasserstein distance in segmentation formulation.

Usually, two different types of texture images are found in natural images. The first are small scale textures corresponding to a lot of oscillations inside the main object, and the second consists of different flat regions given by large scale textures within the object of interest in the given image. Figure 2 shows two real images with different texture information. Figure 2a, shows *Cheetah* and *Tiger* images, together with their corresponding pixel-valued image (scaled grayscale values) in Fig. 2b, and the computed local cumulative distribution function of the inner region of the main object to be segmented, Fig. 2c, with $r = 10$. As shown, the local cumulative distribution function for the *Cheetah* has an almost convex shape over all the domain, whereas the *Tiger* image has a local cumulative distribution function which oscillates

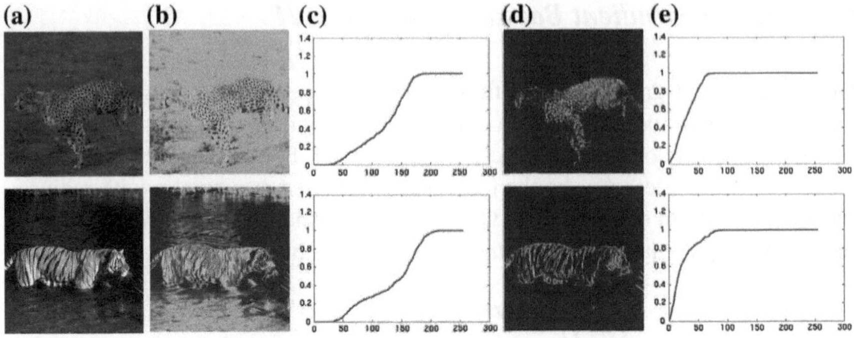

Fig. 2 Local cumulative distribution functions of two images with different texture information. **a** Input images. **b** The scaled pixel-values of the input images showing the nature of texture present. **c** Corresponding local cumulative distribution functions inside the region of interest using $r = 10$. **d** The scaled pixel-values of the gradient image. **e** Corresponding local cumulative distribution functions inside the region of interest in (**d**) using $r = 10$

between convex and concave shapes. This is because the $Tiger$ has a lot of different flat regions inside the body which can be considered as large scale textures. Then, the image gradient norm is used in the computation of local histograms in order to apply the weighted gradient fitting term approach. Figure 2d shows how the image gradient norm recovers oscillations patterns inside the $Tiger$ image. Furthermore, Fig. 2e shows that local cumulative distribution functions corresponding to the image gradient norm have an almost single convex shape over the whole domain.

2.3.1 Some Extensions

Extensions for the input channel (8) are listed below.

• The local histogram computation can also be applied to the image gradient norm instead of the original input image I. That is, $\Psi_{2,|\nabla I|}(\mathbf{x}) = \int_0^L F_{\mathbf{x}}(|\nabla I|, \mathrm{y})\,\mathrm{dy}$ is considered together with the input channel

$$f_4(I)(\mathbf{x}) = \Psi_{2,|\nabla I|}(\mathbf{x}) f_1(I)(\mathbf{x}) = \Psi_{2,|\nabla I|}(\mathbf{x}) |\nabla I(\mathbf{x})|_\sigma, \tag{9}$$

and the corresponding fitting term is

$$\lambda \int_\Omega r_4\big(c_4^{in}, f_4(I)\big)\, u \,\mathrm{d}\mathbf{x} + \lambda \int_\Omega r_4\big(c_4^{out}, f_4(I)\big)\,(1-u)\,\mathrm{d}\mathbf{x}.$$

• By combining (8) and (9), another extension is defined with the data term

$$\lambda \int_{\Omega} \left(r_3\left(c_3^{in}, f_3(I)\right) + r_4(c_4^{in}, f_4(I)) \right) u \, \mathbf{dx} \\ + (1-\lambda) \int_{\Omega} \left(r_3\left(c_3^{out}, f_3(I)\right) + r_4(c_4^{out}, f_4(I)) \right) (1-u) \, \mathbf{dx}, \tag{10}$$

where $0 \leq \lambda \leq 1$.

• The previous extension can be applied to color images using RGB decomposition. For a texture color image $\mathbf{I} = (I_1, I_2, I_3)$, where I_1, I_2 and I_3 represent red, green and blue input channels, respectively, the new fitting terms are

$$\lambda \sum_{j=1}^{3} \int_{\Omega} \left(r_{3_j}\left(c_{3_j}^{in}, f_3(I_j)\right) + r_{4_j}\left(c_{4_j}^{in}, f_4(I_j)\right) \right) u \, \mathbf{dx} \\ + (1-\lambda) \sum_{j=1}^{3} \int_{\Omega} \left(r_{3_j}\left(c_{3_j}^{out}, f_3(I_j)\right) + r_{4_j}\left(c_{4_j}^{out}, f_4(I_j)\right) \right) (1-u) \, \mathbf{dx}, \tag{11}$$

where $r_{i_j}\left(c_{i_j}^{in}, f_i(I_j)\right) = \left(f_i(I) - c_{i_j}^{in}\right)^2$ and $r_{i_j}\left(c_{i_j}^{out}, f_i(I_j)\right) = \left(f_i(I) - c_{i_j}^{out}\right)^2$.

3 Numerical Solution for the Proposed Model

A two-step methodology is implemented for solving the proposed texture segmentation approach (1). In the first step, u is fixed and the minimization with respect to $\mathbf{c}$ is computed. Then, $\mathbf{c}$ is fixed and the minimization with respect to u is performed. Although the functional $G(\mathbf{c}, \cdot)$ is convex in u, the minimization is carried out over a binary set. Following the same approach as in Chan et al. [12], it is proposed to use soft smooth membership function $u \in [0, 1]$. The new convex minimization problem is

$$\min_{u \in [0,1]} G(\mathbf{c}, u), \tag{12}$$

for which it is guaranteed the existence of a global minimizer. Moreover, if u is a minimizer of the convex relaxed problem (12), then for *a.e.* $s \in [0, 1]$, the function $\hat{u} = \mathbb{1}_{\{\mathbf{x} \in \Omega : u(\mathbf{x}) > s\}}$ is a minimizer of the original binary problem (1). The minimization of (12) can be efficiently solved using the dual minimization approach of the TV term [6, 10].

3.1 Fast Dual Minimization

A fast numerical algorithm applying the methods in Aujol et al. [4] and Bresson et al. [6] is implemented for solving the minimization problem (12). First, it should be noted that solving the minimization problem (12) is equivalent to solve

$$\min_{u \in [0,1]} \left\{ \tilde{G}(\mathbf{c}, u) = \int_\Omega |\nabla u| \, d\mathbf{x} + \sum_{i=1}^{n} \int_\Omega \left(\lambda_i^{in} r_i(c_i^{in}, f_i(I)) - \lambda_i^{out} r_i(c_i^{out}, f_i(I)) \right) u \, d\mathbf{x} \right\}.$$

In order to solve an unconstrained minimization problem, the convex constrained minimization problem is replaced with the following unconstrained minimization problem

$$\min_u \left\{ \tilde{G}(\mathbf{c}, u) + \alpha \int_\Omega \nu(u) \, d\mathbf{x} \right\}, \tag{13}$$

where

$$\alpha > \frac{1}{2} \| \sum_{i=1}^{n} \left(\lambda_i^{in} r_i(c_i^{in}, f_i(I)) - \lambda_i^{out} r_i(c_i^{out}, f_i(I)) \right) \|_{L^\infty(\Omega)}$$

and

$$\nu(\xi) := \max\{0, 2|\xi - \frac{1}{2}| - 1\}.$$

The solution of (13) is addressed by decoupling the TV term and the fitting terms. A new variable v is introduced to replace u in the fitting term. The term $\frac{1}{2\theta}\|u - v\|^2_{L^2(\Omega)}$ should also be added to the formulation so that v is forced to be close enough to u. Then, the minimization problem is

$$\begin{aligned} \min_{u,v} \Bigg\{ \tilde{G}_{decoupled}(u, v) = & \int_\Omega |\nabla u| \, d\mathbf{x} + \frac{1}{2\theta} \|u - v\|^2_{L^2(\Omega)} \\ & + \sum_{i=1}^{n} \int_\Omega \Big(\lambda_i^{in} r_i(c_i^{in}, f_i(I)) \\ & - \lambda_i^{out} r_i(c_i^{out}, f_i(I)) v + \alpha \nu(v) \Big) d\mathbf{x} \Bigg\}, \end{aligned} \tag{14}$$

where θ is chosen to be small.

The solution of the minimization problem (14) is given by the following coupled problems:

1. Fixing v, the minimization problem in u is:

$$\min_u \left\{ \int_\Omega |\nabla u| \, d\mathbf{x} + \frac{1}{2\theta} \|u - v\|^2_{L^2(\Omega)} \right\}. \tag{15}$$

The solution of (15) is given by $u = v - \theta \operatorname{div} \mathbf{p}$ where $\mathbf{p} = (p_1, p_2)$ satisfies $\nabla(\theta \operatorname{div} \mathbf{p} - v) - |\nabla(\theta \operatorname{div} \mathbf{p} - v)| p = 0$, which is solved using a fixed point method: $\mathbf{p}^0 = 0$ and

$$\mathbf{p}^{n+1} = \frac{\mathbf{p}^n + \delta t \nabla(\theta \operatorname{div}(\mathbf{p}^n) - v/\theta)}{1 + \delta t |\nabla(\theta \operatorname{div}(\mathbf{p}^n) - v/\theta)|}.$$

2. Fixing u, the minimization problem in v is:

$$\min_v \left\{ \frac{1}{2\theta} \|u - v\|^2_{L^2(\Omega)} + \sum_{i=1}^{n} \int_\Omega \Big(\lambda_i^{in} r_i\big(c_i^{in}, f_i(I)\big) - \lambda_i^{out} r_i\big(c_i^{out}, f_i(I)\big)\, v + \alpha \nu(v) \Big) \mathbf{dx} \right\}, \tag{16}$$

and the solution is found as

$$v = \min\left\{ \max\left\{ u - \theta \sum_{i=1}^{n} \Big(\lambda_i^{in} r_i\big(c_i^{in}, f_i(I)\big) - \lambda_i^{out} r_i\big(c_i^{out}, f_i(I)\big) \Big), 0 \right\}, 1 \right\}.$$

It is important to note that in the fast dual approach the constants c_i^{in} and c_i^{out} are updated every few iterations of the algorithm above using the equations

$$c_i^{in} = \frac{\int_\Omega f_i(I) u \, \mathbf{dx}}{\int_\Omega u \, \mathbf{dx}} \quad \text{and} \quad c_i^{out} = \frac{\int_\Omega f_i(I)(1-u) \, \mathbf{dx}}{\int_\Omega (1-u) \, \mathbf{dx}}.$$

4 Related Models for Comparison

The proposed model with previously described input channels for texture image segmentation can be compared with other very well-known models. This section, briefly describes texture segmentation approximations implemented by Wang et al. [37], Ni et al. [32] and Bao et al. [5], which will be compared with the current gradient based fitting terms I and II, respectively. Following the arguments from the previous section, the minimization of the extended structure tensor model and the local histogram segmentation (using the Wassertein distance) can be solved using a two-step methodology, where u is allowed to take values in [0, 1]. At the first step, u is fixed, and the corresponding constant and local histograms according to the considered model are computed. Then in the second step, the solution of $u \in [0, 1]$ is computed.

4.1 The Extended Structure Tensor on Local Windows

In Wang et al. [37], the authors have introduced an efficient CV model for texture image segmentation by adding local terms to the original CV formulation [15]. In the main framework of Nikolova et al. [12], the problem is

$$
\min_{\substack{u\in\{0,1\}\\(\mathbf{c},\mathbf{d})}} \Big\{ E_1(\mathbf{c},\mathbf{d},u) := \int_\Omega |\nabla u|\, \mathrm{d}\mathbf{x}
+ \int_\Omega \left(\lambda_{in}|I_{input} - c_{in}|^2 + \overline{\lambda}_{in}|g_k * I_{input} - I_{input} - d_{in}|\right) u\, \mathrm{d}\mathbf{x}
+ \int_\Omega \left(\lambda_{out}|I_{input} - c_{out}|^2 + \overline{\lambda}_{out}|g_k * I_{input} - I_{input} - d_{out}|\right) (1-u)\, \mathrm{d}\mathbf{x} \Big\}, \tag{17}
$$

where g_k is an averaging convolution operator with $k \times k$ size window, and $\mathbf{c} := (c_{in}, c_{out})$ and $\mathbf{d} := (d_{in}, d_{out})$ are unknown averages of I_{input} and $g_k * I_{input} - I_{input}$, inside and outside the unknown segmentation curve, respectively. Constants λ_{in}, λ_{out}, $\overline{\lambda}_{in}$, $\overline{\lambda}_{out}$ are non-negative fixed parameters weighting fitting terms. For the extended structure tensor approximation, equations involving the computation of vectors $\mathbf{c}$ and $\mathbf{d}$ are:

$$
c_{in}(u) = \frac{\int_\Omega I_{input}\, u\, \mathrm{d}\mathbf{x}}{\int_\Omega u\, \mathrm{d}\mathbf{x}}, \qquad c_{out}(u) = \frac{\int_\Omega I_{input}\ (1-u)\ \mathrm{d}\mathbf{x}}{\int_\Omega (1-u)\ \mathrm{d}\mathbf{x}}
$$

$$
d_{in}(u) = \frac{\int_\Omega (g_k * I_{input} - I_{input})\, u\, \mathrm{d}\mathbf{x}}{\int_\Omega u\, \mathrm{d}\mathbf{x}}, \quad d_{out}(u) = \frac{\int_\Omega (g_k * I_{input} - I_{input})\ (1-u)\ \mathrm{d}\mathbf{x}}{\int_\Omega (1-u)\ \mathrm{d}\mathbf{x}}.
$$

Then, it follows the minimization with respect to u by keeping the vectors $\mathbf{c}$ and $\mathbf{d}$ fixed. The local information for the minimization problem (17) is given by the input channel $g_k * I_{input} - I_{input}$, where it is expected that for pixels with higher values the model will keep a higher intensity inside the local window g_k, making the intensity region different from the rest of the image.

For segmentation of images with texture information in Wang et al. [37], the texture representation is completely described using a smoothed version of the extended structure tensor. It is an extension of the classical structure tensor (6). Given a scalar image I, the extended structure tensor is defined by the matrix

$$
\begin{pmatrix} G_\sigma * I_x^2 & G_\sigma * I_x I_y & G_\sigma * I_x I \\ G_\sigma * I_y I_x & G_\sigma * I_y^2 & G_\sigma * I_y I \\ G_\sigma * I I_x & G_\sigma * I I_y & G_\sigma * I^2 \end{pmatrix}.
$$

For the minimization model described in (17), the new input channel for the algorithm is

$$
I_{input} = \frac{1}{9} G_\sigma * \left(I_x^2 + I_x I_y + I_x I + I_y I_x + I_y^2 + I_y I + I I_x + I I_y + I^2\right).
$$

As noticed by the authors Wang et al. [37], their model can be extended to color images using the CV model for vector-valued images [13]. Under a RGB image decomposition, the extended structure tensor is computed in each color component.

4.2 Local Histograms with the Wassertein Distance

A region-based active contour model for texture image segmentation with local histograms has been proposed by Ni et al. (see [32]). It is an improvement of their previous model developed in Chan et al. [11]. The new texture image approximation uses the local histogram notion to differentiate between the object texture and the background. In their new approach, the problem is

$$\min_{\substack{u\in\{0,1\}\\(P_1,P_2)}} \left\{ E_2(P_1, P_2, u) := \int_\Omega |\nabla u|\,d\mathbf{x} + \lambda \int_\Omega W_1(P_1, P_\mathbf{x}) u\,d\mathbf{x} + \lambda \int_\Omega W_1(P_2, P_\mathbf{x})(1-u)\,d\mathbf{x} \right\}.$$

where P_1 and P_2 are constant histograms approximating local histograms inside and outside some optimal region, respectively. The parameter λ is a constant weighting the fitting term. W_1 is the Wasserstein distance with exponent 1. Given two histograms P and Q and their corresponding cumulative distribution functions F_P and F_Q, the Wasserstein distance between P and Q is defined as

$$W_1(P, Q) = \int_0^L \left|F_P(\mathrm{y}) - F_Q(\mathrm{y})\right| \mathrm{dy}.$$

Minimization with respect to F_1 and F_2 gives

$$\int_\Omega u \frac{F_1(\mathrm{y}) - F_\mathbf{x}(\mathrm{y})}{|F_1(\mathrm{y}) - F_\mathbf{x}(\mathrm{y})|} d\mathbf{x} = 0 \quad \text{and} \quad \int_\Omega (1-u) \frac{F_2(\mathrm{y}) - F_\mathbf{x}(\mathrm{y})}{|F_2(\mathrm{y}) - F_\mathbf{x}(\mathrm{y})|} d\mathbf{x} = 0, \tag{18}$$

respectively, for every $y \in [0, L]$, where the solutions to the equations in (18) are

$$F_1(\mathrm{y}) = \text{weighted (by } u\text{) median of} F_\mathbf{x}(\mathrm{y})$$

$$F_2(\mathrm{y}) = \text{weighted (by } 1-u\text{)median of } F_\mathbf{x}(\mathrm{y}),$$

respectively. Then, fixing P_1 and P_2 leads a convex minimization problem with respect to u.

4.3 Variational Color Image Segmentation via Chromaticity-Brightness (CB) Decomposition

A variational model for color image segmentation which extends the local histograms model previous discussed were proposed by Bao et al. [5]. Considering that the essential geometrical information is contained in the gray level of color images, color and textures information are treated separately in their segmentation model [8, 25]. Utilizing the chromoticity–brightness (CB) decomposition of a color image and the vectorial CV model [13], the problem to solve is

$$\min_{\substack{u\in\{0,1\}\\(P_1,P_2)\\(\mu_1,\mu_2,\mu_3)}} \left\{ E_3(P_1,P_2,u) := \int_\Omega |\nabla u|\,\mathbf{dx} + \int_\Omega R_{in} u\,\mathbf{dx} + \int_\Omega R_{out}(1-u)\,\mathbf{dx} \right.$$
$$\left. \gamma \sum_{j=1}^{3} \left((|\mu_{j,in}|-1)^2 + (|\mu_{j,out}|-1)^2 \right) \right\}, \tag{19}$$

where

$$R_{in} = \lambda_B W_1(P_{in}, P_{\mathbf{x}}) + \lambda_C \sum_{j=1}^{3} (C_j - \mu_{j,in})^2,\; R_{out} = \lambda_B W_1(P_{out}, P_{\mathbf{x}})$$
$$+ \lambda_C \sum_{j=1}^{3} (C_j - \mu_{j,out})^2.$$

The local histograms computations are done over the brightness component of a color image, while the images C_i correspond to the components of the color space define by the chromaticity. Given an RGB image $I = (I_1, I_2, I_3)$, the brightness and chromaticity components are defined by $|I|$ and $I/|I|$ respectively. Minimization with respect differents μ_i gives:

$$\mu^{n+1}_{j,in}(u) = \frac{\gamma \frac{\mu^n_{j,in}}{|\mu^n_{j,in}|} + \lambda_C \int_\Omega C_j\, u\,\mathbf{dx}}{\gamma + \lambda_C \int_\Omega u\,\mathbf{dx}},\quad \mu^{n+1}_{j,out}(u) = \frac{\gamma \frac{\mu^n_{j,out}}{|\mu^n_{j,out}|} + \lambda_C \int_\Omega C_j\,(1-u)\,\mathbf{dx}}{\gamma + \lambda_C \int_\Omega (1-u)\,\mathbf{dx}}.$$

5 Numerical Experiments

The proposed texture segmentation models with weighted gradient fitting terms are implemented in MATLAB 7 R2009a, on a laptop with Intel Core2 Duo, with 2.20 GHz. In all experiments, 80 iterations in points 1. and 2. of the fast dual minimization algorithm have been implemented. The parameters $\delta t = 1/8$ and the smoothing parameter of Gaussian kernel $\sigma = 10$ are fixed.

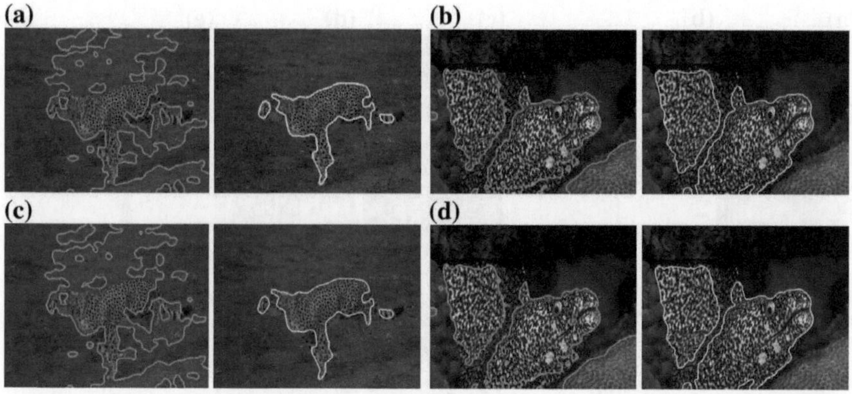

Fig. 3 Comparison of segmentation results for different texture images. *First row* In each subfigure segmentation results of (*left*) Wang et al. [37] and (*right*) propose approach with (4) ($f_2(I) = (|\nabla I|I)_\sigma$) are shown. *Second row* Color extension of Wang et al. [37] (with *green* contour) and the proposed model (*yellow* contour) using the RGB image decomposition

5.1 Segmentation Results for the Weighted Gradient Based Fitting Terms I

For the weighted gradient based fitting terms by means of the original image (see Sect. 2.2), the final segmentation results take about 3 s to be computed for a 321×481 texture image. The parameter θ is equal to 1, and the value of the parameter λ is equal to 0.1.

Figure 3 shows segmentation results for different grayscale and color real images implementing the proposed model. The weighted fitting term using the original image improve the extended structure tensor segmentation results [37]. As can be seen, the new input term leads to good texture segmentation. It can be visualized under the yellow contour that the proposed model is able to identify the main object in the different images while the extended structure tensor model (green contour) can not distinguishes between two different texture regions.

5.2 Segmentation Results for the Weighted Gradient Based Fitting Terms II

The segmentation model combining the image gradient norm and local histogram information is now implemented. For all reported experiments, values $r = 10$ and $\theta = 1$ are fixed. The parameter λ is specified in each experiment. In this approach, final segmentation results take about 3 min to be computed for a 321×321 texture image.

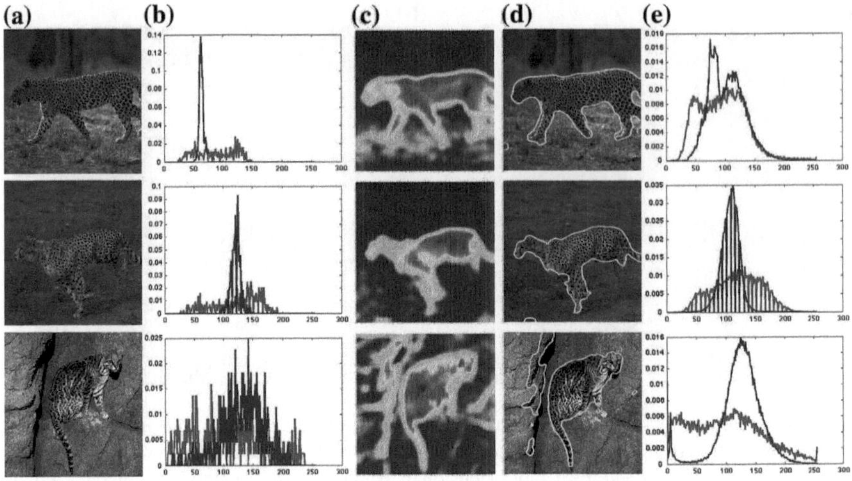

Fig. 4 Segmentation results for real grayscale images using the input channel (8). **a** Input images. **b** Neighborhood histograms where *red* and *blue* histograms correspond to the the foreground (*inside*) and background (*outside*) information of the image, respectively, using $r = 10$. **c** Weighted gradient based term $f_4(I)(\mathbf{x}) = \Psi_{2,I}(\mathbf{x})|\nabla I(\mathbf{x})|_\sigma$ input channels, where higher values are indicated in *red* and lower in *blue*. **d** Segmentation results with 80 iterations and $\lambda = 0.1$. **e** Histograms after segmentations

Figure 4 shows segmentation results for different real grayscale images using the input channel (8). The original grayscale images are displayed in the first column, Fig. 4a. The second column, Fig. 4b, shows image histograms, where red and blue histograms correspond to foreground (inside) and background (outside), respectively, using $r = 10$. Third, fourth, and fifth columns, Fig. 4c, d and e, represent input channels given by $f_4(I)(\mathbf{x}) = \Psi_{2,I}(\mathbf{x})|\nabla I(\mathbf{x})|_\sigma$, the segmentation results and the corresponding histograms after segmentations, respectively. Comparing neighborhood histograms before and after segmentation, shows that a smoother histogram separation is obtained and that the weighted gradient based input image provides a good segmentation.

Figure 5 shows similar segmentation results for the extension given in Eq. (9). The neighborhood histograms of the gradient norm image (without smoothing) is given in Fig. 5b, and input channels $f_5(I)(\mathbf{x}) = \Psi_{2,|\nabla I|}(\mathbf{x})|\nabla I(\mathbf{x})|_\sigma$ are given in Fig. 5c. The corresponding segmentation results in Fig. 5d and e show histograms after segmentation. As can be seen, the proposed extension gives good segmentation overall.

The approach combining the original image, the image gradient norm and the local histograms information as described in (10) (with $\lambda = 0.5$), and the local histogram based model from Ni et al. [32] are compared. Segmentation results given in Fig. 6 show the advantage of using balanced weighted information based on local histograms with smoothed gradients. First row shows segmentation results for the *Cheetah* image in Fig. 6a. A better segmentation is given using the proposed

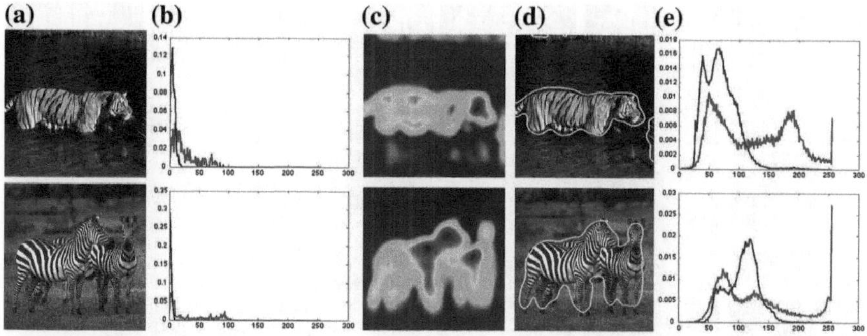

Fig. 5 Segmentation results for real grayscale images using (9). **a** Input images. **b** Neighborhood histograms where *red* and *blue* histograms correspond to the foreground (*inside*) and background (*outside*) information of the image gradient norm, respectively, using $r = 10$. **c** Weighted gradient based term $f_5(I)(\mathbf{x}) = \Psi_{2,|\nabla I|}(\mathbf{x})|\nabla I(\mathbf{x})|_\sigma$ input channels, where higher values are indicated by *red* and lower by *blue*. **d** Segmentation results with 80 iterations and $\lambda = 0.1$. **e** Histograms after segmentations

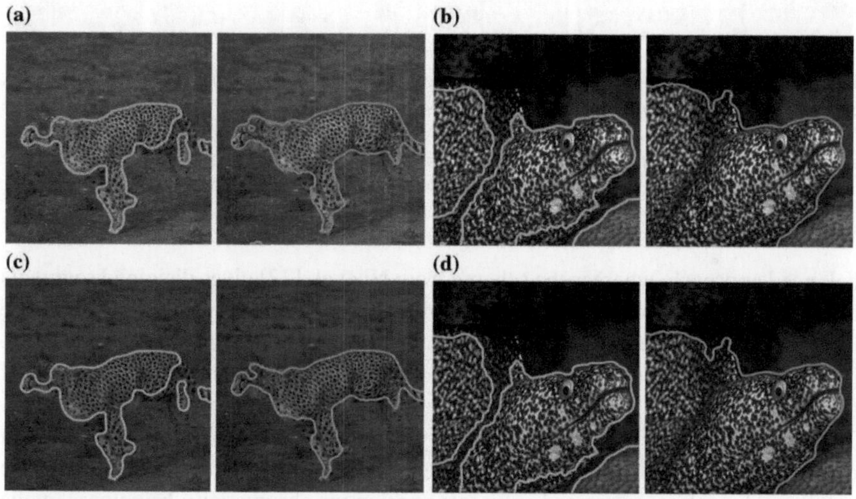

Fig. 6 Comparison of segmentation results for different texture images. *First row* In each sub-figure segmentation results of (*left*) Ni et al. [32] and (*right*) proposed approach with (10) are shown. *Second row* In each sub-figure segmentation results of (*left*) Bao et al. [5] and (*right*) proposed *color* approach with (11) are shown

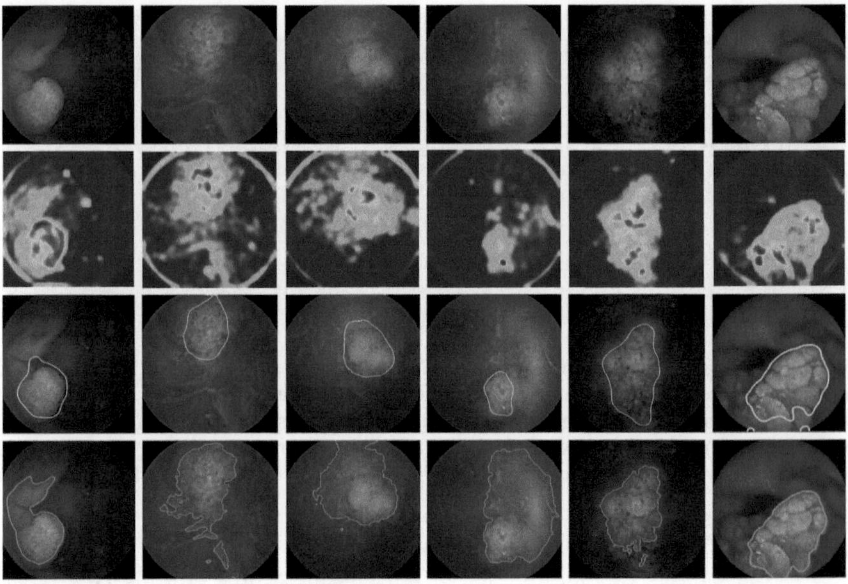

Fig. 7 Segmentation results for wireless capsule endoscopic images. *First row* Original images. *Second row* Input channels computed with Eq. (4) ($f_2(I) = (|\nabla I|I)_\sigma$), where higher values are indicated in *red* and lower in *blue*. *Third row* Segmentation result with 200 iterations, $\theta = 0.1$ and $\lambda = 0.000001$. *Fourth row* Segmentation result using Wang et al. approach (extended structure tensor) [37]

balanced approach, whereas the scheme from Ni et al. [32] gives disjoined segments of the *Cheetah*'s body, see for example the tail part. Similarly, in the *Fish* image in Fig. 6b, a single unified segment is obtained, whereas the model from Ni et al. [32] gives spurious segments at the left hand side of the image. Color extension of the proposed model through the fitting term (11) are displayed in Fig. 6c and d. The proposed color model represented by yellow contour shows better segmentation result compared with the model proposed by Bao et al. [5] where authors have combined local histograms and color information via chromaticity-brightness image decomposition.

5.3 Wireless Capsule Endoscopy Images

The segmentation of colonic polyps from wireless capsule endoscopic images are considered, as an application of the proposed segmentation algorithms. Wireless capsule endoscopy (WCE) is a new modality in gastroenterology, which acquires digital photographs of the intestine tract using a swallowable miniature divide LED flash lights (see [1, 17, 21, 24, 26, 27]). The captured images are then analyzed by medical doctors, who should detect abnormal features or lesions usually named polyps, in order to carry out diagnostic assessments. One major problem with this new WCE technology is that it generates a huge number of images per exam. Therefore, it is very relevant to design a computerized and also fast method for the inspection of WCE images. Wireless capsule images consist of two major regions. One is the lumen, the intermediate region where the capsule moves. The other part is the mucosa, which is a mucus-secreting membrane lining the lumen cavities. Abnormal tissues and lesions, like ulcers and polyps, are usually seen as exterior parts of the mucosa, and the lumen is filled with intestinal juices of the human digestive system. Polyps seems to have texture information represented by large scale textures given by big flat regions. Utilizing the texture information on polyps regions the variational segmentation model with input channel defined by the smoothed product of the image with its gradient magnitude ($f_2(I) = (|\nabla I|I)_\sigma$) is used for detecting polyps in WCE.

First row displays different wireless capsule endoscopic images with polyps (Fig. 7). All the images show texture information as well as planar regions. In the second row, the weighted gradient of the grayscale WCE images are shown. The different polyp regions are highlighted from the rest of the mucosa region. The segmentation results presented in the third row indicates the proposed approach singles out the polyp successfully against a turbid liquid background, in contrast to the segmentations trough the extended structure tensor on local windows algorithm [37] and local histograms with Wassertein distance approach [32] as it can be noticed in fourth and fifth rows.

6 Conclusions

In this work, new variational texture image segmentation models based on the CV segmentation approach have been proposed using input channels defined weighting the image gradient norm with global and local information. The proposed models take advantage of discontinuity points lying in different regions by means of the image gradient norm over gray scale images. The global information is defined with original intensity image values, and local information is provided using local histogram information around each pixel allowing to extract the most important features related to texture data embedded in a image. Color extension of the proposed models have been also implemented in this chapter. Experiments on real images implementing the dual minimization of the TV term have demonstrated the desired segmentation performance of the proposed models. Comparison with some previous well-known segmentation algorithms also demonstrate that the current texture segmentation approaches show better results. In addition, theoretical issues related to the existence of solutions to the main minimization approaches have been established.

Acknowledgments This work was partially supported by the research project UTAustin/MAT/0009/2008 of the UT Austin | Portugal Program (http://www.utaustinportugal.org/) and by CMUC and FCT (Portugal), through European program COMPETE/FEDER. The author was supported by FCT

(Portugal) under the PhD grant SFRH/BD/33370/2008. Special thanks to Dr. Pedro Figueiredo (Department of Gastroenterology, University Hospital of Coimbra, Portugal) for providing the medical images.

References

1. Adler DG, Gostout CJ (2003) Wireless capsule endoscopy. Hosp Physician 2003:14–22
2. Aubert G, Barlaud M, Faugeras O, Jehan-Besson S (2003) Image segmentation using active contours: calculus of variations or shape gradients? SIAM J Appl Math 63(6):2128–2154
3. Aubert G, Kornprobst P (2006) Mathematical problems in image processing: partial differential equation and calculus of variations. Springer, New York
4. Aujol J-F, Gilboa G, Chan T, Osher S (2006) Structure-texture image decomposition—modeling, algorithms and parameter selection. Int J Comput Vis 67(1):111–136
5. Bao Z, Liu Y, Peng Y, Zhang G (2010) Variational color image segmentation via chromaticity-brightness decomposition. In: Advances in multimedia modeling (MMM), Chongqing. Lectures notes in computer science, vol 5916. Springer, pp 295–302
6. Bresson X, Esedoglu S, Vandergheynst P, Thiran J, Osher S (2007) Fast global minimization of the active contour/snake model. J Math Imaging Vis 28(2):151–167
7. Brox T, Rousson M, Deriche R, Weickert J (2003) Unsupervised segmentation incorporating color, texture and motion. In: Computer analysis of images and patterns (CAIP), Groningen. Lectures notes in computer science, vol 2756. Springer, pp 353–360
8. Caselles V, Coll B, Morel J-M (2002) Geometry and color in natural images. J Math Imaging Vis 16(2):89–105
9. Caselles V, Kimmel R, Sapiro G (1997) Geodesic active contours. Int J Comput Vis 22(1):61–79
10. Chambolle A (2004) An algorithm for total variation minimization and applications. J Math Imaging Vis 20(1–2):89–97
11. Chan TF, Esedoglu S, Ni K (2007) Histogram based segmentation using wasserstein distances. In: First international conference on scale space methods and variational methods in computer vision (SSVM), Ischia. Lectures notes in computer science, vol 4485. Springer, pp 697–708
12. Chan TF, Esedoglu S, Nikolova M (2006) Algorithms for finding global minimizers of image segmentation and denoising models. SIAM J Appl Math 66(5):1632–1648
13. Chan TF, Sandberg BY, Vese LA (2000) Active contours without edges for vector-valued images. J Vis Commun Image Represent 11(2):130–141
14. Chan TF, Shen J (2005) Image processing and analysis: variational, PDE, wavelet, and stochastic methods. Society for Industrial and Applied Mathematics, Philadelphia
15. Chan TF, Vese LA (2001) Active contours without edges. IEEE Trans Image Proc 10(2):266–277
16. Cremers D, Rousson M, Deriche R (2007) A review of statistical approaches to level set segmentation: integrating color, texture, motion and shape. Int J Comput Vis 72(2):195–215
17. Delvaux M, Gay G (2008) Capsule endoscopy: technique and indications. Best Pract Res Clin Gastroenterol 22(5):813–837
18. Figueiredo IN, Moreno JC, Prasath VBS, Figueiredo PN (2010) A segmentation model using image gradient information and applications to endoscopic images. Technical report 30, DMUC, pp 10–30
19. Figueiredo IN, Moreno JC, Prasath VS, Figueiredo PN (2012) A segmentation model and application to endoscopic images. In: Image analysis and recognition (ICIAR), Aveiro. Lectures notes in computer science, vol 7325. Springer, pp 164–171
20. Figueiredo PN, Figueiredo IN, Surya Prasath VB, Tsai R (2011) Automatic polyp detection in pillcam colon 2 capsule images and videos: preliminary feasibility report. Diagn Ther Endos 2011:7 (Article ID 182435)

21. Gerber J, Bergwerk A, Fleischer D (2007) A capsule endoscopy guide for the practicing clinician: technology and troubleshooting. Gastroentest Endosc 66(6):1188–1195
22. Hong B-W, Ni K, Soatto S (2012) Entropy-scale profiles for texture segmentation. In: Third international conference on scale space methods and variational methods in computer vision (SSVM), Ein-Gedi. Lectures notes in computer science, vol 6667. Springer, pp 243–254
23. Houhou N, Thiran J-P, Bresson X (2009) Fast texture segmentation based on semi-local region descriptor and active contour. Numer Math Theory Methods Appl 2(4):445–468
24. Iddan G, Meron G, Glukhovsky A, Swain F (2000) Wireless capsule endoscopy. Nature 405(6785):417
25. Maenpaa T, Pietikainen M (2004) Classification with color and texture: jointly or separately? Pattern Recogn 37(8):1629–1640
26. Moglia A, Menciassi A, Dario P (2008) Recent patents on wireless capsule endoscopy. Recent Pat Biomed Eng 1(1):24–33
27. Moglia A, Menciassi A, Dario P, Cuchieri A (2009) Capsule endoscopy: progress update and challenges ahead. Nature Rev Gastroenterol Hepatol 6(6):353–361
28. Morel J-M, Solimini S (1994) Variational methods in image processing. Birkhauser, Boston
29. Moreno JC (2012) Contributions to variational image segmentation. Ph.D. thesis, Department of Mathematics, Coimbra
30. Moreno JC, Figueiredo IN, Prasath VBS (2011) Texture image segmentation using higher order derivatives. In: Proceeding of the congress on numerical methods in engineering (CMNE), Coimbra, p 10
31. Mumford D, Shah J (1989) Optimal approximations by piecewise smooth functions and associated variational problems. Commun Pure Appl Math 42(5):577–685
32. Ni K, Bresson X, Chan T, Esedoglu S (2009) Local histogram based segmentation using the Wasserstein distance. Int J Comput Vis 84(1):97–111
33. Paragios N, Deriche R (2002) Geodesic active regions: a new paradigm to deal with frame partition problems in computer vision. J Vis Commun Image Represent 13:249–268
34. Prasath VBS, Palaniappan K, Seetharaman G (2012) Multichannel texture image segmentation using local feature fitting based variational active contours. In: Proceedings of the eighth Indian conference on computer vision, craphics and image processing, ICVGIP '12, pp 78:1–78:6
35. Rousson M, Brox T, Deriche R (2003) Active unsupervised texture segmentation on a diffusion based feature space. In: Proceedings of the 2003 IEEE computer society conference on computer vision and pattern recognition (CVPR), Madison, pp 699–704
36. Sandberg B, Chan TF, Vese L (2002) A level-set and Gabor-based active contour algorithm for segmenting textured images. Technical report 02-39, UCLA CAM
37. Wang X-F, Huang D-S, Xu H (2010) An efficient local Chan-Vese model for image segmentation. Pattern Recogn 43(3):603–618

Study of the Prognostic Relevance of Longitudinal Brain Atrophy in Post-traumatic Diffuse Axonal Injury Using Graph-Based MRI Segmentation Techniques

Emanuele Monti, Valentina Pedoia, Elisabetta Binaghi and Sergio Balbi

Abstract Diffuse axonal injury is a kind of brain lesion on a microscopic level produced by the mechanism or rapid acceleration-deceleration of the head. It is characterized by a widespread damage throughout the brain with no focalization, but with prevalent involvement of some areas; it implies a state of coma of sudden onset followed by a recovery the entity of which may vary according to the amount of sustained damage. This traumatic pattern differs from focal lesion because it does not result in focal neurological deficit related to a particular brain area, but it interferes with more sophisticated functions relying upon brain networks, being damaged from a diffuse white matter shearing. For patients who recover from unconsciousness, disability is characterized by cognitive impairments with domains of memory and attention being mainly affected. When the patient is in coma clinicians has no proper instrument to predict the clinical evolution except the qualitative evaluation of lesions depicted on MRI scan. Delayed brain atrophy, measured on seriated MRI volumetric scans may represents an useful biomarker to predict the prognosis of these patients because data coming from recent observations show relevant correlations between the amount of WM atrophy and prognosis assessed by neuropsychological tests. Here we present a new graph-based method for MRI brain segmentation, and its application to our problem of WM atrophy estimation for prognostic inference.

Keywords Diffuse axonal injury · Neuropsychological test · MRI · Segmentation · Graph searching · Graph cut

E. Monti · S. Balbi
Dipartimento di Biotecnologie e Scienze della Vita,
Università degli Studi dell'Insubria, Varese, Italy

V. Pedoia (✉) · E. Binaghi
Dipartimento di Scienze Teoriche e Applicate—Sezione Informatica,
Università degli Studi dell'Insubria, Varese, Italy
e-mail: valeped83@yahoo.it

P. Di Giamberardino et al. (eds.), *Computational Modeling of Objects Presented in Images*, Lecture Notes in Computational Vision and Biomechanics 15,
DOI: 10.1007/978-3-319-04039-4_14,

1 Diffuse Axonal Injury in Traumatic Brain Injury

In this Chapter we argue about a particular kind of brain lesion consequent to head trauma and on the application of non conventional MRI image analysis techniques for studying the correlation between information extracted from images and the physical state of the patient. Traumatic Brain Injuries(TBI) may be classified as:

- Focal: contusion, laceration, hemorrhage (intra-parenchymal, subdural, epidural).
- Diffuse: *Diffuse Axonal Injury(DAI)*, diffuse vascular injury, hypoxic/ ischemic damage, brain swelling.

Diffuse axonal injury is one of the most common and important pathological features of traumatic brain lesion characterized by widespread disruption of white matter fibers induced by shear-strain forces originated by the mechanism of rapid acceleration-deceleration of the head, as happens in a motor-vehicle crash [34].

Generally it is present in association with other mechanisms of brain damage such as contusion, anoxia, intracerebral hemorrhage and penetrating cerebral trauma, but it may also be the unique pathological feature.

This traumatic pattern accounts as a main feature in 40–50% of traumatic brain injuries requiring hospital admission in the United States. It is characterized by microscopic damage with prevalent involvement of the interface between region of the brain with different tissue density, as the white-grey matter junction; in particular at the level of the parasagittal white matter of the cerebral cortex, corpus callosum, and the pontine- mesencephalic junction adjacent to the superior cerebellar peduncles [39].

After previous histological observation conducted by Strich (23) in 1956 in patients who died from a severe TBI following a motor-vehicle crash, the term "diffuse axonal injury" was first introduced, in the early 1980s by Gennarelli and coworkers as a patho-physiological descriptor of a clinical condition characterized by a rapid progression to coma after head trauma in the absence of specific focal lesions [24]. They discovered in a primate model, in which monkeys were exposed to acceleration and deceleration in the oblique, lateral and sagittal planes, that this kind of diffuse brain injury may be the sole contributor to post-traumatic unconsciousness [24].

Subsequently as the concept of axonal damage and diffuse axonal injury matured, the leading hypothesis held by neuroscientist became that a spectrum of injuries occurred , all due to the same axonal pathology, but differing in amount.

It was therefore postulated that to a progressive physiological disturbances of function, there was a corresponding progressive amount of axonal damage, delineating a continuum of events. From concussive syndromes to most severe form of brain impairment characterized by persistent vegetative state or death [23].

A component of DAI is believed to be present in all motor-vehicle crashes where the patient has lost consciousness, and even in sport-related injuries formerly ascribed to concussion. The microscopic features of DAI, characterized by disruption of the neuro-filament subunits within the cytoskeleton, depend on the length of time after injury; but within a day or so after injury, there is evidence of damage to axons in the form of axonal bulbs. This is because DAI is not caused only by primary axotomy from mechanical forces but also from secondary axotomy triggered by biochemical factors. The microscopic features correspond to Wallerian-type axonal degeneration. There is a slow progression from axonal swelling to axonal bulbs and, weeks later to the development of small clusters of microglia throughout the parasagittal white matter, the corpus callosum, the internal capsule, and the deep gray matter that usually continues for months to years. Many of the injured neurons may survive, but it may take weeks for them to be restored to normal physiologic function, including action potential propagation. The phase just described correspond to neurological recovery that we observe in our patients.

In the first 2 years after DAI there is active myelin degeneration, which represents the final stage of the process. The traumatic injury to the axons leads to the disconnection of various target sites, which is assumed to translate into the resultant morbidity [50].

The Adams classification is used to categorize the degree of DAI as mild, moderate or severe according to the extension of damage from more superficial to deeper region of the brain, as the brainstem, that represents the fulcrum for the forces being applied to the cerebrum during head trauma. Because the definitive diagnosis of DAI can be established only at autopsy, it has been consistently underestimated as a mechanism of TBI.

1.1 Radiological Diagnosis of Diffuse Axonal Injury

With sensitive MRI technique, DAI has been shown to be an important part of the brain injury in surviving patients with moderate and severe TBI, and even in mild cases. Traumatic axonal injury is grossly underestimated by CT, that nevertheless remains the initial imaging study of choice for head trauma patients, because is readily available, fast and sensitive in detecting hemorrhage; in contrast MRI allows the nature and extent of both hemorrhagic and non-hemorrhagic cerebral tissue injuries to be determined at higher resolution especially within the posterior fossa and deep white matter.

Therefore, in recent years MRI has become the image modality of choice in this clinical setting [5].

Recent advanced techniques, such as the diffusion tensor imaging, have consistently demonstrated loss of axonal integrity in TBI patients compared with controls, but normative data for diagnostic use in individual patients are not yet sufficiently developed. Therefore, conventional MRI sequence is still considered to be the standard imaging method in the routine clinical evaluation of TBI patients, in the sub-acute and chronic phase of TBI. MRI takes longer time than CT, and often the patients are too unstable to have an MRI upon initial presentation.

In most severe cases of DAI axonal pathology is often accompanied by intraparenchymal hemorrhage, which is clearly visible on CT, but when used to evaluate mild to moderate DAI, MRI is demonstrably superior to CT scanning in detecting petechial hemorrhages and non-hemorrhagic lesions. T2 gradient echo (T2 GRE) sequences are sensitive to iron in blood breakdown product and depict hemorrhagic Traumatic Axonal Injury (TAI) lesions, while fluid attenuated inversion recovery (FLAIR) also depicts non- hemorrhagic lesions by reducing signal interference from cerebrospinal fluid. Early MRI findings after injury have been associated with clinical outcome; however it may be challenging to perform MRI during the first weeks post-injury in patients who are unstable or do not cooperate. One study has demonstrated that hemorrhagic TAI lesions appear less conspicuous with time. However both CT and MRI probably underestimate the extent of axonal damage as most of this damage is microscopic [43].

Some advanced techniques that appears to be more sensitive than conventional MRI in detecting DAI, as Diffuse Weighted Imaging (DWI) have been recently used In DAI, because this leads to an alteration of local water diffusion.

In DAI regions there is an evolution with time from restricted diffusion to unrestricted diffusion (vaso-genic edema). In addition to these modalities there is Diffusion Tensor Imaging (DTI) that may be more sensitive in identifying DAI specifically in certain neuroanatomical locations such as white matter bundles. The recent development of high resolution Susceptibility Weighted Imaging (SWI) has resulted in another tool to evaluate post-traumatic pathology.

1.2 Clinical Manifestations

A patient who sustains a diffuse traumatic axonal injury generally rapidly lapses into coma; this loss of consciousness may last few hours to a longer period, and sometimes it may be permanent, according to the severity of the underlying damage. Axonal injury in the brainstem, appears to be one of the primary factors responsible for the generation of coma in DAI, particularly when the reticular activating system, that is a band of tissue connecting the upper brainstem reticular core to the cortex through synaptic relays in thalamic nuclei, is involved. Injuries to the brainstem are often associated with poor outcome [57].

After this kind of lesion, the cognitive domains of memory, executive functions and processing speed are commonly affected; difficulties with encoding and retrieving new information, accompanied by problems in information processing and executive skills are very common [51]. This is likely due to the fact that abilities such as memory and cognitive functions depend on the coherent activity of widely distributed brain networks; nodes in these networks are connected by long white matter tracts that may be damaged in traumatic brain injury as a result of diffuse axonal injury. Then white matter disruption is a critical factor in the development of cognitive impairment after traumatic brain injury, but conventional neuroimaging underestimates its extent. Positive correlation has been established between the duration of unconsciousness and the extension of damage.

1.3 Clinical Course

DAI is a particular kind of brain lesion that dose not require surgical treatment because brain damage underlying the described syndrome occurs at a microscopic level, throughout the whole brain with prevalent involvement of some areas.

Usually patients with DAI lesion not complicated by other conditions like hypossia or edema do not show elevated intracranial pressure values. In the most severe case, recovery of consciousness can take several weeks or the patient may not even recover at all [69].

Here it is important to stress the concept that persistent disability in these kind of patients depends particularly from cognitive impairments. Clinical scales like GCS are useful in general in brain trauma because are related to the outcome, but in the particular subgroup of DAI patient, as we experiment, it does not seem to be true, because for the same level of depthness of coma at the arrival in ICU, sometimes different trajectories of recovery are followed by different patients [20].

1.4 Progressive Atrophy

Cerebral atrophy is a common sequela of TBI, and it is postulated that volume loss occurs due to direct injury to neuronal cell bodies, ultimately resulting in cytotoxic or apoptotic cell death, or loss of cerebral volume may be the result of TAI with secondary wallerian degeneration and delayed neuronal cell death rather than primary somal injury. Blatter et al. [7] for example studied cerebral atrophy cross- sectionally in 123 TBI patients grouped according to time between injury and MRI scanning, concluding that there was a progressive decrease in total brain volume starting 3 weeks after moderate to severe TBI and reaching significance at 8–12 months later. Subsequent brain volume loss continued at a rate greater than that seen with normal aging for up to three years after injury. In our preliminary result we found a general agreement with literature reports [18, 44].

The association between post-traumatic global atrophy and functional outcome is more complex, but in general, cerebral atrophy in the chronic phase is better related to the injury severity than functional outcome. The relationship between brain volume and intelligence has been a topic of a scientific debate since at least the 1830s. In 1836, Frederick Tiedmann wrote that there exists an indisputable connection between the size of the brain and the mental energy displayed by the individual man [38]. Nowadays this sounds ironic, but in literature there is a growing number of works trying to address the task to establish some sort of correlation between reduction of global or regional brain volumes and sophysticated brain functions assessed by neuropsychometric tests [31]. Cerebral atrophy has been widely used as a gross neuro-pathological hallmark of diffuse injury, especially in the sub-acute (<30 days after injury) and chronic (>6 months later) phases. Therefore when an human brain undergoes a TBI, the resulting effect seems to be that of a neurodegenerative disease with progressive WM and GM re-absorption. The greatest part of this disruption, called delayed atrophy [**?**], occurs later under apoptotic cellular signal, being driven by neuronal deafferentation and axonal damage; the resulting effect on a macroscopic level is that of a progressive brain matter atrophy, measurable as brain volume reduction [44].

Some recent studies showed that post-traumatic atrophy is not uniformly diffuse throughout subcortical structures, but involves with the highest rates, the amygdala, hippocampus, thalamus and putamen; loss of volume in the amygdala and hippocampus may contribute to various behavioral and cognitive difficulties that commonly affect head-injured patients, such as lability of mood, heightened irritability, and difficulties with memory and learning. Considering subcortical white matter, we note that a variety of regions experienced marked atrophy, with the most dramatic volume loss occurring in the temporal lobes, superior frontal lobes, precuneus and paracentral lobules. The atrophy seems therefore to have a preferential spatial distribution (regional selectivity. Recent works show that regional morphometry may hold value as a biomarker for recovery after trauma [71].

1.5 Clinical Relevance of Outcome Prediction

A concern of families, physicians and neuroscientist involved in the care of patient who sustain a traumatic brain injury is the limited ability to predict long-term neuropsychological and social consequences of such injuries for a given patient [52].

Since most survivors are young and have near normal life expectancy, the possibility of predicting the final outcome of a patient with diffuse axonal injury, assumes great importance because this information can feedback the rehabilitative process with increasing scientific evidence of outcome modulation, when conducted in a proper temporal window.

Therefore there is the need of a clinical biomarker related to the amount of diffuse brain damage, that could be measured in the sub-acute period when the patient is still recovering; the importance of such an indicator is not just to predict the possibility of consciousness restoration, but also to infer about the entity of recovery of higher cerebral functions not contemplated by classical outcome scales, but dramatically related to social functioning of an individual.

1.6 Brain Volume as a Biomarker: From Benchmark to Bedside

Quantitative measurement of change in brain size and shape (e.g., to estimate atrophy) is an important current area of research. New methods of change analysis attempt to improve robustness, accuracy, and extent of automation. In december 2002 A.G. Sorensen, Director of the MGH Martinos NMR Center, introduce the term Neurovolumetrics to emphasize the importance of volumetric image analysis for diagnosis and therapy of neurological diseases. Decision in the setting of clinical neurology mostly rely on qualitative (i.e. visual) interpretation of structural brain images. On visual assessment, for example, global brain atrophy is recognized by an increase of cerebrospinal fluid spaces and shrinkage of parenchymal structures. However such an assessment can detect only macroscopic changes with a rather low level of inter-observer agreement. MRI permits in vivo quantification of brain compartment volume, and has many applications in cognitive, clinical and comparative neuroscience. Quantitative assessment of brain volumes, obtained through volumetric MRI has been increasingly applied in recent years to a wide range of neurologic conditions due to advances in computational technology. Its role should be complementary to that of visual assessment of brain structural images, with the specific aim of improving detection of focal and subtle brain pathology. Volumetric methods are mainly based on brain segmentation, that is the separation of the intracranial content into parenchymal and non-parenchymal tissue classes. We know that recovery trajectory is under the influence of different moderators, such as age, pre-morbid I.Q., years of school education; parameters which are related to cerebral plasticity and connectivity and more in general to the concept of functional reserve. The concept of brain volume as a biomarker for neurodegenerative diseases emerged relatively recent in time and represents a challenging instrument for clinical research.

1.7 Monitoring the Recovery

Based on the experimental assumption that after a mechanical inertial load is brought to axons part of fibers are torn with no possibility to recover while the remaining substain subcritical damage of different entity leading to progressive delayed atrophy [44], we set up a longitudinal multicentric study oriented to track the trajectory of brain volume reduction with respect to the functioning of the brain as measured by neuropsychological tests. Our aim is to collect a great amount of clinical and morphometric data of patient victim of traumatic brain injury (DAI type) in order to find out statistical correlations that would allow us to infer about clinical prognosis. Collecting and analyzing many data would lead us to the realization of a prognostic algorithm, helping us to decide the correct timing and intensity of rehabilitation process. In a previous retrospective study conducted at our institution we analyzed perspectives of using brain volume as a predictor of clinical recovery after TBI with pure DAI pattern, finding statistically significant correlation between cognitive performance scores on tests and reduction of brain WM between two time points.

2 MRI Brain Segmentation

Proper and accurate quantitative measurement of change in brain size and shape can be achieved through the use of segmentation procedures that minimize the user interaction. Automatic segmentation of the brain in Magnetic Resonance Images is a key task in many neuroscience and medical studies either because the brain is the final anatomical structure of interest or because the automatic extraction facilitates further analysis [2, 30]. Whole brain segmentation is a task available in software such as Brain Visa [72], FSL [58] and Brainsuite [55], however in most cases they give poor results especially in case of tumors located on the border of the brain [30].

The problem of segmenting all or part of the brain in MRI imagery continues to be investigated giving rise to a variety of approaches attempting to satisfy the high accuracy demand in diversified clinical and neuroimaging applications [2, 3, 15, 30]. The rationale behind this effort is to improve upon existing early methods suffering from incorrect detection due to noise, difficulties in assigning threshold in the edge image and over and under estimation. The proposed solutions make use of a single, gray scale 2D or 3D image or multiple MR images with different gray scale contrast [15]. Focusing on whole brain segmentation from gray scale images, the early most intuitive approach proposed is automatic thresholding. The application of this approach to MR brain image segmentation includes works based on iterative, knowledge guided thresholding [13, 65] and histogram analysis [1] complemented in some cases with image processing techniques such as morphological filtering [36]. The solutions proposed suffers in general from the difficulty in setting threshold values and present strong limitations in the presence of inhomogeneity, image artefact and anatomical variability.

The Region Growing approach extends thresholding by combining it with connectivity. Methods within this approach need an operator for manual setting of seed for each region and their results depend on the heuristic assessment of thresholding for homogeneity [17, 45]. As a consequence, suitable accuracy is achieved only detecting the contour in slices where the brain is one homogeneous region without pathological alterations and inhomogeneity.

Supervised statistical pattern recognition approaches are proposed in MR image segmentation to circumvent the problem of explicitly and analytically describing the specific segmentation procedure and related parameters, lying to a learning stage the charge of inducing the classifier from supervised data available. Parametric and non parametric methods are proposed showing a competitive behavior in reducing the effect of Radio Frequency (RF) inhomogeneity but requiring some interaction to provide tissue training pixels and to perform post processing adjustments [16, 28]. The parametric probabilistic classification is sensitive to accurate estimation of the probability density function (PDF) [60]. Nonparametric approaches obtain the parameters of the PDF from data without any assumptions, so these approaches are accurate but expensive [14, 40]. Computational complexity and low generalization of trained classifiers limit their applicability. Unsupervised methods employed for MR brain image segmentation include K-Means and its fuzzy equivalent Fuzzy c-Means (FCM) [25]. From a viewpoint of reproducibility, unsupervised methods are clearly desirable. Many algorithms are introduced to make FCM robust against noise and inhomogeneity but most of them still present low accuracy [26, 73]. Other pattern recognition methods such as neural networks and template matching have been also applied to MR brain image segmentation [26, 68].

Edge-based segmentation approaches have been widely investigated to segment MR images of the head [8, 15, 19]. Base methods apply local operations to every point of the input picture, in order to extract short edge elements. Some of these operations are very simple, like the gradient or the Laplacian, whereas other operations are more complex and allow the elimination of most of the local noise [4]. When small edge elements have been obtained, edge following strategies are applied to connect them to form borders. Snell et al. use an active surface template to find the intracranial boundary in MRI volumes of the head [59]. The method is based on the active contour model algorithm "Snakes" [29]. However the resulting procedure requires user interaction to provide a good initial contour for subsequent snake contour refinement. The Bayesian dynamic contour (BDC) model [35] shows advantages over the snakes active contour as the energy functions used to find the boundary can be more generally based on information about the whole region, rather than just the local boundary characteristics. The results are promising for the central slices of multispectral images presented, but have yet to be developed for isolating the whole brain. Contour-based deformable models are applied successfully to MRI brain segmentation although the approach suffer from the difficulty of determining the initial contour and tuning parameters [1, 30]. Khotanlou et al. [30] explicitly propose a segmentation method based on deformable models and asymmetry analysis. Proceeding from the assumption that in normal brain the symmetry plane of the head is approximately equal to the symmetry plane of the segmented brain, a MRI brain segmentation algorithm robust in presence of tumor has been developed. Results obtained are satisfactorily but they heavily depend from the validity of the symmetry assumption.

2.1 Graph-Based Segmentation

A boundary tracing method using dynamic programming for noisy brain sections with vague boundaries, is proposed but successful application for global segmentation of MR images remains to be demonstrated since a good initial guess for the boundaries is required [70]. Of the many techniques available for automated border detection, those based on graph searching principles [37] have been successful in several applications.

The value of graph search method lies in robustness which derives from the property typical of the optimization methods of embedding global information about edges and the structure of object in a figure of merit allowing accurate border detection from noisy pictures [41]. Graph searching has become one of the best investigated segmentation tool for medical image data with applications to coronary angiography, ultrasound and cardiac MRI imaging [21, 62, 64, 67]. However, to the best of our knowledge the application of this technique to MRI brain segmentation has not yet investigated. In early works the analysis of the entire volume of data was usually accomplished by applying 2D contour detection strategy slice-by-slice, conceiving individual slices independent and without incorporating interrelation information of the spatial sequence of images [27].

Graph searching has become one of the best investigated segmentation tool for 2D medical image data [21, 49, 64]. The application of graph search to contour detection was first published in [37] presenting a method for detecting edges and contours in noisy pictures. The overall detection process is transformed into the search for the optimal path in a weighted graph, that connects two specific nodes, the starting and ending nodes. The procedure can then be seen as an edge following procedure that uses global information. The value of graph search segmentation methods lies both in robustness and improvements in computing time. Robustness derives from the fact that it inherits the property of optimization methods of embedding global information about edges and structure of object in a figure of merit, allowing accurate border detection from noisy pictures [41]. The formulation of the optimization problem as a search of the shortest path, allows to use heuristic information to speed up the search, leading to improvements in computing time with respect to other optimization [61].

When dealing with volumetric segmentation, the application, slice-by-slice of 2D graph searching techniques for the identification of 3D object boundary suffers of some limitations essentially due to lack of contextual spatial information.

In recent years, we assist to a wide spread utilization of three dimensional models, often conceived as an extension of previously defined 2D solutions [27]. Unfortunately, standard implementation of graph searching for optimal path cannot be directly applied to perform on optimal surface search. All path-based methods are limited to 2D applications because object boundary in 3D volumes can not be represented by a path. The topic of extending the graph-searching techniques to a direct volumetric medical image segmentation has been investigated in literature [22, 63, 66, 67] giving rise to two main approaches, one acting on graph representation in order to take advantage from the existing search techniques, and the other acting on search algorithm that directly performs an optimal surface determination. Both of them attempt to create a balance between two opposite criteria: to limit the computational complexity and to reach a global optimality. In particular Thedens et al. [67] proposes a method of graph searching belonging to the first category. To make the method efficient, the proposed transformation of the lattice representing the graph imposes the restriction that the number of points to which a single point within the lattice is linked, should be very small and secondly, one dimension of the lattice should be small compared to the other two. The first requirement is satisfied by imposing a smoothness constraint, the second, unfortunately, prevents the applicability of the method to several imaging such as volumetric brain MRI Imaging in which voxels are isotropic and the volume dimensions in the three axis are comparable. The method, applied to MRI cardiac imagery, is computational expensive [2].

A graph cut segmentation method for optimal hypersurface detection was developed by Li et al. [33]. The solution proposed is based on the representation of the problem in terms of a geometric graph and on the computation of a minimum *s-t cut* in a derived directed graph of reduced complexity [12]. The Graph Cut framework for segmentation is based on an implicit representation of object boundaries. Thus, it allows the same flexible topological properties of segments as in techniques where the edge properties are explicit, level-sets for example [54]. Since the introduction of the approximation energy minimization via Graph Cut proposed by Boykov et al.

[12] and the subsequent technique formalization for solving segmentation problem on N-D Images [9, 10], many methods have been proposed to solve problems or emphasize features of the classic Graph Cut.

The Graph Cut has undergone evolutions in different directions: some with the aim of improving the interactivity [53], other incorporating other techniques as watershed or gaussian mixture model [6, 48] and other integrating high-level contextual information [32]. In this Chapter we address two MRI Brain Segmentation tasks adopting different graph-based segmentation methods. The first task consists in the fully automatic whole brain segmentation from MRI volume. We derive our method from the edge-based approach adopting Graph Searching tecnique [37] for 2D boundary detection. The solutions investigated in this paper are an extension of those adopted in a previous work [41] from which we inherit the graph searching model. The MRI volume is processed slice by slice, the overall segmentation procedure is made fully automatic and easily reproducible by the automatic detection of frames including eyes and by computing the internal main parameters directly from the image data in this Chapter are reported the salient aspect of the method are reported all the details are reported in [46, 47].

The second task concerns the segmentation of the different brain tissues White Matter, Gray Matter and Cerebral Spinal Fluid in order to be able to study if the atrophy of these tissues are biomarkers for neurodegenerative diseases. For achieving this task a modified Graph Cut method is used that incorporates in the energy function a component related to a-priori information on the spatial distribution of tissues already used by the authors in [42].

3 Proposed Multidisciplinary Study

Our multidisciplinary study recruites patients with pure DAI lesion pattern on MRI, being in a state of coma of sudden onset, whit no history of psychiatric disease, alcohol or drugs abuse, previous head trauma or brain intervention, with no incompatibility for MRI examination. The first MRI is performed for clinical need of making diagnosis of DAI that could explain the counsciosness impairment in the absence of focal brain lesion on CT examination. Then, after submittion of written informed consent by the relatives, the patient is MRI-scanned at four time points : 1 month post-trauma, 6 month, 1 and 2 years later. The acquisition sequence is 3D T1 MP-RAGE isotropic with voxel of 1 mm^3. Then we post-elaborate these sequences with graph-based morphometry analysis techniques in order to segment 26 the brain tissues and measure WM, GM and CSF volumes. The cognitive recovery is monitored by neuropsychologic evaluation performed 6 month, 1 and 2 years post-trauma (according to patient clinical condition) Our tests battery is composed by Mini Mental State Examination (MMSE), Trail making test (TMTA, TMTB), Frontal Assessment Battery (FAB), Wisconsin card sorting test (WCST), phonemic and semantic fluencies, Token test, Rey Auditory Verbal Learning Test (RAVLT), Rey figure, Story recall test, Raven progressive matrix , stroop test, beck depression

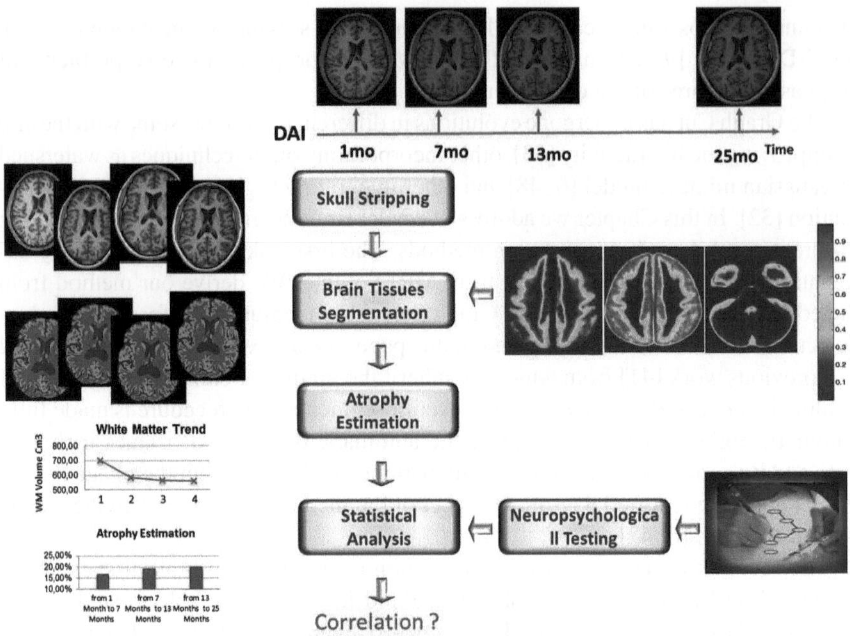

Fig. 1 Scheme of the proposed multidisciplinary study for for evaluating the prognostic relevance of longitudinal brain atrophy estimation in post-traumatic DAI

inventory. The brain volume trajectory and cognitive neuropsychometric trajectory are then coupled and analyzed together to find out correlations on a patient level and on a population level. The overall scheme of our procedure is shown in Fig. 1

3.1 Graph-Based Brain Tissues Volumety

The overall procedure to extract the volume changes of White Matter (WM), Gray Matter (GM) and Cerebral Spinal Fluid (CSF) is composed of two essential steps. The aim of the first phase is to segment the whole brain from the head MRI and the aim of the second phase is to cluster WM, FM and CSF for examining separately the changes in volume over time of the three classes.

3.1.1 Whole Brain Segmentation

We briefly describe the key points of this strategy.

A contour of radial shape can be conveniently treated by using polar coordinates. Working in polar space, the radial boundary of a given object can be represented by a transformation $\rho = f(\theta)$ characterized by the following feasibility constraints:

Boundary as a Function $f(\theta)$ is single valued and the value ρ exists for each θ with $1 \leq \theta \leq N$.
Connectivity Constraint $|f(\theta+1) - f(\theta)| \leq 1$ for $1 \leq \theta \leq N-1$.
Closing Constraint $|f(1) - f(N)| \leq 1$ imposing that the first and last pixels satisfy the connectivity constraint.

Each feasible function $f(\theta)$ is a candidate object boundary. The goal is then to find the minimum cost boundary subject to the feasibility constraints. The boundary detection task within the graph searching framework is modeled by embedding the properties of the boundary in a cost function and formulating the boundary extraction as the problem of minimizing this function subject to the feasibility constraints. The boundary cost is defined as follows:

$$B_c = \sum_{\theta=1}^{N} C(\theta, f(\theta)) \tag{1}$$

where $C(\theta, f(\theta))$ is a cost image. The value of each pixel in the cost image must be inversely related to the likelihood that an edge is present at that point. The likelihood is usually determined by the application of a low-level local edge operator [67]. In general, the definition of this cost function depends on a priori knowledge on the object to be segmented. The boundary cost allows to express both local and global information that can be incorporated within the constrained minimization strategy for optimal boundary detection. The 2D brain segmentation is accomplished in the three following phases.

Phase 1 Polar Conversion The image is converted in polar coordinates, both the correct number of sampling angles both the brain's centroid are automatically computed
Phase 2 Skull Boundary Detection The cost image is computed using vertical Sobel filter and the graph searching technique is applied, finding the skull boundary. A binary mask is computed distinguishing between pixels with ρ less and greater than the edge. This mask is applied to cost image and it is inverted for finding a new cost image for the second step: the actual brain segmentation.
Phase 3 Brain Boundary Detection The strategy is again applied on this new cost image. The minimal path in the graph is the brain boundary in the polar space. The last step is the conversion in cartesian coordinates of the detected boundary.

The value of graph search method lies both in robustness and improvements in computing time. Robustness derives from the fact that it inherit the property of optimization methods of embedding global information about edges and the structure of object in a figure of merit allowing accurate border detection.

3.1.2 White Matter, Gray Matter, Cerebral Spinal Fluid Segmentation

After the whole brain segmentation phase the WM, GM and CSF are segmented in the entire volume. We address this task choosing within the graph searching framework the min-cut technique [9, 10, 12]. The Graph Cut framework offers a globally optimal object extraction method for N-dimensional images [9].

This strategy, belongs to the category of the energy minimization methods that, formalize the segmentation problem in terms of optimization, defining an energy function whose the minimization is the solution of the segmentation. A fairly general cost function that can include both region and boundary properties of segments and certain types of topological constraints are described. These components naturally fit into the global optimization framework. The main technical novelty of the object extraction approach of the Graph Cut is that segmentation energy is formalized over binary variables whose values only indicate whether the pixel is inside or outside the object of interest. In contrast to the earlier path-based combinatorial methods [22, 63, 66, 67], this can be seen as a region-based approach to encode image segments [10]. In fact, the difference between path-based and region-based representations of segments on a discrete graph is analogous to the difference between explicit contour representation, e.g. snakes, and the implicit level-sets approach.

Moreover, Boykov and Kolmogorov have studied the practical efficiency of combinatorial min-cut/max-flow algorithms on applications in computer vision [11]. It was shown that some max-flow techniques could solve 2D and 3D segmentation problems in close to real-time using regular PCs. The Graph Cut framework for segmentation is based on an implicit representation of object boundaries. Thus, it allows the same flexible topological properties of segments as in level-sets techniques. The segmentation results may have isolated objects which may also contain holes. However, it may be useful to impose some topological constraints reflecting certain high-level contextual information about the object of interest. Graph cut can incorporate some types of topological constraints. For example, the hard constraints can indicate some image pixels a priori known to be a part of the object or background [9].

The aim of a volumetric segmentation problem is to assign to each voxel $v \in V$ a label that says the membership of the voxel to a specific region L_i d the goal is to find the optimal labeling.

We assume that each voxel v of the brain volume V has three cost values concerning the association of the specific voxel to the White Matter $R_v(O_{WM})$ to the Gray Matter $R_v(O_{GM})$ and to the Cerebral Spinal Fluid $R_v(O_{CSF})$. Moreover, we assume each pair of adjacent voxels $v, w \in N$ has a cost $B_{v,w}$ associated with the fact that the pair of voxel has different labeling, where N is a set of pairs of 3D neighboring voxel. Our goal is to find the optimal labeling $L = (L_{WM}, L_{GM}, L_{CSF})$ in assigning each voxel v to the brain tissues by the minimization of the following cost function:

$$E(L) = \lambda R(L) + B(L) \tag{2}$$

where

$$R(L) = \sum_{v \in V} R_v(O_v) \tag{3}$$

is called *Regional Term* and

$$B(L) = \sum_{v,w \in N} B_{v,w} \delta_{L_i,L_j}; \tag{4}$$

where $\delta_{L_i,L_j} = 0$ if $L_i = L_j$ and $\delta_{L_i,L_j} = 1$ if $L_i \neq L_j$ is called *Boundary Term.*

In our application the Regional Term is the euclidian distance between each voxel and the centroid of the three clusters (WM, GM and CSF) computed with the K-means algorithm and the Boundary Term is computed with gradient function. The segmentation problem can be formulated as finding the optimal set of voxel belonging to a desired 3D objects; considering the translation of the segmentation problem in an optimization problem solvable with 3D graph $G\{V, E\}$, we have to look for the partition of the graph that minimizes the cost of the cut.

Each $v \in D$ becomes a graph node V that is connected to the 26, 3D neighbors with a link called *n-link.* There are also three specially designated terminal nodes, that represent WM, GM and CSF prototypes. Each node is also connected to both the terminal node with a link called *t-link.* To every link both *t-links* and *n-links* is given a weight. Weight assigned to *n-link* represents the distance between two neighbor nodes, thus the Boundary term $B_{v,w}$ and the weight assigned to *t-link* represents the distance between nodes and both the terminal nodes, thus the Regional terms $R_v(O_{WM})$, $R_v(O_{WM})$ and $R_v(O_{CSF})$. An s-t cut is a subset of edges such that the terminal nodes become completely separated on the graph. The cost of a cut is sum of all the weight crossed by the cut. The segmentation goal is to identify the cut that minimize the cost using the max-flow/min-cut algorithm [11, 12]. The min-cut Graph Cuts framework offers a globally optimal object extraction method for N-dimensional images. A fairly general cost function is described that can include both region and boundary properties of segments and certain types of topological constraints that naturally fit into our global optimization framework.

In the present work a specific problem dependent solution has been introduced within the general min-cut technique which is suggested by regularity of the spatial distribution of WM, GM, CSF. By exploiting the flexibility in the description of the energy function that allows to take into account a-priori information, work we consider a modified version of equation 2 by including a new term:

$$E(L) = \lambda R(L) + \mu A(L) + B(L) \tag{5}$$

where $A(L) = \sum_{v \in D} A_v(O_v)$ is an Atlas Term. We assume that each voxel v of the brain volume V has three a-priori cost values concerning the association of the specific voxel to the White Matter $A_v(O_{WM})$, to the Gray Matter $A_v(O_{GM})$ and to the Cerebral Spinal Fluid $A_v(O_{CSF})$. These costs are derived using a brain tissue

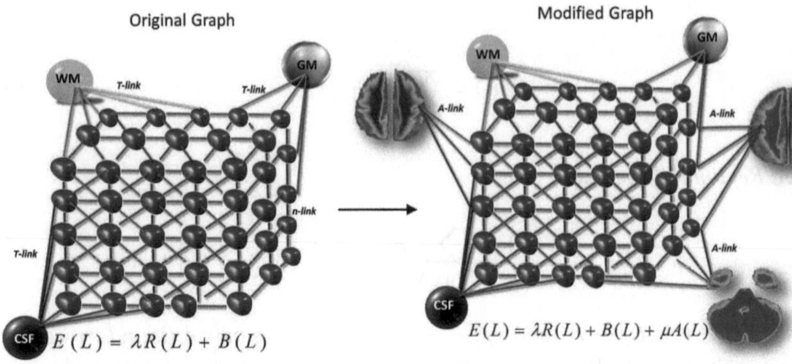

Fig. 2 3D Graph topology for classical graph cut and the proposed atlas based graph cut

probabilistic atlas, made available from the Laboratory of Neuroimaging (LONI) of the UCLA University [56]. The atlas consists of three volumes, which the value of each voxel indicates the probability that this belongs to the WM, GM and CSF respectively. In the 3D lattice structure, besides the classic *n-links* and *n-links*, the *a-links* for each tissue are added. The weight of these connections is given by the a priori probability that the voxel belongs to a class, which is found in the probabilistic atlas. The min-cuts of this new graph are the 3D boundaries of the WM, GM and CSF. In Fig. 2 shows the original and modified graph.

3.2 Atrophy Estimation

After the brain tissues segmentation the atrophy rate of the White Matter along time can be computed with the follow:

$$Athrophy(t) = \frac{Vol_{WM}(t_0) - Vol_{WM}(t)}{Vol_{WM}(t_0)} \quad (6)$$

Analyzing the atrophy rate, computed for the four time point scans, we note that this phenomenon is grossly influencing the early 7 months period; once past this point the curve slopes down as atrophy rate progressively reduces,tending to normal value and atrophy rate progressively reduces according to its average age-dependent trend. Therefore, we realized the importance of focusing on this particular period of post-traumatic recovery, in order to characterize white matter decrease trajectory in the tract where the curve may greatly vary from one patient to another according to the damage sustained. This is the most informative tract because the patient is usually still recovering in. In Fig. 3 the results obtained for four patients are shown. In our opinion if we introduced one ore more further time point between 1st and 2nd ones (i.g. 2 months post-trauma)we would be able to better infer about the recovery

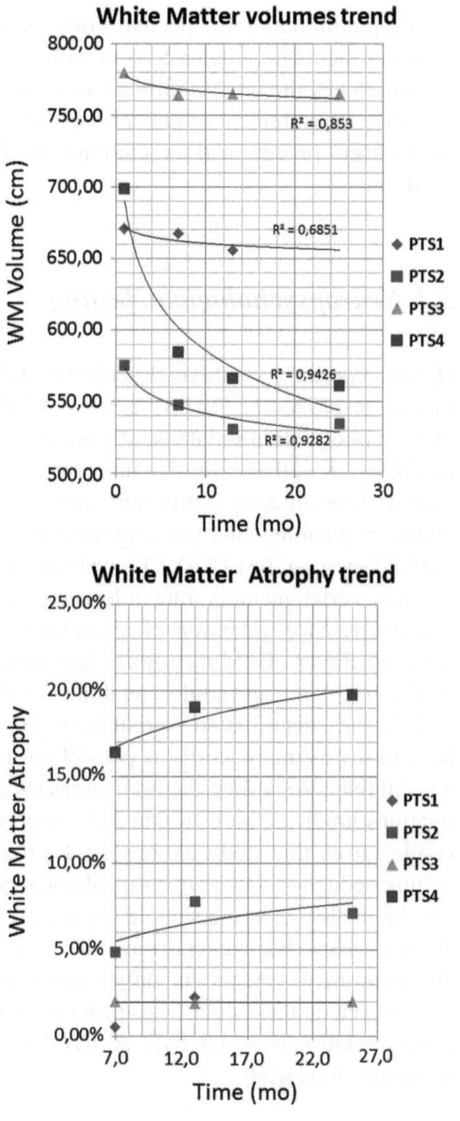

Fig. 3 Trend of the atrophy rate computed for the four time point scans

progress during the phase in which we generally have no proper instruments to predict the clinical evolution of the patient. The basis of such a study consist in systematically studying the atrophy phenomenon with respect to its timing, and correlation to patient prognosis. We decided to perform first MRI examination 1 month post-trauma, not to take into account early brain volume variations related to inflammation and affine phenomena. We set up a battery of neuropsychological tests tailored on these patients to evaluate the cognitive domains mainly affected by traumatic DAI.

In a preliminary retrospective work conducted at our institution we applied these tests to patients finding agreement with what medical literature reports. So now we submitted just the most significant ones from them. The key concept is to get some objective measurement of patient cognitive status allowing us to define numerically the recovery process and its relation with the loss of white matter fibers caused by head trauma.

3.3 Neuropsychological Testing

Here is reported a synthetic description of the tests performed by the patients. Trail making test (TMTA, TMTB): is a test of visual attention and task switching. It can provide information about visual search speed, scanning, speed of processing, mental flexibility, as well as executive functioning. Rey-Osterrieth Complex Figure: this test permits the evaluation of different functions, such as visual-spatial abilities, memory, attention, planning, and working memory (executive functions). The Rey Auditory Verbal Learning Test (RAVLT) evaluates a wide diversity of functions: short-term auditory-verbal memory, rate of learning, learning strategies, retroactive, and proactive interference, retention of information, and differences between learning and retrieval. Ravens CPM measures clear-thinking ability; is used to assess the degree to which children and adults can think clearly, or the level to which their intellectual abilities have deteriorated. Verbal fluency tests are a kind of test in which participants have to say as many words as possible from a category (semantic or phonemic) in a given time. Regarding the brain areas used in this task, neuropsychological investigations implicate both frontal and temporal lobe areas. Analyzing the initial data coming from this study we observed a trend of correlation between white matter volume reduction and neuropshycological performance assessed by tests. Considering the small size of the sample, we are not allowed to perform a robust parametric statistics. However, we report in Table 1 the Pearson correlation values for each test. We are aware of the fact that only a larger number of cases may confirm or refute the thesis made on these data. These encouraging results agree with statistically significant correlation between TMT A, RAVLT, phon. flu. and WM volume as we found in our previous study.

4 Application Examples

In this section some examples of the application of our segmentation strategies are shown. In [46, 47] an extensive evaluation phase of the brain segmentation strategy used in this context and in [42] some experiments for assessing the performance of the Atlas based Graph Cut are provided respectively.

In Fig. 4 two example of brain segmentation results are shown. The segmentation are judged satisfactory by a group of medical experts. Looking at the brain/extra-

Table 1 Evaluation of the coupling between the white matter atrophy and the patients tests performance

PTS	Time	WM atrophy (%)	TMTA	TMTB	RAV LTi	RAV LTd	fReyc	fReyi	Raven CPM	phon. flu.	sem. flu.
1	6 M.	0.51	14.0	278.0	NP	NP	24.4	12.6	23.8	21.0	30.0
2	6 M.	4.86	48.0	126.0	25.2	0.0	31.2	1.8	27.6	NP	NP
3	6 M.	2.00	59.0	137.0	54.1	9.5	33.4	25.9	30.2	32.0	16.0
4	6 M.	16.40	NP	NP	15.1	19.0	29.7	NP	31.0	7.8	31.5
4	12 M.	19.01	89.0	190.0	14.3	3.2	33.0	26.0	31.0	7.8	31.5
Pearson correlation			**0.854**	−0,1194	**−0.8498**	0.264	0.39	0.465	0.720	**−0.885**	0.587

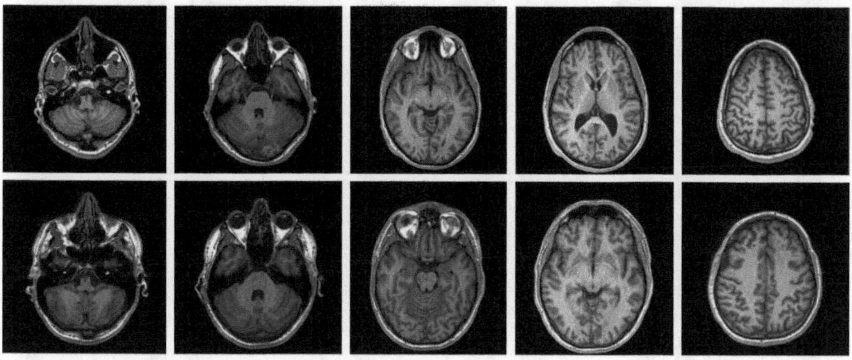

Fig. 4 Examples of whole brain segmentation

brain boundaries seem that proposed performed a correct classification of voxels in all cases even in complex situations such as in slices including eyes and in the area located in the posterior cranial fossa.

Figure 5 shows some examples of the WM/GM/CSF segmentation. In the first row of the image the original slices are shown, in the second, third and fourth rows the superimposing between the original MRI and the segmented White Matter, Gray matter and Cerebral Spinal Fluid are shown respectively. In the last row all the tissue segmentation results are shown together, the slices shown have been randomly chosen in our dataset. Our medical staff visually inspected all the results of segmentation procedure finding that the general qualitative level was good; critical issues of manual segmentation such as to distinguish between deep nuclei of GM and surrounding WM tracts, and between cortex and subcortical WM, were solved without evident inaccuracies. Also the interface between CSF and other two tissues has been delineated correctly.

All volumetric images in our database has a good quality and there are no particular inhomogeneities. However, when dealing with this kind of medical problem, there is no proper way to validate a segmentation system like that we have developed, because it is not possible to create a phantom to work on.

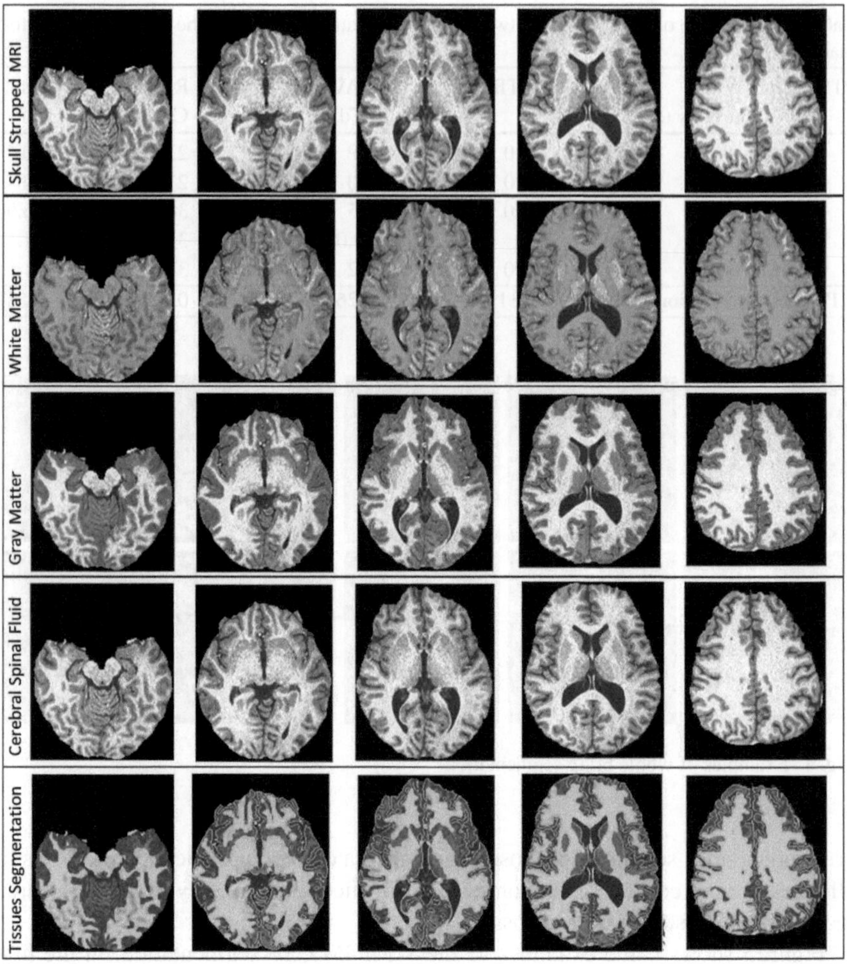

Fig. 5 Examples of brain tissues segmentation

5 Conclusion

The present work addresses the problem of providing a quantitative strategy for brain volume tracking and use it as biomarker for neurodegenerative diseases. In this contest the assessment of an accurate prognosis has both ethic and clinico-economical values because it could regulate the intensity of therapeutic rehabilitative intervention in function of what it is assumed to be achievable on the basis of a sophisticated characterization of brain damage, substrate of patient disability. Our hope is that characterizing brain pathology by means of a clinical biomarker will lead us to better interpret the clinical condition of the patient and its potential evolution.

The assessment of an accurate prognosis has an ethic valence, besides of clinico -economical and logistic one, because it could regulate the intensity of therapeutic rehabilitative intervention in function of what it is assumed to be reachable on the basis of a sophisticated characterization of brain damage, substrate of patient disability. An early clinico-radiological follow up represents therefore an important prognostic moment. We record the satisfaction of patients, relatives and caregivers, and this highlights the social value of this kind of intervention. We record the satisfaction of patients, relatives and caregivers, and this highlights the social value of this kind of intervention. Preliminary results are presented in this work. Future plan contemplates further investigation with more robust medical cases.

References

1. Aboutanos GB, Dawant BM (1997) Automatic brain segmentation and validation: image-based versus atlas-based deformable modelsn. In: Proceedings of the SPIE-medical imaging, vol 3034. pp 299–310
2. Atkins MS, Mackiewich B, Whittall K (1998) Fully automatic segmentation of the brain in MRI. IEEE Trans Med Imaging 17(1): 98–107
3. Balafar M, Ramli A, Saripan M, Mashohor S (2010) Review of brain MRI image segmentation methods. Artif Intell Rev 33:261–274. doi:10.1007/s10462-010-9155-0
4. Bankman IN (2008) Handbook of medical image processing and analysis. Academic press
5. Beretta L, Gemma M, Anzalone N (2008) The value of MR imaging in posttraumatic diffuse axonal injury. J Emerg Trauma Shock 1(2):126–127
6. Blake A, Rother C, Brown M, Perez P, Torr PHS (2004) Interactive image segmentation using an adaptive gmmrf model. In: eighth European conference on computer vision, Springer, Prague, pp 428–441
7. Blatter D, Bigler E, Gale S, Johnson S, Anderson C, Burnett B, Ryser D, Macnamara S, Bailey B (1997) Mr-based brain and cerebrospinal fluid measurement after traumatic brain injury: correlation with neuropsychological outcome. Am J Neuroradiol 18(1):1–10
8. Bomans M, Hohne KH, Tiede U, Riemer M (1990) 3-D segmentation of MR images of the head for 3-D display. IEEE Trans Med Imaging 9(2):177–183
9. Boykov Y, Funka-Lea G (2006) Graph cuts and efficient n-d image segmentation. Int J Comput Vision 70:109–131
10. Boykov Y, Jolly MP (2001) Interactive graph cuts for optimal boundary and region segmentation of objects in n-d images. In: proceedings of the eighth IEEE international conference on computer vision, vol 1. pp 105–112
11. Boykov Y, Kolmogorov V (2004) An experimental comparison of min-cut/max-flow algorithms for energy minimization in vision. IEEE Trans Pattern Anal Mach Intell 26:1124–1137
12. Boykov Y, Veksler O, Zabih R (2001) Fast approximate energy minimization via graph cuts. IEEE Trans Pattern Anal Mach Intell 23:1222–1239
13. Li C, Goldgof DB, Hall LO (1993) Knowledge-based classification and tissue labeling of MR images of human brain. IEEE Trans Med Imaging 12:740–750
14. Chang PL, Teng WG (2007) Exploiting the self-organizing map for medical image segmentation. In: 20th IEEE symposium on computer-based medical systems, pp 281–288
15. Clarke L, Velthuizen R, Camacho M, Heine J, Vaidyanathan M, Hall L, Thatcher R, Silbiger M (1995) MRI segmentation: methods and applications. Magn Reson Imaging 13(3):343–368
16. Clarke L, Velthuizen R, Phuphanich S, Schellenberg J, Arrington J, Silbiger M (1993) MRI: stability of three supervised segmentation techniques. Magn Reson Imaging 11(1):95–106

17. Cline H, Lorensen W, Kikinis R, Jolesz F (1990) Three-dimensional segmentation of MR images of the head using probability and connectivity. J Comput Assist Tomogr 14(6):1037–1045
18. Cowie CJA (2012) Quantitative magnetic resonance imaging in traumatic brain injury. University of Newcastle, Tyne
19. Dellepiane S (1991) Image segmentation: errors, sensitivity, and uncertainty. In: proceedings of the annual international conference of the IEEE Engineering in Medicine and Biology Society, vol 13. pp 253–254
20. Dressler J, Hanisch U, Kuhlisch E, Geiger KD (2007) Neuronal and glial apoptosis in human traumatic brain injury. Int J Legal Med 121(5):365–375
21. Falcao A, Udupa J, Miyazawa F (2000) An ultra-fast user-steered image segmentation paradigm: live wire on the fly. IEEE Trans Med Imaging 19(1):55–62
22. Falcao AX, Udupa JK (2000) A 3d generalization of user-steered live-wire segmentation. Med Image Anal 4(4):389–402
23. Gennarelli TA (1996) The spectrum of traumatic axonal injury. Neuropathol Appl Neurobiol 22(6):509–513
24. Gennarelli TA, Thibault LE, Adams JH, Graham DI, Thompson CJ, Marcincin RP (1982) Diffuse axonal injury and traumatic coma in the primate. Ann Neurol 12(6):564–574
25. Gerig G, Martin J, Kikinis R, Kubler O, Shenton M, Jolesz FA (1992) Unsupervised tissue type segmentation of 3d dual-echo MR head data. Image Vis Comput 10:349–360
26. Hall L, Bensaid A, Clarke L, Velthuizen R, Silbiger M, Bezdek J (1992) A comparison of neural network and fuzzy clustering techniques in segmenting magnetic resonance images of the brain. IEEE Trans Neural Netw 3(5):672–682
27. Heimann T, Meinzer H-P (2009) Statistical shape models for 3D medical image segmentation: a review. Med Image Anal 13(4):543–563
28. Bezdek JC, Hall LO, Clarke LP (1993) Review of MR image segmentation techniques using pattern recognition. Med Phys 20(4):1033–1048
29. Kass M, Witkin A, Terzopoulos D (1988) Snakes: active contour models. Int J Comput Vis 1:321–331. doi:10.1007/BF00133570
30. Khotanlou H, Colliot O, Atif J, Bloch I (2009) 3d brain tumor segmentation in mri using fuzzy classification, symmetry analysis and spatially constrained deformable models. Fuzzy Sets Syst 160:1457–1473
31. Kinnunen KM, Greenwood R, Powell JH, Leech R, Hawkins PC, Bonnelle V, Patel MC, Counsell SJ, Sharp DJ (2010) White matter damage and cognitive impairment after traumatic brain injury. Brain 134:449–463
32. Kumar PM, Torr PHS, Zisserman A (2005) Obj cut. In: CVPR'05: proceedings of the 2005 IEEE Computer Society conference on computer vision and pattern recognition (CVPR'05), vol 1. IEEE Computer Society, Washington, DC, USA, pp 18–25
33. Li K, Wu X, Chen DZ, Sonka M (2006) Optimal surface segmentation in volumetric images-a graph-theoretic approach. IEEE Trans Pattern Anal Mach Intell 28:119–134
34. Li XY, Feng DF (2009) Diffuse axonal injury: novel insights into detection and treatment. J Clin Neurosci 16(5):614–619
35. Lundervold A, Storvik G (1995) Segmentation of brain parenchyma and cerebrospinal fluid in multispectral magnetic resonance images. IEEE Trans Med Imaging 14:339–349
36. Brummer ME, Mersereau RM, Eisner RL, Lewine RRJ (1993) Automatic detection of brain contours in MRI data sets. IEEE Trans Med Imaging 12:153–166
37. Martelli A (1972) Edge detection using heuristic search methods. Comput Graph Image Process 1(2):169–182
38. Mcdaniel MA (2005) Big-brained people are smarter: a meta-analysis of the relationship between in vivo brain volume and intelligence. Intelligence 33(4):337–346
39. Meythaler JM, Peduzzi JD, Eleftheriou E, Novack TA (2001) Current concepts: diffuse axonal injury[ndash] associated traumatic brain injury. Arch Phys Med Rehabil 82(10):1461–1471
40. Mitchell JR, Karlik SJ, Lee DH, Fenster A (1994) Computer-assisted identification and quantification of multiple sclerosis lesions in MR imaging volumes in the brain. J Magn Reson Imaging 4(2):197–208

41. Montanari U (1971) On the optimal detection of curves in noisy pictures. Commun ACM 14:335–345
42. Monti E, Pedoia V, Binaghi E, De Benedictis A, Balbi S (2012) Graph based MRI analysis for evaluating the prognostic relevance of longitudinal brain atrophy estimation in post-traumatic diffuse axonal injury. In: proceedings of computatioanl modelling of object presented in images: fondumnentals, methods and application, CompIMAGE, pp 297–302
43. de Morais DF (2006) Clinical application of magnetic resonance (MR) imaging in injured patients with acute traumatic brain injury. Arq Neuropsiquiatr 64:1051–1051
44. Ng K, Mikulis DJ, Glazer J, Kabani N, Till C, Greenberg G, Thompson A, Lazinski D, Agid R, Colella B, Green RE (2008) Magnetic resonance imaging evidence of progression of subacute brain atrophy in moderate to severe traumatic brain injury. Arch Phys Med Rehabil 89(12, Suppl):S35–S44. (<>Special issue on traumatic brain injury from the Toronto Rehabilitation Institute TBI recovery study: patterns, predictors, and mechanisms of recovery plus new directions for treatment research<>)
45. Pannizzo F, Stallmeyer MJB, Friedman J, Jennis RJ, Zabriskie J, Plank C, Zimmerman R, Whalen JP, Cahill PT (1992) Quantitative MRI studies for assessment of multiple sclerosis. Magn Reson Med 24(1):90–99
46. Pedoia V, Binaghi E (2012) Automatic MRI 2D brain segmentation using graph searching technique. Int J Numer Method Biomed Eng (in press)
47. Pedoia V, Binaghi E, Balbi S, De Benedictis A, Monti E, Minotto R (2011) 2d MRI brain segmentation by using feasibility constraints. In: proceedings of the vision and medical image processing, VipIMAGE, pp 251–256
48. Peng Y, Liu R (2010) Object segmentation based on watershed and graph cut. In: 3rd international congress on image and signal processing (CISP), vol 3. pp 1431–1435
49. Pope DL, Parker DL, Clayton PD, Gustafson DE (1985) Left ventricular border recognition using a dynamic search algorithm. Radiology 155:513–518
50. Povlishock J, Katz D (2005) Update of neuropathology and neurological recovery after traumatic brain injury. J Head Trauma Rehabil 20(1):76–94
51. Scheid R, Walther K, Guthke T, Preul C, von Cramon D (2006) Cognitive sequelae of diffuse axonal injury. Arch Neurol 63(3):418–424
52. Robertson IH (2008) Traumatic brain injury: recovery, prediction, and the clinician. Arch Phys Med Rehabil 89(12, Suppl):S1–S2. (<>Special issue on traumatic brain injury from the Toronto Rehabilitation Institute TBI recovery study: patterns, predictors, and mechanisms of recovery plus new directions for treatment research<>)
53. Rother C, Kolmogorov V, Blake A (2004) "Grabcut": interactive foreground extraction using iterated graph cuts. ACM Trans Graph 23(3):309–314
54. Ho S, Bullitt E, Gerig G (2002) Level set evolution with region competition: automatic 3-d segmentation of brain tumors. Proc Int Conf Pattern Recognit 1:523–535
55. Shattuck DW, Leahy RM (2002) Brainsuite: an automated cortical surface identification tool. Med Image Anal 6(2):129–142
56. Shattuck DW, Mirza M, Adisetiyo V, Hojatkashani C, Salamon G, Narr KL, Poldrack RA, Bilder RM, Toga AW (2008) Construction of a 3d probabilistic atlas of human cortical structures. NeuroImage 39(3):1064–1080
57. Shaw NA (2002) The neurophysiology of concussion. Prog Neurobiol 67(4):281–344
58. Smith SM (2002) Fast robust automated brain extraction. Hum Brain Mapp 17(3):143–155
59. Snell JW, Merickel MB, Ortega JM, Goble JC, Brookeman JR, Kassell NF (1994) Segmentation of the brain from 3d mri using a hierarchical active surface template. In: proceedings of the SPIE conference on medical imaging, pp 2–9
60. Song T, Jamshidi M, Lee R, Huang M (2007) A modified probabilistic neural network for partial volume segmentation in brain MR image. IEEE Trans Neural Networks 18(5):1424–1432
61. Sonka M, Hlavac V, Boyle R (1993) Image processing, analysis and machine vision, 3rd edn. Chapman and Hall, London
62. Sonka M, Winniford M, Collins S (1995a) Robust simultaneous detection of coronary borders in complex images. IEEE Trans Med Imaging 14(1):151–161

63. Sonka M, Winniford M, Collins S (1995b) Robust simultaneous detection of coronary borders in complex images. IEEE Trans Med Imaging 14(1):151–161
64. Sonka M, Zhang X, Siebes M, Bissing M, Dejong S, Collins S, McKay C (1995c) Segmentation of intravascular ultrasound images: a knowledge-based approach. IEEE Trans Med Imaging 14(4):719–732
65. Suzuki H, ichiro Toriwaki J (1991) Automatic segmentation of head MRI images by knowledge guided thresholding. Comput Med Imaging Graph 15(4):233–240. (<>NMR image processing and pattern recognition<>)
66. Thedens D, Skorton D, Fleagle S (1990) A three-dimensional graph searching technique for cardiac border detection in sequential images and its application to magnetic resonance image data. In: proceedings of computers in cardiology, pp 57–60
67. Thedens D, Skorton D, Fleagle S (1995) Methods of graph searching for border detection in image sequences with applications to cardiac magnetic resonance imaging. IEEE Trans Med Imaging 14:42–55
68. Tian D, Fan L (2007) A brain MR images segmentation method based on som neural network. In: proceedings of the 1st international conference on bioinformatics and biomedical engineering (ICBBE'07), pp 686–689
69. Wada T, Kuroda K, Yoshida Y, Ogawa A, Endo S (2005) Recovery process of immediate prolonged posttraumatic coma following severe head injury without mass lesions. Neurol Med Chir (Tokyo) 45(12):614–619. (discussion 619–620)
70. Waks A, Tretiak OJ (1990) Recognition of regions in brain sections. Comput Med Imaging Graph 14(5):341–352. (<>Progress in imaging in the neurosciences using microcomputers and workstations<>)
71. Warner MA, Marquez De La Plata C (2010) Assessing spatial relationships between axonal integrity, regional brain volumes, and neuropsychological outcomes after traumatic axonal injury. J Neurotrauma 27(12):2121–2130
72. Cointepas Y, Mangin JF, Garnero L, Poline JB, Benali H (2001) Brain visa: software platform for visualization and analysis of multi-modality brain data. Neuroimage 6:339–349
73. Zhang DQ, Chen SC (2004) A novel kernelized fuzzy c-means algorithm with application in medical image segmentation. Artif Intell Med 32(1):37–50

The Development of a Hybrid Solution to Replacement of Clouds and Shadows in Remote Sensing Images

Ana Carolina Siravenha, Danilo Sousa and Evaldo Pelaes

Abstract Nowadays, many works are dedicated to improve the research results, previously achieved manually, by computational solutions. On light of this, the presented work aims to overcome a common problem in many satellite images, which is the presence of undesirable atmospheric components such as clouds and shadows at the time of scene capture. The presence of such elements hinders the identification of meaningful information for applications like urban and environmental monitoring, exploration of natural resources, etc. Thus, it is presented a new way to perform a hybrid approach toward removal and replacing of these elements. The authors propose a method of regions decomposition using a nonlinear median filter, in order to map regions of structure and texture. These types of regions will explain which method will be applied to region redefinition. At structure region, will be applied the method of inpainting by a smoothing based on DCT, and at texture one, will be applied the exemplar-based texture synthesis. To measure the effectiveness of this proposed technique, a qualitative assessment was presented, at the same time that a discussion about quantitative analysis was made.

Keywords Inpainting · Texture synthesis · Replacement of clouds and shadows

A. C. Siravenha (✉) · D. Sousa · E. Pelaes
Federal University of Para, Belém, Brazil
e-mail: siravenha@ufpa.br

D. Sousa
e-mail: danilofrazao@ufpa.br

E. Pelaes
e-mail: pelaes@ufpa.br

P. Di Giamberardino et al. (eds.), *Computational Modeling of Objects Presented in Images*, Lecture Notes in Computational Vision and Biomechanics 15,
DOI: 10.1007/978-3-319-04039-4_15,

1 Introduction

It is noticeable that remote sensing images are susceptible to the undesirable presence of the atmospheric interferences, such as clouds, hazes and shadows, and that a major precondition for a efficient analysis of soil observation data is the provision of information free from external influences and disturbances. These occurrences are largely present in equatorial and tropical warm-to-hot regions and changes the brightness values of pixels at different levels of saturation, which can corrupt the visual representation of the covered land surface. The presence of such elements affect, in many ways, the image processing in an environmental or urban monitoring, and also the segmentation and/or classification methods that are the mainly responsible for the image information extracting.

Experts worldwide carried out many studies in order to find an effective method to reduce or eliminate the impact of clouds [10, 20]. Algorithms dedicated to the satellite images processing should be robust in the sense that this sort of image usually has large dimensions and large spectral variations (very heterogeneous). In this sense, the encouragement to develop new alternatives for image interpretation and improvement of efficient known techniques is remarkable.

To remove dense clouds and shadows is commonly related the use of reference images or by the estimative of the covered areas. The first strategy can use a multi-temporal analysis [20] or can use another image of the same scene, captured by a different sensor, as a SAR image [10], both aims to replace the region affected by a non-affected area. This technique is also know as substitution. It is a simple way to replace regions, but are mandatory some calibrations and corrections of the images. The differences between the DN it is from factors as atmospheric conditions, sun-target-sensor geometry and soil moisture [9] and the adjustments allow the digital numbers (DN) become equivalent between images. It is important to note that in substitution task, a completely cloud free image cannot be guaranteed, since certain pixels may be hider by clouds in all images used to compose the result.

The estimative of covered area, can also be made by an interpolation method called inpainting [11, 13]. Many methods use derivations of this method in order to fill up some damaged regions or to remove large objects. However, there is evidence that it effectiveness is rather for small or homogeneous regions, because this kind of methods can be regarded as approximation of unknown values within an arrangement of known values [19]. Another method employed to redefine regions is the texture synthesis [12, 15]. Generally working in blocks, reach better results for areas that contains some textural pattern in heterogeneous regions.

Some studies has exploring hybrid solutions, observing both texture synthesis and inpainting effectiveness by Bugeau and Bertalmio [4]. In that investigation, each approach is responsible for redefine the texture and structure regions separately, ensuring images with no interferences and with real textures. Another example of hybrid study in this way were performed by Bertalmio et al. [2].

Inserted into the context of hybrid solutions, this paper presents a novel hybrid approach using inpainting by smoothing based on multidimensional DCT as proposed by Garcia [7] and an exemplar-based texture synthesis as proposed in Criminisi et al. [5]. The structure and texture mapping was based in Vese and Osher [18] through a novelty approach using nonlinear median filter. As noted in literature, to replace the interference located in homogeneous regions will be used the inpainting technique, whilst the texture synthesis will be applied to fill in the spots located at texture regions.

The following sections will present the algorithm developed, Sect. 2, sectioned in four steps: Regions Detection Algorithm (Sect. 2.1), Image Decomposition (Sect. 2.2), Inpainting by Smoothing (Sect. 2.3) and Texture Synthesis (Sect. 2.4).

2 Methodology

2.1 Regions Detection Algorithm

Before apply the filling algorithm, described further, it is important identify the regions that will be processed. The algorithm used in this proposal was first presented in Hau et al. [8] and lately expanded in Siravenha [16]. Here, the different image features are identified and separated into four classes: dense cloud, thin cloud, shadow and not affected area. To this, statistical measures of image average value and standard deviation are computed, and the classification is possible.

Besides, [16] added the capability of shadows detection, was also added two parameters called cp and sp (cloud parameter and shadow parameter, in the order given), increasing the algorithm flexibility. The equation that describes this operation is:

$$m(x,y) = \begin{cases} f(x,y) < sp \times f_{av-sd}, & f(x,y)\varepsilon 0, \\ f_{av-sd} < f(x,y) < f_{av}, & f(x,y)\varepsilon 1, \\ f_m < f(x,y) < cp \times f_{av+sd}, & f(x,y)\varepsilon 2, \\ f(x,y) > cp \times f_{av+sd}, & f(x,y)\varepsilon 3. \end{cases} \tag{1}$$

where $f(x, y)$ is the pixel value, f_{av} is the average value of image pixels, f_{av+sd} is the sum of the average value pixels and the standard deviation value of the image and f_{av-sd} is the subtraction of the average value by the standard deviation pixels.

The region labeled as 0 represents a shadow region, labeled as 1 means region not affected by atmospheric interference, while regions labeled as 2 represents thin clouds, and dense cloud are labeled as 3. For images with multiple bands these labels are assigned if and only if the rule is valid for all bands.

To complete this process, it is applied a morphological opening operation that aims to remove very small objects that can cause mistakes in following steps.

2.2 Image Decomposition

The method proposed by Vese and Osher [18] decomposes an image into two sub-images, each representing the components of structure or texture, thus, a better image redefinition can be made. On the structured part, should be applied the technique of inpainting based on DCT, whilst into texture portions and heterogeneous areas is suitable to use texture synthesis.

The generalized model is defined as:

$$f = u + v, \tag{2}$$

where f is the input image, u is the structure image and v is the texture image. So, given these sub-images one can reconstruct the original image. However, in practice it is observed that the original image can be only approximately reconstructed. The goal of the method is to have a structure image u that preserves all strong edges with smoothed internal regions, and an image v that contains all the texture and noise information.

The method used to construct the structured image u is based on the assumption that u is a $2D$ function and in attempt to minimize this function in the space of all Bounded Variation functions (BV). Functions in BV space are functions whose total variation are limited by some constant value less than infinity. Minimizing u in BV space ensures resulting in a stable image and without infinite values. It should be noted, however, that this space allows for functions which have very large derivatives (although non-infinite), thereby ensuring that strong edges are preserved.

Taking in mind the intuition described above, the minimization problem should logically have two terms. One of them will be the fidelity, responsible for maintaining the difference between f and u small. This term ensure that data of the input image are kept on result. The other one imply a smoothing over u, although not necessarily in all u components. The minimization is computed as [14]:

$$F(u) = \left[\left(\int |\nabla u| \right) + \left(\lambda \int |f - u|^2 \right) \right] dxdy, \tag{3}$$

with $u \in BV$ and ∇ representing the gradient operator. The second term is the data term and the first one is a regularization term to ensure a relatively smooth image. λ is a tuning parameter. As can be seen, this seeks find the optimal u and ignores the v image. The reason is that, in Vese and Osher [18], the authors had considered the v image to be noise, and therefore to be discarded.

There is an unique result to this optimization problem, and methods exist for finding the solution. Noting that $v = f - u$ it is possible to easily modify the above equation to incorporate v:

$$F(u) = \int |\nabla u| + \lambda \int \| v \|^2 dxdy, \tag{4}$$

(still $u \in BV$). Which yields the Euler-Lagrange equation $u = f + \frac{1}{2\lambda}div(\frac{\nabla u}{|\nabla u|})$. Making the right manipulation $v = f - u = -\frac{1}{2\lambda}div(\frac{\nabla u}{|\nabla u|})$. At this point it is useful to break v into its x and y components respectively. It will be denoted as g_1 and g_2, where:

$$g_1 = -\frac{1}{2\lambda}div(\frac{\nabla u_x}{|\nabla u|}) \text{ and } g_2 = -\frac{1}{2\lambda}div(\frac{\nabla u_y}{|\nabla u|}). \quad (5)$$

This allows us to write v as: $v = div\mathbf{g}$ where $\mathbf{g} = (g_1, g_2)$. It can be seen that $g_1^2 + g_2^2 = \frac{1}{2\lambda}$, so that $\| \sqrt{g_1^2 + g_2^2} \| = \frac{1}{2\lambda}$.

This allows us to rewrite v as:

$$v(x, y) = div\mathbf{g} = \partial_x g_1(x, y) + \partial_y g_2(x, y). \quad (6)$$

And leads to the final minimization problem ($u \in BV$):

$$\begin{aligned} G(u, v1, v2) &= \int |\nabla u| + \lambda \int |f - u - \partial_x g_1 \\ &\quad -\partial_y g_2|^2 dxdy + \mu \int \sqrt{g_1^2 + g_w^2} dxdy. \end{aligned} \quad (7)$$

Solving the minimization problem (Eq. 7) yields the Euler-Lagrange equations:

$$u = f - \partial_x g_1 - \partial_y g_2 + \frac{1}{2\lambda}div(\frac{\nabla u}{|\nabla u|}) \quad (8)$$

$$\mu \frac{g_1}{\sqrt{g_1^2 + g_2^2}} = 2\lambda[\frac{\partial}{\partial_x}(u - f) + \partial_{xx}^2 g_1 + \partial_{xy}^2 g_2] \quad (9)$$

$$\mu \frac{g_2}{\sqrt{g_1^2 + g_2^2}} = 2\lambda[\frac{\partial}{\partial_y}(u - f) + \partial_{xy}^2 g_1 + \partial_{yy}^2 g_2] \quad (10)$$

2.3 *Inpainting by Smoothing Based on Multidimensional DCT*

This method was proposed by Garcia [7], and so as in Bertalmio et al. [1], is based on the information propagation by smoothing. The specificity of this approach is related to the use of the Discrete Cosine Transform (DCT) to simplify and to solve linear systems, to an efficient smoothing.

2.3.1 Smoothing by Penalized Least Squares Regression

In statistics and data analysis, smoothing is used to reduce experimental noise or information and keeping the most important marks of the data set. Considering the following model for the one-dimensional noisy signal y from the Eq. 11.

$$y = \hat{y} + \varepsilon, \tag{11}$$

where ε represents a Gaussian noise with zero mean and unknown variance, and $\hat{y}$ is the so-called smoothing, i.e., has continuous derivatives up to some order (usually ≥ 2) throughout the domain. The smoothing of y depends on the best estimate of $\hat{y}$ and this operation is usually performed by a parametric or nonparametric regression.

A classic approach to smooth is the Penalized Least Squares Regression. This technique minimizes a criterion that balances the data fidelity, measured by the Residual Sum-of-Squares (RSS) and by a penalty term (P), which reflects the robustness of the smoothed data. Another simple and straightforward approach to express the robustness is by using a Second-order Divided Difference ($SoDD$), which produces an one-dimensional array of data.

Now, using RSS and the $SoDD$, the minimization of $F(\hat{y})$ results in a linear system, expressed in Eq. 12, which allows the smoothed data determination.

$$(I_n + sD^T D)\hat{y} = y, \tag{12}$$

where I_n is the identity matrix $n \times n$, s is a positive real scalar that controls the grade of smoothing, so that, as it increases, the degree of smoothing of $\hat{y}$ increases too; and D^T represents the transpose of D. Its important to note that $(I_n + sD^T D)$ is a penta-diagonal symmetric matrix, and the last equation can be solved numerically in a computationally efficient way.

2.3.2 Smoothing Equally Spaced Data

Equation 12 can be solved using the left division matrix applied to sparse matrices [7]. Solving this linear system, however, can be a lot of time expensive for a large amount of data. But, this algorithm can be simplified and accelerated, since the data are evenly spaced, in images where pixels are equally spaced, resulting in the following equation for multidimensional data:

$$\hat{y} = IDCT(\Gamma DCT(y)), \tag{13}$$

where *DCT* and *IDCT* refer to the Discrete Cosine Transform and its inverse, respectively. Γ is represented by:

$$\Gamma_{i,j} = [1 + s(2 - 2\cos((i-1)\pi/n))^2]^{-1}. \tag{14}$$

It is more convenient to use an algorithm based on Eq. 13, instead of Eq. 12, when the data are equidistant. DCT has a computational complexity of $O(n\log(n))$, while Eq. 12, which requires a Cholesky factorization, has computational complexity of $O(n^3)$.

As described in Garcia [7], the task of smoothing can be performed by an multi-dimensional iterative process to ensure greater convergence of the process, as shown in Eq. 15.

$$\hat{y}_{k+1} = IDCTN(\Gamma^N \circ DCTN(y_k)). \tag{15}$$

where $DCTN$ and $IDCTN$ refers to the N-dimensional DCT and its inverse, respectively. k is the number of iterations, N is the number of dimensions, $\circ$ is the Schur product (element by element) and Γ^n represents a tensor of rank N defined by:

$$\Gamma^n = 1^N \div (1^N + s \wedge^n \circ \wedge^n). \tag{16}$$

Here, the operator $\div$ symbolizes the division element by element, and 1^N is a tensor of rank N composed by 1's. $\wedge$ is the following tensor of rank N [3]:

$$\wedge^N_{i_1,\ldots,si_N} = \sum_{j=1}^{N} \left(-2 + 2\cos\frac{(i_j - 1)\pi}{n_j} \right), \tag{17}$$

where n_j denotes the size of $\wedge^n$ along the $j - th$ dimension.

Can also be observed that when there are undefined values in the image, smoothing is also responsible for interpolation of data, functioning as an inpainting method. In order to accelerate the convergence, the process starts performing nearest neighbor interpolation on the image to be restored.

Summarizing, for the inpainting performing in this work, initially is applied the nearest neighbor interpolation, following is used iteratively the Eq. 15 for two-dimensional data, i.e., $N = 2$. The smoothing parameter is set at 3, for which we obtain better results, as proposed in Garcia [7], where can be seen more details about technique explanation.

2.4 Texture Synthesis

The texture synthesis has been an intensive field of study because its purpose variety. It can be applied in objects fill-in tasks, image recovery, video compression, foreground removal and others. In the computational literature, the classes that one can describe the texture are regular and stochastic. Regular texture is composed by elements that are repeated in a region, whilst in stochastic textures there aren't repeated texture elements. However, in general, in a real application, the textures are located in a middle region between this classes and should be represented in just one model, which is an important question in this field.

One can define texture as a visual pattern in a $2D$ infinite plan that, at some scale, has a steady distribution, then, naturally, one can obtain a finite sample of textures present in this plan in order to synthesize other samples from the same texture. This finite sample can be extracted from an uncountable different textures, and it is an

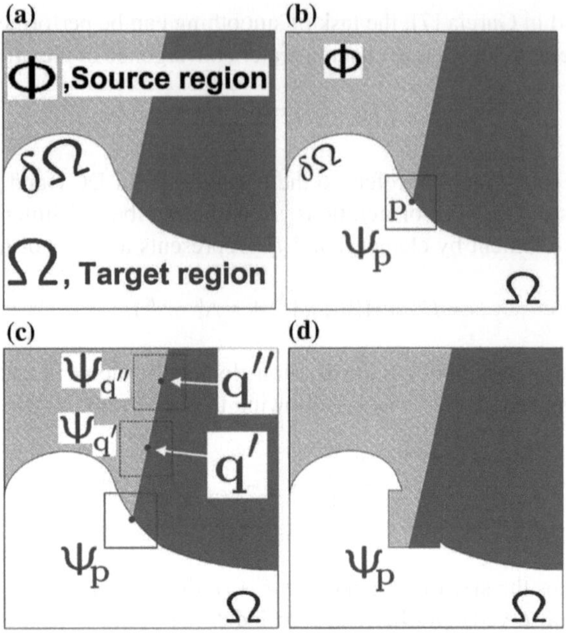

Fig. 1 Model based texture synthesis. **a** Original image. **b** Ψ_p fragment centralized in $p \in \Phi$. **c** The most probable candidates $\Psi_{q'}$ e Ψ_q''. **d** The most probable candidate is propagated to the target fragment

ill-posed situation. To contour this, the assumption is that the sample is larger enough to capture the textural stead distribution of the image where the texture elements scale is known [6]. Furthermore, the texture synthesis is responsible for merging continuous regions with minimal imperfection and perception of the operation, ensuring the visual quality.

The approach proposed by Criminisi et al. [5], aims to remove or redefine larges objects in a digital image with the neighborhood information. This method uses the texture synthesis to fill in regions that contains two-dimensional textural patterns with moderated stochasticity. For this, generates new sampling textures from a source image and make a simple copy to the target areas.

In Fig. 1, is presented the Criminisi [5] algorithm for texture synthesis, in a simplified form. Suppose an image where there is a target region (Ω) contoured by $\delta\Omega$ and completed by a source region Φ, clearly distinguishable (Fig. 1a). The objective is synthesize the area delimited by the fragment named Ψ_p, which is centralized on the $p \in \Phi$ point, illustrated in Fig. 1b. Then, it is counted the most probable candidates to fill Ψ_p presented in $\delta\Omega$, for example $\Psi_{q'}$ and Ψ_q'' in Fig. 1c. Among the candidates, there is one that has the better corresponding to the target fragment, and this candidates is copied to the Ψ_p fragment. This process is repeated until the full fill of Ω. In Fig. 1d can be noted that the texture, as well the structure (the line that apart the light and dark gray regions), are propagated to the Ψ_p fragment.

Fig. 2 Notation diagram of an image and its components according the synthesis texture

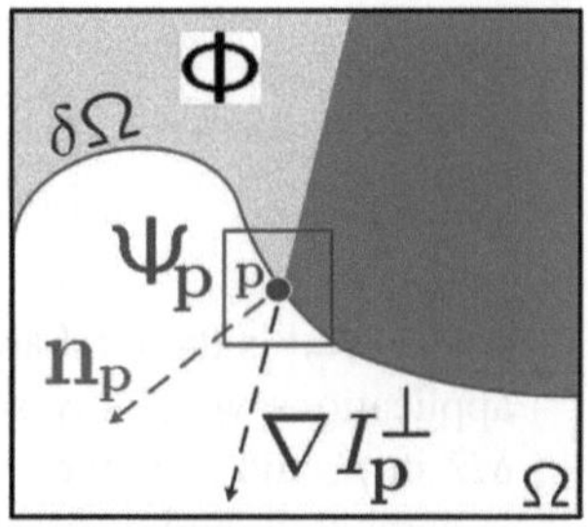

The fill in order is influenced by the linear structures adjacent from the target region. Thus, the model based texture synthesis algorithm with propagation along the isophotes direction of the image, presents efficiency and qualitative performance respecting the restrictions imposed by the linear structures.

2.4.1 Fill in Regions Algorithm

Taking a source image with a target region Ω to be redefined and a source region Φ, that can be expressed as the subtraction of the image f by the target region ($\Phi = f - \Omega$), one must define the window size to the model called Ψ. It is very common use a window with 9×9 dimension, but it is recommended that the size are lager than the biggest distinguishable textural element in the source region.

In this algorithm, each pixel maintain a color value (or NaN, if is an undefined pixel to be filled) and a confidence value, which reflects the confidence in the color value since the pixel is filled [5]. During the algorithm execution, the fragments located in $\delta\Omega$ contour receive temporary priority value, defining the order to be filled. Hence, an interactive process is executed in the following sequence:

(1) *Computing fragments priority*: Because the texture synthesis works with priorities, the strategy called *best-first* fill in the regions according the priority levels and becomes tendentiously to the regions that a) are on strong continuity borders or b) are surrounded by high confidence pixels.

The Fig. 2 shows an image to be processed, and given the fragment Ψ_p, n_p is the normal to the contour $\delta\Omega$ of the target region and $\nabla I_p^{\perp}$ is the isophote at point p. The isophote represents the direction and intensity in that point.

The priority ($P(p)$) is defined as a product of the confidence term ($C(p)$) and the data terms ($D(p)$), that are defined as:

$$C(p) = \frac{\sum_{q \in \Psi_p \bigcap (f-\Omega)} C(q)}{|\Psi_p|} \tag{18}$$

and

$$D(p) = \frac{|\nabla I_p^{\perp} \cdot n_p|}{\alpha}, \tag{19}$$

where $|\Psi_p|$ is the total area of Ψ_p, α is the normalization factor (255 in typical applications with gray scale images), n_p is an unit vector orthogonal to the $\delta\Omega$ in p, and $\perp$ is the orthogonal operator. For each border fragment a $P(p)$ is computed, and every distinct pixel represents a fragment on a target region border. During the initialization, taking the $C(p)$ equals to 0 for all point p in the target region and $C(p)$ equals to 1 for all point in source region.

The confidence represents the measure of trusted information surrounding a pixel. Thus, the algorithm aims to fill, firstly, those most reliable fragments, including those with more redefined pixels or fragments whose pixels were never part of the target region.

The $D(p)$ term defines the isophotes strength on $\delta\Omega$ in every iteration and it is responsible by increases the confidence of the linear structures, making a safely filling.

(2) *Structure and texture spread informations*: Once the priorities are computed, the $\Psi_{\hat{p}}$ high confidence fragment is found and filled by the information extracted from Φ source region more similar to that region. Formally

$$\arg \min_{\Psi_q \in \Phi} d(\Psi_{\hat{p}}, \Psi_q), \tag{20}$$

where the distance $(d(\ldots))$ between fragments Ψ_a and Ψ_b is defined as a Sum of Squared Differences (SSD) of the pixels that contains information in these fragments (possible already filled pixels). The ideal fragment to fill in one region is that one who minimizes the SSD.

Having found the source model, every pixel value $(p'|p' \in \Psi_{\hat{p}\cap\Omega})$ is copied to the correspondent target region inside $\Psi_{\hat{q}}$.

(3) *Updating the confidence values*: After $\Psi_{\hat{p}}$ receive this new values it is redefined the confidence values

$$C(p) = C(\hat{p}) \forall p \in \Psi_{\hat{p}} \cap \Omega. \tag{21}$$

This simple rule to update the confidence values allows the measure of the relative confidence even without any specific image information. It is expected that the confidence values decay during the filling process, this indicates there are less assurance about the pixels color values that are near the center of the target region.

2.4.2 Implementation Proposed in this Work

In this study was not used the addition of each component obtained above (Sect. 2.2), since this approach results in considerable error generated at the image reconstruction and also due to the difficulty in establishing appropriate parameters for an acceptable image decomposition. Instead, a strategy was proposed for mapping structure and texture areas of an image based on the decomposition process.

This process begins transforming the component that contains the texture information, i.e. image v, in a binary image with values 1 for texture heterogeneous areas and 0 for structure areas. Then a nonlinear median filter is applied to make homogeneous (smoothed) areas where small gaps of a given feature are surrounded by predominant regions of another sort. The threshold is defined according the mask (kernel, a square matrix) used in the filter and it will change for each image in an empirical way, depending on the image analyst decision.

This step is critical due to the presence of clouds and shadows in the image, and is performed in order to correctly define the techniques to be employed for each region. This happens because clouds and shadows will always be structure components, so to define which technique use to remove them, one must observe the surrounding regions. Therefore, as a result of application of the filter, those regions to be redefined are mapped in the binary image to the texture or structure regions, to finally apply inpainting or texture synthesis on the input image, respectively.

3 Results and Discussions

A major problem in literature is the lack of quantitative evaluation methods for inpainting algorithms. Along this work was tested the evaluation measures PSNR (local and global), Kappa and the Sum of Absolute Differences (SAD). It was concluded that none of them appropriately evaluate different approaches to redefine regions. For example, certain results from hybrid approach, and even just using texture synthesis, visually performs a region filling which appears more consistently than those resulting from inpainting (sometimes showing large blurs). However, looking to the quantitative evaluations cited, it is common that the inpainting approach achieve better results.

According Taschler [17], the only explanation for this discrepancy is that the texture synthesis can reach more faithful results to the goal, but some elements are not located at the corresponding position in the reference image, i.e., if the difference is one or two pixels, it's led to a lower PSNR value for the entire region. Another explanation can be given because these metrics and inpainting are pixel-by-pixel performed, while texture synthesis commonly is block-by-block, taking some disadvantage in evaluation.

With regards to qualitative assessment, Fig. 3a has an image affected by the presence of dense clouds and shadows over texture (urban) and structure (dense vegetation) areas. In Fig. 3b is illustrated a red mask containing these regions to be

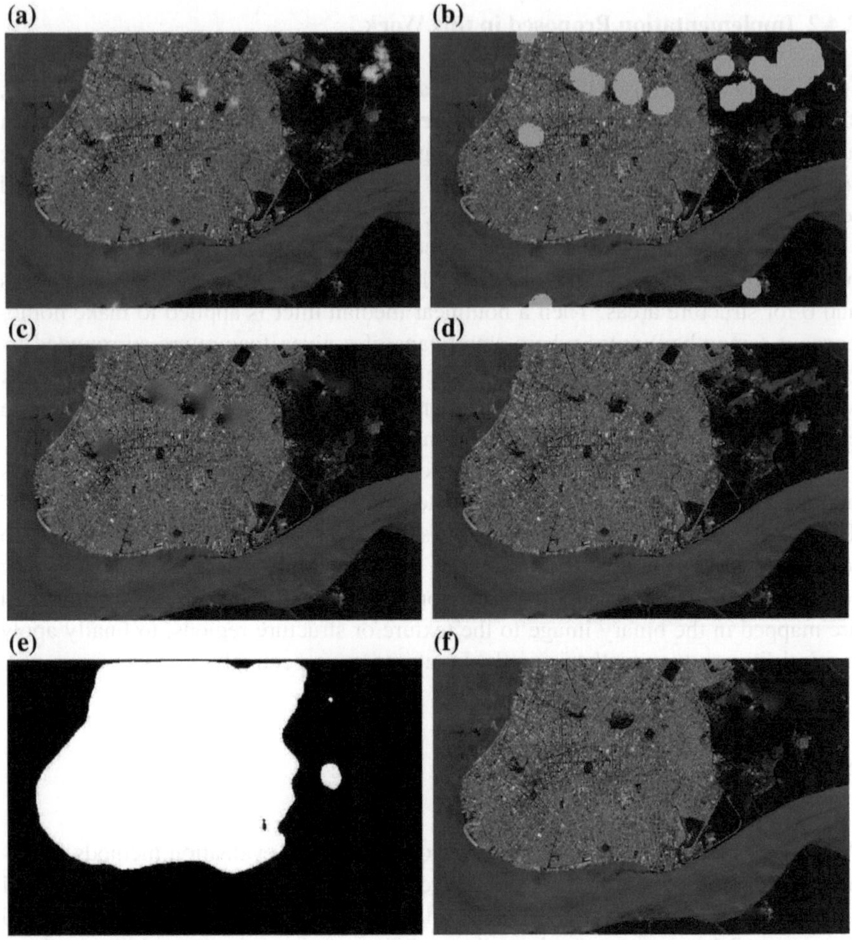

Fig. 3 Process of clouds and shadows removal applied over an image of the city of Belém-Brazil. **a** Original image. **b** Mask from regions detection. **c** Inpainting result. **d** Texture synthesis result. **e** Binary image representing proposed image decomposition. **f** Proposed hybrid approach results

redefined. This mask was produced by the algorithm cited in Sect. 2.1. The Fig. 3c, d shows the isolated results of inpainting and texture synthesis, respectively. As previously discussed are visible blurs generated by smoothing performed in urban areas (Fig. 3c) and the erroneous replacement of the texture synthesis in areas of dense vegetation (Fig. 3d). From these results, then it is decided to apply the hybrid approach. Fig. 3e shows a binary image after passing v image through the median filter, containing texture (white) and structure (black) regions. From this mapping, Fig. 3f shows the hybrid approach result, where becomes clear the union of advantages of the techniques applied in suitable regions thereof, thereby visually overcoming other methods.

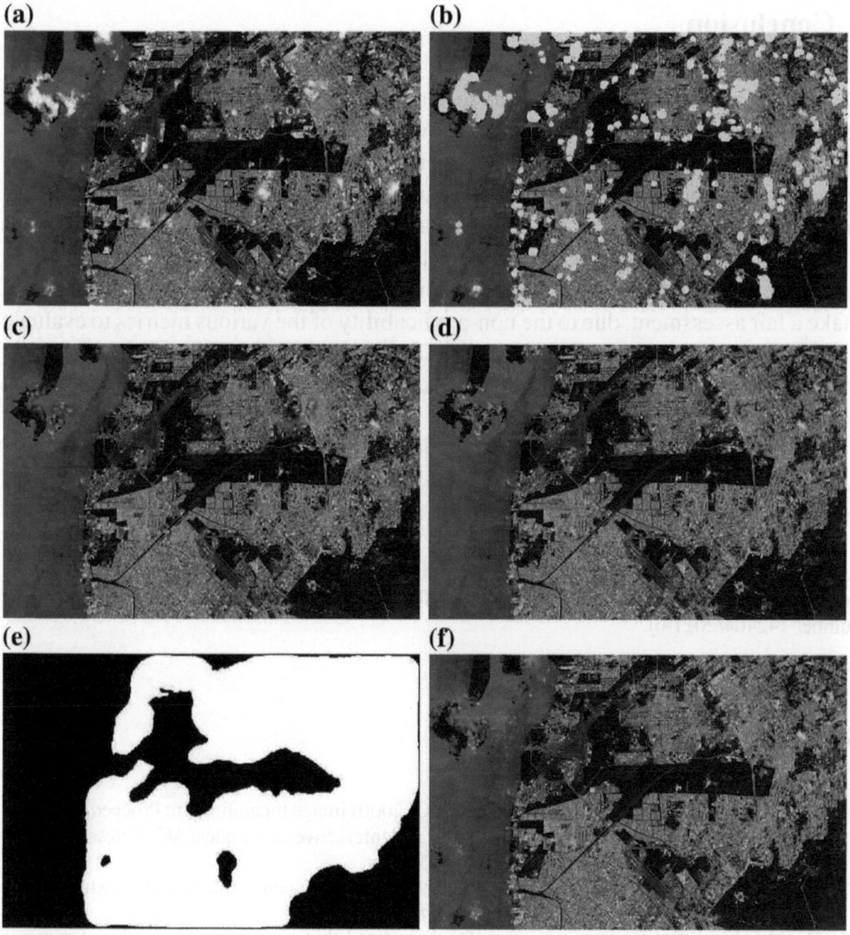

Fig. 4 Process of clouds and shadows removal over another image of Pará-Brazil. **a** Original image. **b** Mask from regions detection. **c** Inpainting result. **d** Texture synthesis result. **e** Binary image representing proposed image decomposition. **f** Proposed hybrid approach results

Following the qualitative assessment, the Fig. 4a has another image from the same region, but captured by other kind of sensor, that also is affected by the presence of dense clouds and shadows over texture (urban) and structure (dense vegetation) areas and in Fig. 4b is illustrated a red mask with the regions to be redefined. As previously, in the Figs. 4c, d are shows the isolated results of inpainting and texture synthesis, respectively. As previously discussed are visible blurs generated by smoothing performed in urban areas and unreal textures on another areas. The Fig. 4f, preceded by the image with binary image (Fig. 4e), shows the hybrid result of this image, clarifying the effectiveness of the proposed method.

4 Conclusion

This work aimed to present a new way to perform a hybrid approach toward detection, removal and replacing of clouds and shadows areas in satellite images. The approach proposes a regions decomposition method using a nonlinear median filter in order to map structure and texture regions, where was be applied the methods inpainting by smoothing based on DCT and exemplar-based texture synthesis, respectively.

In qualitative evaluation was evident that the hybrid approach overcomes the use of the techniques in a separated way. In the quantitative tests was not possible to make a fair assessment, due to the non-applicability of the various metrics to evaluate different approaches to redefine regions. Like as in Fig. 3, when applied to the other images, the hybrid method overcome the isolated approaches and due the free-space available these results was omitted.

Actually, we are interested in use quantitative approaches with a more reasonable justification, using not only information of pixel value, but also the context, shape and other attributes that are similar to the subjective evaluation of human eyes.

Acknowledgments This work was supported by the Amazon Research Foundation/Vale S/A [grant number 021/2010]; and the National Council of Technological and Scientific Development [grant number 142404/2011-0].

References

1. Bertalmio M, Sapiro G, Caselles V, Ballester C (2000) Image inpainting. In: Proceedings of the 27th annual conference on computer graphics and interactive techniques. ACM Press/Addison-Wesley Publishing Co, New York, pp 417–424
2. Bertalmio M, Vese L, Sapiro G, Osher S (2003) Simultaneous structure and texture image inpainting. IEEE Trans Image Process 12(8):882–889
3. Buckley M (1994) Fast computation of a discretized thin-plate smoothing spline for image data. Oxf Biometrika 81:247–258
4. Bugeau A, Bertalmio M (2009) Combining texture synthesis and diffusion for image inpainting. In: Ranchordas A, Araújo H (eds) VISAPP 2009—Proceedings of the fourth international conference on computer vision theory and applications, vol 1. INSTICC Press, Lisboa, pp 26–33
5. Criminisi A, Perez P, Toyama K (2004) Region filling and object removal by exemplar-based image inpainting. IEEE Trans On Image Process 13(9):1200–1212, IEEE Computer Society
6. Efros A, Leung T (1999) Texture synthesis by non-parametric sampling. In: International conference on computer vision. IEEE Computer Society, Washington, pp 1033–1038
7. Garcia D (2010) Robust smoothing of gridded data in one and higher dimensions with missing values. Comput Stat Data Anal 54(4):1167–1178 (Elsevier, Maryland Heights)
8. Hau CY, Liu CH, Chou TY, Yang LS (2008) The efficacy of semi-automatic classification result by using different cloud detection and diminution method. The international archives of the photogrammetry, remote sensing and spatial information sciences
9. Helmer E, Ruefenacht B (2005) Cloud-free satellite images mosaics with regression trees and histgram matching. Photogram Eng Remote Sens 32(9):1079–1089
10. Hoan NT, Tateishi R (2008) Cloud removal of optical image using SAR data for ALOS applications. Experimenting on simulated ALOS data. The international archives of the photogrammetry, remote sensing and spatial information sciences, Beijing

11. Liu H, Wang W, Bi X (2010) Study of image inpainting based on learning. In: proceedings of the international multi conference of engineers and computer scientists. Newswood Limited, Hong Kong, pp 1442–1445
12. Liu Y, Wong A, Fieguth P (2010) Remote sensing image synthesis. In: Geoscience and remote sensing symposium (IGARSS). IEEE International, Honolulu, pp 2467–2470
13. Maalouf A, Carre P, Augereau B, Fernandez Maloigne C (2009) A bandelet-based inpainting technique for clouds removal from remotely sensed images. IEEE Trans Geosci Remote Sens 47(7):2363–2371
14. Rudin LI, Osher S, Fatemi E (1992) North-Holland nonlinear total variation based noise removal algorithms. Phys D 60:259–268
15. Sarkar S, Healey G (2010) Hyperspectral texture synthesis using histogram and power spectral density matching. IEEE Trans Geosci Remote Sens 48(5):2261–2270
16. Siravenha A (2011) Um método para classificação de imagens de satélite usando Transformada Cosseno Discreta com detecção e remoção de nuvens e sombras. Universidade Federal do Pará, In Dissertação de mestrado
17. Taschler M (2006) A comparative analysis of image inpainting techniques. Technical report. The University of York, New York
18. Vese LA, Osher SJ (2002) Modeling textures with total variation minimization and oscillating patterns in image processing. J Sci Comput 19:553–572 (Plenum Press, New York)
19. Webster R, Oliver M (2007) Geostatistics for environmental scientists, 2nd edn. Wiley, West Sussex
20. Zhang X, Qin F, Qin Y (2010) Study on the thick cloud removal method based on multi-temporal remote sensing images. In: Conference international on multimedia technology (ICMT). IEEE, Ningbo, pp 1–3

Echocardiographic Image Processing

Massimiliano Pedone

Abstract The image sequences elaboration, which represent our main topic, concerns the identification of contours of an object for segmentation and study of its movement over time. A newer dynamic approach to the well-known static variational method for the time-series medical echocardiographic images is presented, and a graphic software applications for synchronization between cardiac movement and electric signals (ECG) are developed. Many approaches have been proposed to process time-series of digital images, and it is difficult establish the most effective one. Here we focus on PDE-based and variational methods. The first is based on snake model for image segmentation and the second by Mumford-Shah (M-S) Functional minimization for image enhancing and a new dinamic approach for movie processing.

1 Ventricular Area Recognition

Our pourposes is the automatic detection of the internal area of the ventricular cavity from echocardiographics images. This suggest us to perform the curve evolution as an initial value problem.

A typical results that represent our goal is presented in the Fig. 1.

In the next part we focus the attention concerning the choice of the filter function for the edge-detection and the related applicability of the speed term formulation in the continuous model problem.

M. Pedone (✉)
Sapienza University of Rome, P.le Aldo Moro, 5, Rome, Italy
e-mail: massimiliano.pedone@uniroma1.it

P. Di Giamberardino et al. (eds.), *Computational Modeling of Objects Presented in Images*, Lecture Notes in Computational Vision and Biomechanics 15,
DOI: 10.1007/978-3-319-04039-4_16,

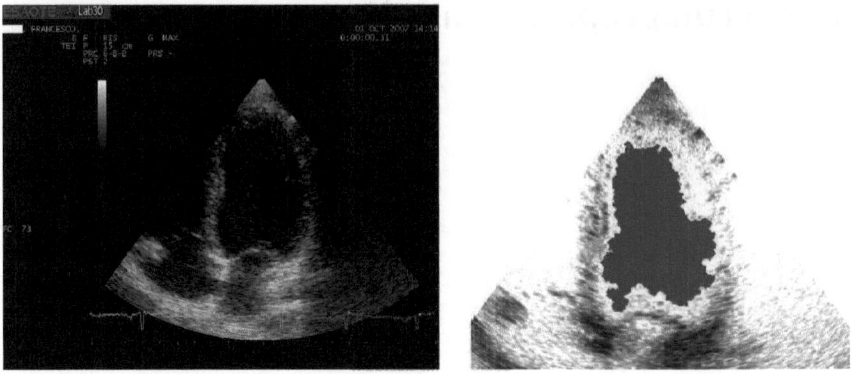

Fig. 1 Echocardiographic frame and its recognized Area

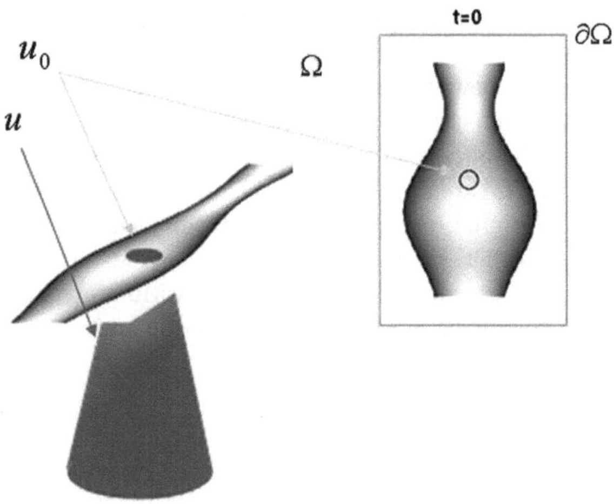

Fig. 2 Curve at isolevel at $t = 0$

1.1 The Segmentation Problem

The aim of segmentation is to find a partition of an image into its costituent parts. For front evolution the *level—set* standard model is adopted [1–3](Fig. 2).

A curve in $\mathbb{R}^2$ can be represented as the zero-level line of a function in higher dimension. More precisely, let us suppose that there exists a function $u : \mathbb{R}^2 \times \mathbb{R}^+ \rightarrow \mathbb{R}$ solution of the initial value problem:

$$\begin{cases} u_t(x,t) - g_I(x)|\nabla u(x,t)| = 0 & x \in \Omega,\ t \geq 0 \\ u(x,0) = u_0(x) & x \in \Omega \end{cases} \tag{1}$$

which is the model of **eikonal equation for front evolution** for segmentation problem, typically involved in the detection for edges of objects contained in an image. We have to note that the evolving function $u(x, t)$ always remains a function as long as g_I is smooth. So we choose a different expression for the speed terms in order to limit the loss of image definition of Gaussian smoothing and by new approach with functional minimization to preserve this property. For ours purposes we intend enough smooth a function $C^2(\Omega)$, [4–12].

1.2 Edge-Detection

Given an image, in particular an echocardiographic image, we need to automatically detect the internal contour of object for clinical pourposes. We focus ours attention to a ventricular cavity. We consider a closed subset Ω of $\mathbb{R}^2$, having $\partial\Omega$ as the external edge of the rectangular image and being $I : \Omega \to [0, 1]$ the brightness intensity. The "edge-detector" (detector of contours) for segmentation of the image is a positive real coefficient, which is dependent of $I(x)$'s gradient at every point of the curve [2, 13].

In particular, the model is represented by a filter function such that

$$g : \mathbb{R}^+ \longrightarrow \mathbb{R}^+$$

where

$$g(z) = \frac{1}{1 + z}$$

decreasing with z and

$$\lim_{z \to \infty} g(z) = 0$$

such that $0 \leqslant g$ and $g(0) = 1$.

1.3 Speed Choice for Image Processing

The speed term is dependent of the brightness intensity at every pixel and is directed along the outward normal, starting from an initial elliptic profile E centered in Ω.

Insofar we define the composite function

$$g_I(|\nabla I(x)|) = g(|\nabla(G_\sigma * I(x))|) = \frac{1}{1 + |\nabla(G_\sigma * I(x))|}, \tag{2}$$

where $G_\sigma * I(x)$ is the convolution of the image $I(x)$ with a regularizing operator G_σ whose algorithmic implementation we are going to explicit later. The operator G_σ

is a filter that allows, by heat equation, to calculate the brightness-intensity gradient of the image in the presence of discontinuous data.

The discretization of the problem is performed by building a rectangular lattice, which is made fine-grained according to image's pixel definition. The curve is parametrized by means of a Lipschitz function. Therefore, the differential problem to be numerically solved will look as follows:

Considering the built-in function $u_0(x)$ such that $E = \{x \in \mathbb{R}^2 : u_0(x) = 0\}$

$$\begin{cases} u_t - g_I(|\nabla I(x)|)|\nabla u| = 0 & x \in \Omega \subset \mathbb{R}^2 \times [0, T] \\ u(x, 0) = u_0(x) & x \in \Omega \subset \mathbb{R}^2 \end{cases} \tag{3}$$

where T is the time horizon.

In the numerical tests the algorithm predicts a stop of the evolving curve at a threshold value th for the speed term, such that, if $g_I(x) \leqslant th \Rightarrow g_I(x) = 0$, then the threshold parameter allows curve evolution to stop in the presence of different gradient values for the regularized image.

2 New Approach to Regularize and Enhance Image

Analysis of images through variational methods finds application in a number of fields such as robotics, elaboration of satellite data, biomedical analysis and many other real-life cases. By segmentation is meant a search for constituent parts of an image, rather than an improving of its quality or characteristics. Our aim is to develop a criterium for enhancing movie frame in two possible ways by functional minimization. First, we adopt the M-S functional and its approximated form proposed by Ambrosio and Tortorelli [14] to regularize data frame for curve evolution method, instead of Gaussian regularization.

We call it "classic functional" since the function space the variational integral converges over contains functions that have the regularity needed for image gradient calculus. Second, we present a numerical scheme, where a time-dependent parameter is inserted, precisely in the second integral part of functional distinguished by a "time gradient", for enhancing the internal moving parts of the object.

A detailed analytical treatment and a numerical scheme for minimization of the functional, which involves some delicate conjectures and refined mathematical steps, can be found in [15]. In the following section we recall in brief the essential formulation of the model problem used to regularize and enhance image. Other particular on numerical approximation and function space are explained in the next parts and in references. The reader can look up, for a complete review, the book by Morel and Solimini[16].

2.1 Ambrosio-Tortorelli Algorithm ('90)

This section refers to M-S algorithm for the approximation of $F(u, K)$ with a sequence F_ε of regular functionals defined on a Sobolev space. We focus our attention on the Ambrosio-Tortorelli approximation, which is among the most used in image analysis. In this particular approach, the set K (or S_u) is replaced by an auxiliary variable S (a function) which approximates the characteristic function $(1 - \chi_K)$.

$$F_\varepsilon(u, S) = \int_\Omega (u-g)^2\,dx + \int_\Omega S^2 \mid \nabla u \mid^2 dx \quad + \int_\Omega \left(\varepsilon \mid \nabla S \mid^2 + \frac{1}{4\varepsilon}(1-S)^2 \right) dx$$

If $(u_\varepsilon, S_\varepsilon)$ minimizes the functional F_ε, then the following result holds [14]:

$$u_\varepsilon \xrightarrow{\mathscr{L}^2} u \ \text{ ed } S_\varepsilon \longrightarrow 1 - \chi_K \ \text{ per } \varepsilon \longrightarrow 0^+$$

We gather from the problem of minimun related to the Ambrosio-Tortorelli functional, the Euler equations, than by an appropriate approximation will give us an algorithm for minimization.

When we apply Euler equation system, if $u_0 = g$ is chosen, an enough rapid continuation method will give good results even though contours are not well defined.

2.2 Euler Equation of the Approximated Functional

Given

$$\int_\Omega \psi(u, \nabla u)dx,$$

the associated Euler equation is

$$div\left(\nabla_\xi \psi(u, \nabla u)\right) - \left(\frac{\partial \psi}{\partial u}\right) = 0.$$

Using Neumann boundary conditions, we get:

$$F(u) = \mu \int_\Omega (u-g)^2 + \int_\Omega (S^2 + K_\varepsilon) \mid \nabla u \mid^2 dx \quad + \alpha \int_\Omega \left(\varepsilon \mid \nabla S \mid^2 + \frac{1}{4\varepsilon}(1-S)^2 \right) dx.$$

Euler equation system for u, considering that the quadratic gradient $2(S^2 + K_\varepsilon)\nabla u^2$ is transformed into the Laplacian, looks as follows:

$$\begin{cases} div(2(S^2 + K_\varepsilon)\nabla u) = \mu(u-g) & \frac{\partial u}{\partial \mathbf{n}} = 0 \ \text{ in } \partial\Omega \\ \alpha\varepsilon\Delta S = S \mid \nabla u \mid^2 - \frac{\alpha}{4\varepsilon}(1-S) & \frac{\partial S}{\partial \mathbf{n}} = 0 \ \text{ in } \partial\Omega \end{cases}$$

where the non linear terms S^2 and ∇u cause the system to be non-linear and elliptic, with such a structure that, when S is known, the first equation gets linear, while, if it is u to be known, it is the second equation to be linear. This suggests the adoption of a two-stage iterative scheme. Where we fix the discrete step of convergence that is enough to give back a regularized image, enhanced in its content edge, as we present in the next section.

3 Approximation of the Models

We are going to describe, in this section, the numerical approximation of the models introduced above. In details, our aim is to present the semilagrangian scheme for curve evolution by numerical solution of eikonal equation. The standard mollifier is constructed by a Gaussian operator as a numerical scheme for heat eqution in two dimensions. The last section reports the procedure to build the approximation of the Mumford-Shah functional by Ambrosio-Tortorelli scheme.

3.1 Semi-Lagrangian Scheme for Eikonal Equation

Semi-Lagrangian (SL) schemes try to mimic the continuous behavior by constructing the solution at each grid point by back integration along the characteristic trajectory passing through the point and reconstructing the value at the foot of the trajectory by interpolation.

The numeric dependence of the domain contains its continuous dependence without any additional condition on Δt and Δx (space lattice is usually defined for finite differences as the pixel resolution of images). This allow a larger time steps than other schemes where the CFL condition has to be imposed for stability guaranty.

The numerical method for eq. (3) following the semilagrangian scheme by [17]. In our implementation we use a threshold value that has been chosen and discussed in a Master thesis [18].

We construct the protocol step of curve evolution by an oriented adaptation to medical application of HJPACK parallel OpenMp Fortran programming language.

3.2 Ambrosio-Tortorelli Approximation of the M-S Functional

The numerical scheme is made by dividing in two coupled parts with $u_0 = g$ and $S_0 = 1$.

At every step we calculate u_1 for $S_0 = 1$ solving a linear elliptic equation and, this way, we find S_1 from the second equation; this process is repeated for a fixed number of iterations.

3.2.1 System Discretization

We use a numerical scheme based on explicit finite differences, over the rectangle Ω with step h; this way we obtain $(x, y) = (ih, jh)$ for $0 \leqslant i, j \leqslant N$. Reducing Ω to a square of side 1 and taking $h = \frac{1}{N}$, discrete coordinates will become: $u(ih, jh) \cong u_{i,j}$ and $S(ih, jh) \cong S_{i,j}$.

We use an approximated scheme that is enough to enhancing little areas, characteristic of the echographic image. Some scheme for the Ambrosio-Tortorelli segmentation problem [19].

In order to determine the minimum of the functional we adopt the schema given, for a finite element, in [20] to a finite difference meshgrid through the following iterative scheme:
given a maximum number of iteration Nit and a tolerance 'ε, then we construct:

- $S_0 = 1, u_0 = g$
- for $n = 1, 2, ...,$ Nit find u_n, by solving:

$$\begin{cases} div(2(S_{n-1}^2 + K_\varepsilon)\nabla u_n) = \mu(u_n - g) & \text{in } \Omega \\ \frac{\partial u_n}{\partial \mathbf{n}} = 0 & \text{in } \partial\Omega \end{cases}$$

and S_n by solving:

$$\begin{cases} \alpha\varepsilon\Delta S_n = S_n \mid \nabla u_n \mid^2 - \frac{\alpha}{4\varepsilon}(1 - S_n) & \text{in } \Omega \\ \frac{\partial S_n}{\partial \mathbf{n}} = 0 & \text{in } \partial\Omega \end{cases}$$

- stop for $n = Nit$.

From minimization theorem 3.1 Proposition 2.1 [20], it respectively follows that:
S_u is a piecewise C^2 submanifolds of $\mathbb{R}^2$.

For any $n > 1$ there exists u_n an S_n solution of the respective system which satisfy the bounds:

$$\|u_n\|_{L^\infty} \leq \|g\|_{L^\infty}.$$

Then we discretize the equations by finite differences.

3.2.2 The Discreet Divergence

In a numerical scheme a function $u \in \mathbb{R}^2$ can be approximated by finite difference, its first order variation on the x direction is:

$$\frac{\partial u}{\partial x} \cong \frac{u_{i+1,j} - u_{i,j}}{h}$$

and for y direction is:

$$\frac{\partial u}{\partial y} \cong \frac{u_{i,j+1} - u_{i,j}}{h}.$$

The divergence of a function $Z(x, y)$ by second order of centered difference is given by

$$div(Z(x, y)\nabla u(x, y)) \cong$$

$$\cong Z_{i+\frac{1}{2},j}(u_{i+1,j} - u_{i,j}) - Z_{i-\frac{1}{2},j}(u_{i,j} - u_{i-1,j})$$

$$+ Z_{i,j+\frac{1}{2}}(u_{i,j+1} - u_{i,j}) - Z_{i,j+\frac{1}{2}}(u_{i,j-1} - u_{i,j}).$$

where

$$Z_{i+\frac{1}{2},j} = \frac{1}{2}(Z_{i+1,j} + Z_{i,j}) \;\; ; \;\; Z_{i-\frac{1}{2},j} = \frac{1}{2}(Z_{i,j} + Z_{i,-1j})$$

$$Z_{i,j+\frac{1}{2}} = \frac{1}{2}(Z_{i,j+1} + Z_{i,j}) \;\; ; \;\; Z_{i,j-\frac{1}{2}} = \frac{1}{2}(Z_{i,j} + Z_{i,j-1})$$

By applying to the system of Euler equation for the nth approximated item of the sequence of the Ambrosio-Tortorelli functional we obtain: the term $Z(x, y) = (S^2(x, y) + K_\varepsilon)$ become by fixing every direction of the space, with K_ε neglected as in [19], we get: for x

$$\frac{\partial}{\partial x}\left(\left(S^2 + K_\varepsilon\right)\frac{\partial u}{\partial x}\right) \cong$$

$$\frac{1}{2h^2}\left[(S^2_{i+1,j} + S^2_{i,j})(u_{i+1,j} - u_{i,j}) + (S^2_{i,j} + S^2_{i-1,j})(u_{i-1,j} - u_{i,j})\right],$$

for y

$$\frac{\partial}{\partial y}\left(\left(S^2 + K_\varepsilon\right)\frac{\partial u}{\partial y}\right) \cong$$

$$\frac{1}{2h^2}\left[(S^2_{i,j+1} + S^2_{i,j})(u_{i,j+1} - u_{i,j}) + (S^2_{i,j} + S^2_{i,j-1})(u_{i,j-1} - u_{i,j})\right].$$

In Image Processing the lattice has a spatial density which is equivalent to image resolution, so we use here finite differences with node resolution equal to the spatial grid-step, so the discretized equation will look as follows

$$\begin{gathered}(S^2_{i+1,j} + S^2_{i,j})(u_{i+1,j} - u_{i,j}) + (S^2_{i,j} + S^2_{i-1,j})(u_{i-1,j} - u_{i,j}) \\ + (S^2_{i,j+1} + S^2_{i,j})(u_{i,j+1} - u_{i,j}) + (S^2_{i,j} + S^2_{i,j-1})(u_{i,j-1} - u_{i,j}) \\ = \mu h^2(u_{i,j} - g_{i,j}).\end{gathered}$$

The discreet laplacian for a function u

$$\Delta u(x,y) := u_{xx} + u_{yy}$$
$$\cong \frac{1}{h^2}\left[u_{i+1,j} + u_{i-1,j} - 4u_{i,j} + u_{i,j+1} + u_{i,j-1}\right].$$

Within Ω, the second equation, using a five-point stencil, will look

$$\alpha\varepsilon\ (S_{i+1,j} + S_{i-1,j} + S_{i,j+1} + S_{i,j-1} - 4S_{i,j}) = h^2 S_{i,j}|\nabla u|^2_{i,j} - h^2\frac{\alpha}{4\varepsilon}(1 - S_{i,j})$$

Being the problem elliptic, we use a discretization such that we get centered finite differences; therefore for 2 points stencil: let $|\nabla u|^2_{i,j} := |\widetilde{\nabla} u|^2_{i,j}$

$$|\widetilde{\nabla} u|^2_{i,j} \cong \frac{1}{4h^2}\left((u_{i+1,j} - u_{i-1,j})^2 + (u_{i,j+1} - u_{i,j-1})^2\right)$$

for nodes inside Ω. Or by other formulation by 3 points stencil: let $|\nabla u|^2_{i,j} := |\widetilde{\widetilde{\nabla}} u|^2_{i,j}$

$$|\widetilde{\widetilde{\nabla}} u|^2_{i,j} \cong \frac{1}{4h^2}\left(\frac{(u_{i+1,j} - u_{i,j})^2 + (u_{i,j} - u_{i-1,j})^2}{2} + \frac{(u_{i,j+1} - u_{i,j})^2 + (u_{i,j} - u_{i,j-1})^2}{2}\right)$$

then

$$S_{i,j} = \frac{\alpha\varepsilon\ \widehat{S}_{i,j} + \alpha\frac{h^2}{4\varepsilon}}{4\alpha\varepsilon + h^2|\nabla u|^2_{i,j} + \alpha\frac{h^2}{4\varepsilon}}. \tag{4}$$

where $\widehat{S}_{i,j} = S_{i+1,j} + S_{i-1,j} + S_{i,j+1} + S_{i,j-1}$.

The discretized u become:

$$u_{i,j} = \frac{(S^2_{i,j})(u_{i+1,j} + u_{i-1,j} + u_{i,j+1} + u_{i,j-1})}{(\mu h^2 + 4S^2_{i,j} + S^2_{i+1,j} + S^2_{i-1,j} + S^2_{i,j+1} + S^2_{i,j-1})} \tag{5}$$
$$+\frac{(S^2_{i+1,j})(u_{i+1,j}) + (S^2_{i-1,j})(u_{i-1,j}) + (S^2_{i,j+1})(u_{i,j+1}) + (S^2_{i,j-1})(u_{i,j-1}) + \mu h^2 g_{i,j}}{(\mu h^2 + 4S^2_{i,j} + S^2_{i+1,j} + S^2_{i-1,j} + S^2_{i,j+1} + S^2_{i,j-1})}.$$

3.2.3 Boundary Conditions

In this context we impose that Neumann boundary conditions are satisfied at the edge. Null derivatives at the border are generated by introducing dummy nodes along the perimeter, for j = 0 and i = 1, . . . , N with j = −1 and y = −h

$$\begin{cases} u_{i,0} - u_{i,-1} = 0 \\ \qquad\qquad\qquad\qquad i = 1, .., N-1 \\ S_{i,0} - S_{i,-1} = 0 \end{cases}$$

and in the same way for the remaining sides.

The equation is written the same way for nodes on the edge. In this case, symmetrical terms disappear in correspondence to dummy nodes introduced.

A linear algebraic system with $2(N+1)^2$ unknown variables is then obtained. By fixing S first and then U, we would get a system of the type:

$$\begin{cases} AU = b \\ BS = e \end{cases}$$

We use a recurrent two-step algorithm, which uncouples the system at every iterative step and calculates the first equation, replaces it in the second one and then replaces the result back into the first equation.

In summary, an iterative process give us, at one of its step, two equations to compute the non-linear elliptic problem related to the minimum conditions proper of the discrete approximated functionals sequence which converge to fix point.

4 Applicability of Methods

Recent scientific literature suggests several methods for recognition of ventricular area, but most of them are focused on semi-curve evolution from two fixed points, which is only suitable for single images. The method adopted here makes use, instead, of an ellipse as the initial profile, with no fixed points. This choice is justified by the chance of processing a multi-image sequence in order to derive the needed area at every frame. The above-mentioned protocol consists of applying segmentation models and methods to a rhythmically moving object.

We focus on the left ventricle of cardiac muscle since, in some clinical cases, the volume of blood introduced into the arterial net by the ventricle (estimated as its ejection fraction) has to be determined. This low-invasive technique gives us a chance to identify the area delimited by ventricular walls over time. Also expulsion time can be assessed by means of our technique, which proves useful to make new analytical hypotheses about blood internal pressure.

Ventricle internal area can be determined by curve-evolution from an assigned position by means of Hamilton-Jacobi PDE model. Other models, which make use of fixed points near to the atrial valve of the muscle, do not prove suitable to treat image sequences because would force to manually draw fixed points on every image in the sequence, due to variability in probe position and muscle movements. We assign, instead, an initial elliptic profile to the curve, centered in the frame.

We apply here a preprocessing method for frames in order to emphasize ventricle contours. Mumford-Shah functional minimization technique has been chosen due to its processing speed and sophistication, which make it suitable for reconstruction of images and several other real-life applications [21].

4.1 Applicability of the Approximation Methods

As shown above [22], the applicability of the evolutionary method based on curve evolution is conditioned, in the presence of discontinuous data, by restrictive hypotheses the punctual dependence of the speed term. Then the existence of the spatial gradient of the brightness-intensity function requests the convolution, in Ω-domain, with a standard mollifier.

In the approximation of the functional, the sequence of functional minima are iterated by the system by Ambrosio Tortorelli method. The technique to fix every equation arise to a quasi-linear class of elliptic systems explained in the paper [20]. At every iteration we obtain a regularized pair of approximated functions dependent from ε. This suggests to leave Gaussian regularization aside, with smaller loss of details, using the function of the K_ε item of the iteration sequence as the brightness-intensity function for curve evolution. u-function can directly be used in the eikonal equation for front evolution. This technique is used in [23], but optical flow theory is left aside [15]; This choice provides the needed regularity in the fracture [24] that represents the critical points of brightness-intensity function g_I of the given image.

A further step of technique refinement, in order to make ventricular walls get emphasized, consists, as mentioned above, of making the second term of the functional dependent of the gradient over the time [25].

The square gradient is point by point calculated over function u as the difference in brightness intensity between the preceding and the following frame. Globally, the variability of this term is mostly due to movements of ventricular walls. In the presence of a continuous movement in the same "scene", we are in condition to assume regularity for function g_I over time.

4.1.1 Regularity of the Speed Term in the Eikonal Equation

The method of Eikonal equation assures solvability in the presence of discontinuous data by convolution with a regularizing operator to control the gradient explosion of the brightness-intensity function $I(x)$ in the speed term of the eikonal Eq. (1) and the lipschitz continuity of the initial data $u_0(x)$.

$$v(x) = \frac{1}{1 + |\nabla I(x)|},$$

instead of the gaussian convolution

$$v(x) = v(|\nabla(G_\sigma * I(x))|) = \frac{1}{1 + |\nabla(G_\sigma * I(x))|}.$$

As mentioned above, for a Hamiltonian $H(x, \nabla u)$, when the element $u_h(x)$ represents the solution at every step of the elliptic system, the following proposition stands true:

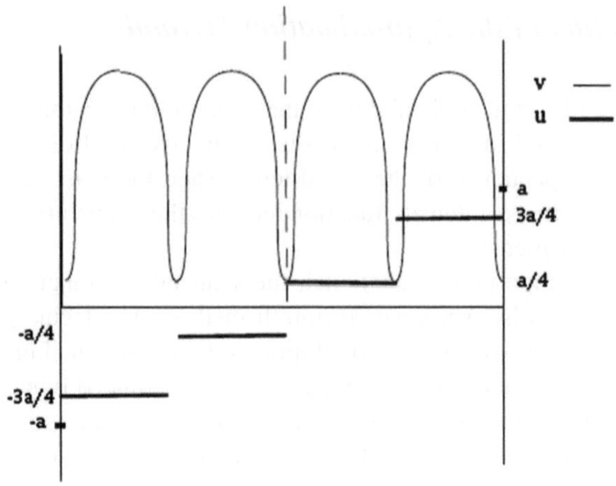

Fig. 3 Approximation of the one dimensional fracture

Prop. If u_{k_ε} represents a solution at kth iteration of the A-T sequence [14] given from alternate solution of the elliptic system for fixed number of iteration, then u_{k_ε} is enough smooth to calculate $|\nabla u_{k_\varepsilon}(x)|$.

Indeed, in the internal points of the domain Ω the amplitude of the fracture is ε's proportional, then we can found, at every step of the iterative solution of AT_ε algorithm, a costant C such that

$$|\nabla u_{k_\varepsilon}(x)| \leq \frac{C}{\varepsilon}$$

then

$$v(x) = \frac{1}{1 + |\nabla u_{k_\varepsilon}(x)|} \geq \frac{1}{1 + \dfrac{C}{\varepsilon}} > 0,$$

we can observe that the function u_{k_ε} has in every direction passing to the internal point $x \in \Omega$, a profile regularized by a C^2 arcs in the fracture as we can see in [24] as explained in the Fig. 3. For the lipschitz continuity needed for the initial condition for the eikonal equation, we choose a regular ellipse centered in the ventricular cavity.

From a computational point of view the discretized image has bounded intensity profile and the difference beetween two neighbor points is at most:

$$\frac{max(I(x_1)) - min(I(x_2))}{|x_1 - x_2|} \leq \frac{256}{1} \quad \forall x_1, x_2 \in \Omega$$

for [0, ..., 255] gray levels images and spatial mesh-grids equal to the image definition.

4.1.2 Convergence and Existence

The extension of existence results for the minimum for the M-S functional, when function u is time-dependent, is currently in progress. Nevertheless, the basic idea consists of considering the fluid change that would ideally result from a continuous movie of some cardiac movement. We try here to reconstruct, from this point of view, the demonstrative steps mentioned above. We are brought to conjecture a tubular neighborhood, on which is based, the Γ-convergence is interpretated as it is in movement; then, for a sufficiently small time, we could imagine that the regularity of u over time is such to assure convergence of the functional sequence to the minimum. Anyway, the analytical problem is still open and, therefore, only some conjectures are allowed [26–29].

In the first tests as to the numerical approximation, for the temporal and spatial gradient calculus, we use the formulation we use the two-point following formula:

$$(|\nabla u|_{i,j}^{(f)})^2 = \frac{1}{4h^2}\left((u_{i+1,j} - u_{i-1,j})^2 + (u_{i,j+1} - u_{i,j-1})^2 + (u_{i,j}^{(f-1)} - u_{i,j}^{(f+1)})^2\right)$$

It has a quite like good performance on the ventricular walls, but a successive application with tree-point stancil, suggested by Professor Stanley Osher evidence a more reliable definition of the pixel, especially in the time dependent elaboration:

$$\begin{aligned}(|\nabla u|_{i,j}^{(f)})^2 = &\frac{1}{4h^2}\left(\frac{(u_{i+1,j} - u_{i,j})^2 + (u_{i,j} - u_{i-1,j})^2}{2}\right)\\ &+ \frac{1}{4h^2}\left(\frac{(u_{i,j+1} - u_{i,j})^2 + (u_{i,j} - u_{i,j-1})^2}{2}\right)\\ &+ \frac{1}{4h^2}\left(\frac{(u_{i,j}^{(f-1)} - u_{i,j}^{(f)})^2 + (u_{i,j}^{(f)} - u_{i,j}^{(f-1)})^2}{2}\right).\end{aligned}$$

This formulation has better results and is adopted to all tests.

5 Echocardiographic Movie Processing

Modern instruments used in hospitals, as well as portable echocardiographic instruments, usually allow data exportation in various video formats (Fig. 4).

The method adopted here makes use of movies in AVI (Audio Video Interleave) format; a typical example of AVI-file characteristics follows:

Filename	'avifilename1.avi'	'avifilename2.avi'
FileSize	134158336	19728384
FileModDate	'25-Jun-2007 14:09:10'	'05-Oct-2007 10:06:14'
NumFrames	1602	1269
FramesPerSecond	27	26
Width	800	800
Height	600	652
ImageType	'truecolor'	'truecolor'
VideoCompression	'Cinepak'	'MP42'
Quality	0	0
NumColormapEntries	0	0

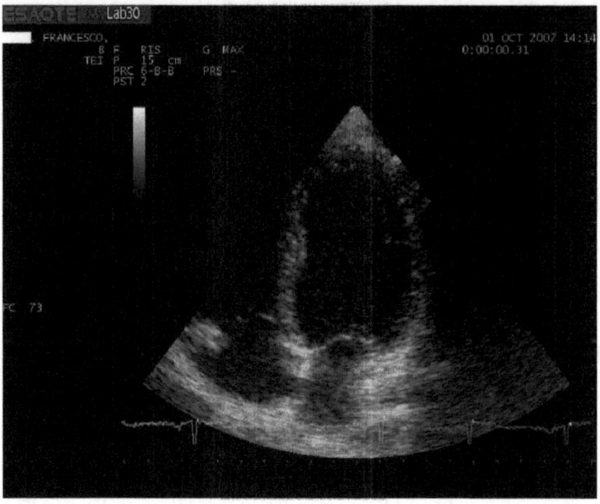

Fig. 4 Entire echo image frame

Data files can be exported and read in DICOM (Digital Imaging and Communication in Medicines) format, the world standard for all medical applications dealing with patient data and further detailed information.

The standard DICOM is composed of different parts and storage levels, suitable for data exchange in the medical context.

At the present level of work, we opt for AVI format in performing image extraction, since, being supported by various operating systems with public licenses, it allows an easiest manipulation of movies. Esaote MyLab30 instrument, currently used by the team lead by Prof. Mario Curione in the Department of Clinical Sciences of "Umberto I" University Hospital, when interfaced with a PC supporting Windows o.s., exports data in different image compression formats, in terms of size and sampling frequency. A single frame looks like:

In particular, sampling frequency (FramesPerSecond:26, 27), allows medical researchers to compare data from areas with the Electro-Cardio-Graphic layout. We shortly mention here the computational protocol that handles the two phases, M-S Preprocessing and H-J Processing of images, which makes use of the well-roundness

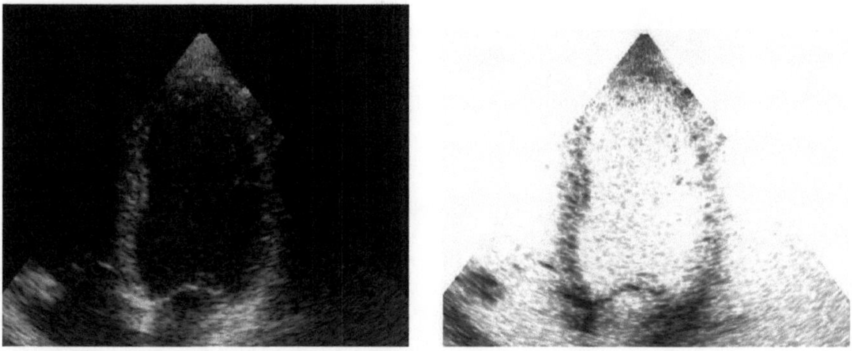

Fig. 5 On the *left* the cropped frame on the *right* its inverse of intensity value

of a MatLab application in the preprocessing stage and of a FORTRAN code with better performance on single frames during processing.

Being the elaboration system implemented on a Linux system, a format conversion algorithm with no video compression is needed (compressed formats are licensed). This involves a further step in preprocessing of the entire file.

5.1 Frame Adaptation

The algorithm selects the part of the image to be cropped ("cropping" step Fig. 5). After gray levels are inverted, brightness intensity difference gets positive in the presence of edges.

This way we obtain the image of the selected frame (Fig. 5 on the right), to be later preprocessed using M-S algorithm with various parameter choices.

5.2 Presence of Edges for H-J PDE

Preprocessed images are then uniformly distributed within the interval [0,1], in terms of gray-tone intensity (double float numerical representation). Curve evolution starts from an initial elliptic configuration u_0, centered in the frame at $t = 0$, and goes on along the external normal direction, with speed proportional to the brightness-intensity gradient of the image at every pixel. The computation of the gradient is corrected by means of a convolution with a regularizing operator called standard Mollifier [22].

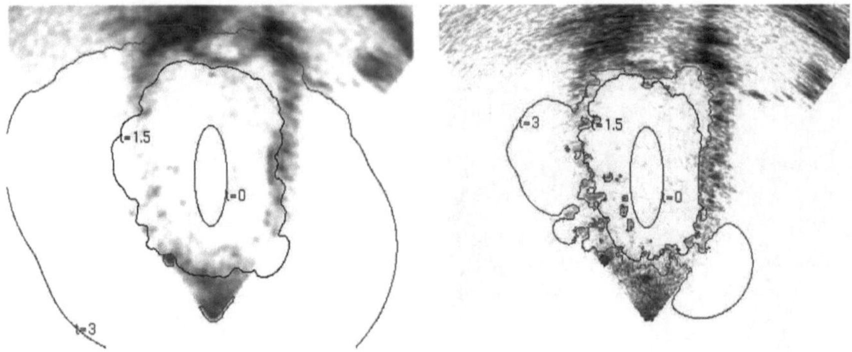

Fig. 6 On the *left* the curve evolved after 10 iteration of Gaussian smoothing, on the *right*

The regularization is made by the diffusion heat equation, this operation is essential for the gradient evaluation, but the image lose important details even with a limited number of iterations, therefore the curve evolution does not found a gradient value to determine its velocity shutdown [23].

To highlight the problem we shown in Fig. 6 the evolution in a frame on which the Gaussian smoothing was repeated for 10 iterations. Clearly, curve evolution is not able to find a gradient value that, in respect to a stopping threshold $th = 0.125$, can cause its stop. Even with a single Gaussian step, the gradient is not able, in some regions of the ventricular contour, to stop curve evolution (see Fig. 6).

5.3 Preprocessing by the M-S Functional

As previously stated, segmentation by solution of H-J equation fails when the probed tissue gives back a small signal represented by a small brightness-intensity gradient. Brightness-intensity gradients along ventricle edges (that is, edge info) could happen not to be visible in all regions of the given frame; in general, small signals come are generated by pixels along ventricular walls, if compared to image noise. Therefore, we decide here to improve the elaboration protocol by introducing a preprocessing phase which makes use of the M-S method. Let us illustrate our attempt to apply the M-S model, whose efficiency strongly depends on the choice of parameters λ, α [28]. This is particularly true for echo-graphic images, probably most due to the density of signal detector in the probe, which causes a limited spatial definition. Consequently, images from each sequence frame show very discontinuous ventricular contours.

5.4 Parameters Involved in the First Step of M-S Application

λ-parameter is directly proportional to smoothness and regularity of u-functions. On the other hand, α-parameter is directly proportional to the size of the selected region along the edge.

The presence of discontinuous and localized signal has suggested us to apply, in a first step, the M-S method to emphasize image details, choosing parameter values which favored small edges (therefore, a small λ and a small α).

Parameter choice proves very important in order to balance selection of image contours in respect to background noise. When small parameter values are chosen, small areas are privileged, thus we can enhance local peculiarities of Echo-Graphic images.

When parameter values are large, ventricle walls are emphasized and larger areas are selected. This suggests, as mentioned above, to perform an iterated search for edges in the preprocessing stage, in order to select small areas first and, subsequently, to reconstruct, starting from previous selection, more regular edges by means of parameters value that privilege smoother and longer contours. Therefore, we choice the following intervals: (0.02 – 0.8) for λ and (0.001 – 0.000001) for α.

5.5 Parameters Involved in the Second Step of M-S Application

After treating images by the above-mentioned choice of M-S parameters, we now go on to treat them again using the same method, but different values. In substance, the procedure is repeated over the jump subset S; this produces the approximation of those parts of the image which are identified as local areas, while the search for longer contours and wider areas is made with the aid of suitable parameters. This way, edges get more evident and continuous, allowing to limit the evolution of H-J model more effectively by using an optimal threshold value. In the course of the second step of M-S application, after some tests, parameters values are taken such that only a direct verification of the out coming images can be used as a measure of goodness of results (in a few words, the method requests to set parameters "with a screwdriver"). Repeated M-S algorithm.

The following paired lines of images report results from the second application of M-S method, in relation to parameter values appearing in image headings.

5.6 Time Dependence

Good results are obtained with prudent choices of parameters, but the presence of some interruptions of the ventricular profile walls results a big obstacle, to the right evolution of the curve, modeled by eikonal equation, avoiding the evolution outside the ventricular border (Fig. 6).

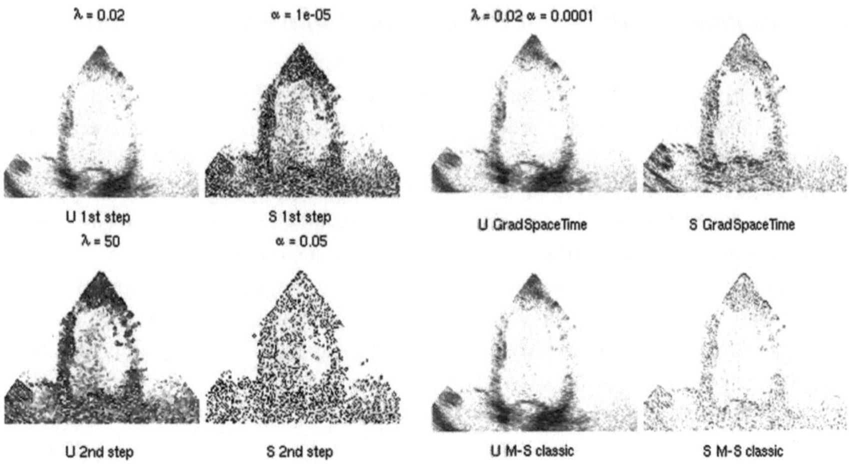

Fig. 7 On the *left* four results of M-S on the *right* four of the grad-time elaboration

Having a whole sequence of consecutive images at our disposal, we make here a sophistication of our scheme in order to enhance moving parts of ventricular walls. Those pixels, which, when comparing two consecutive images, show a variability in terms of brightness intensity, represent moving parts ventricular walls. To this aim, we put dependence on time gradient into the functional, calculated between the frame preceding the one in elaboration and the following.

As to the numerical code, various simplifications have been made in order to directly insert time dependence ∇u_t into the computation of the spatial gradient ∇u. This all has to be demonstrated in analytical terms.

The contribution ∇u_t is inserted into the computation of the gradient of function u at every spatial pixel $(x, y, \bar{t})$.

In the context of finite-difference numerical scheme with time step (frame to frame), the natural choice consists of centering the current frame in respect to those adjacent. Then, for every frame f:

$$(|\nabla u|_{i,j}^{(f)})^2 = \frac{1}{4h^2}\left((u_{i+1,j} - u_{i-1,j})^2 + (u_{i,j+1} - u_{i,j-1})^2 + (u_{i,j}^{(f-1)} - u_{i,j}^{(f+1)})^2\right);$$

with this change gradient value is increased, as well as the minimum, as testified by larger presence of contours. In general, the jump set S finds more contours, mainly located where, proportionally, a greater variability of brightness intensity is present. The practical comparison reveals the emphatization of mobile profiles of ventricular walls.

We can appreciate how edge portions not selected by the classical method are now emphasized. We notice that less mobile parts of the image—for example, pixels near to the vertex of the echographic cone—present a decrease in selection, thus hypothetically proving less representative of moving edges; on the contrary, ventricle walls get emphasized, since characterized by greater time variability in its brightness-intensity square gradient (Fig. 7).

5.7 Elaboration Method Case Schema

The block diagram summarizing the protocol is reported in the figure below.

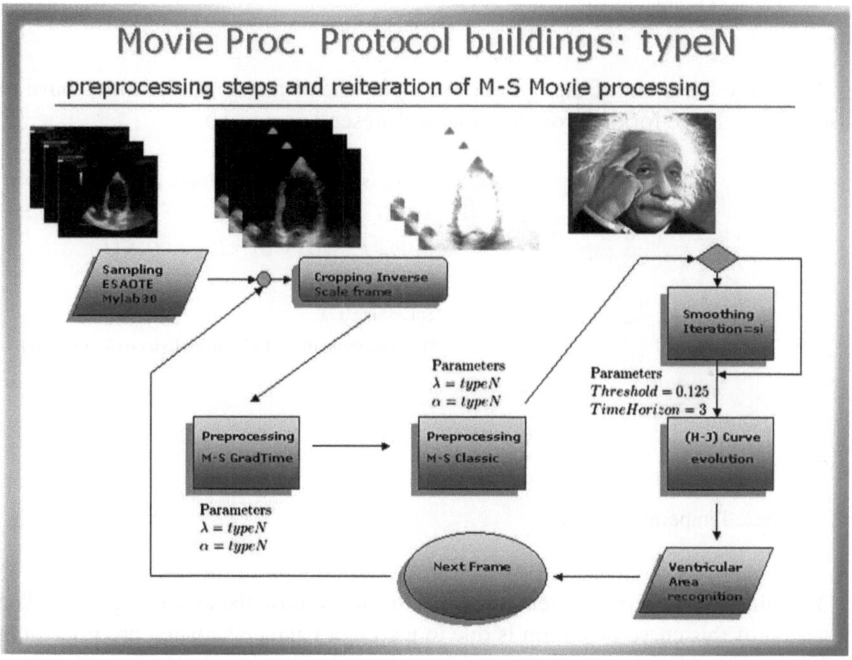

Next section explains the different kinds of preprocessing and the consequent selected area in frame.

5.7.1 Results for Different Processing Choice

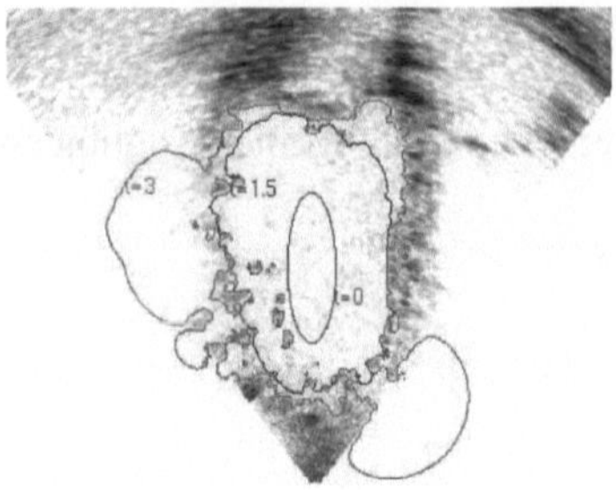

Preprocessing: n/a,

Processing:

Smoothing: eq. Heat 1 iteration

H-J: Threshold (th=0.125) Time-Horizon (3, step 0.03)

Type1: Original image

The curve leaks out of the left and the right side of the ventricle, so we have to discard this choice for the protocol of area representation graph.

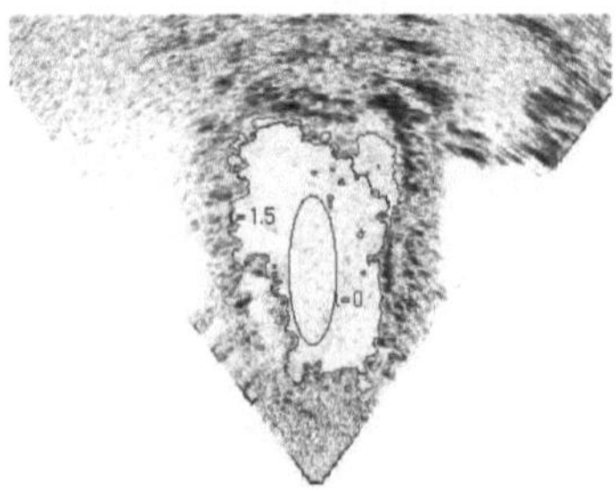

Preprocessing: M-S Grad Temp ($\lambda = 0.02, alpha = 0.0001$)

$(UOrig(f-1, f, f+1)) \rightsquigarrow (Ureg_1(f), S_1(f))$

Processing:

Smoothing: n/a

H-J: Threshold (th=0.125) Time-Horizon (3, step 0.03)

Type2: Temporal gradient

With this choice of parameters we obtain the best ventricular area recognition. The precision of this curve evolution is due to a correct balance between preprocessing and processing phase.

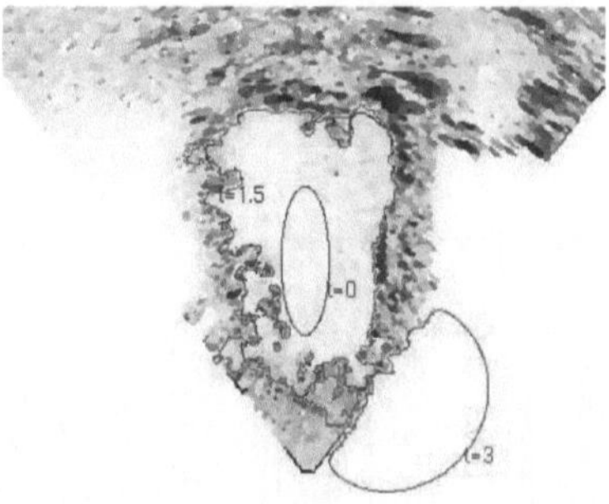

Preprocessing:

Step1, M-S Time Grad ($\lambda = 0.02, \alpha = 0.0001$)

$(UOrig(f-1, f, f+1)) \rightsquigarrow (Ureg_1(f), S_1(f))$

Step2, Classic M-S ($\lambda = 50, \alpha = 0.02$)

$(Ureg_1(f), S_1(f)) \rightsquigarrow (Ureg_2(f), S_2(f))$

Type 3: Classical M-S on original image

In this case we apply M-S Time Grad algorithm and use the preprocessed U for curve evolution. A single step of M-S is made. In this case two steps of M-S algorithm are used with a different choice of parameters at each step. However, the curve evolves outside the ventricular border. Also this choice is not suitable for area recognition.

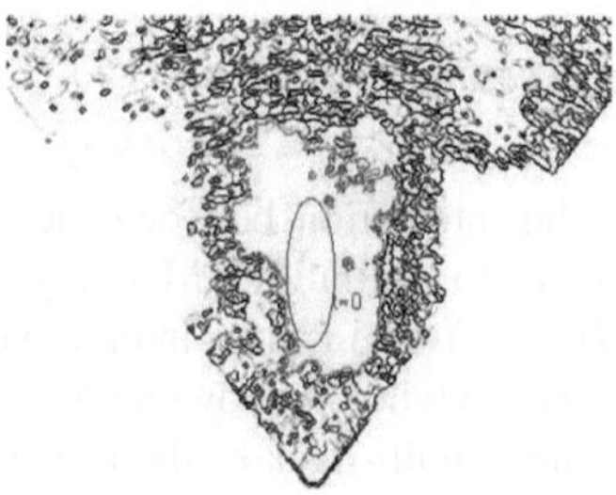

Preprocessing: Step1, M-S Time Grad ($\lambda = 0.02, \alpha = 0.0001$)

$(UOrig(f-1, f, f+1)) \rightsquigarrow (Ureg_1(f), S_1(f))$

Step2 M-S Classic ($\lambda = 50, \alpha = 0.02$)

$(Ureg_1(f), S_1(f)) \rightsquigarrow (Ureg_2(f), S_2(f))$

Processing:

Smoothing: n/a

H-J($S_2(f)$): Threshold (th=0.125) Time-Horizon (3, step 0.03)

Type 4: M-S iterated on the jump set S

Curve evolution has a good performance on the ventricular area, but it not fills the entire cavity. This kind of choice is better than the one presented in Type 2 in the case of low resolution of the image frame. The comparison between these preprocessing methods selects which is the most viable for front evolution. The reported experiments are indicative of suitable methods for ventricular area recognition. Some of the above tests reveal how much edge emphatization is useful for moving edge recognition. The Preprocessing step allows to use small threshold values, so that front evolution fits the ventricular edge in an optimal way. Therefore, we choose to adopt Type2 and Type4 protocol for the analysis of image sequences. A real-case results of ventricular areas by movie of 300 frames (10 s) see Fig. 8.

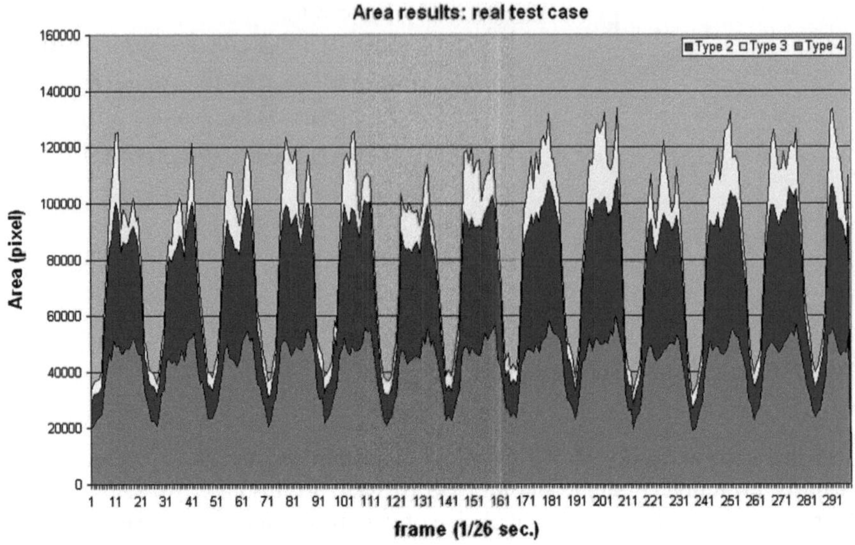

Fig. 8 Areas trends

6 The Graphic Application for Signal Synchronization

Medical research is interested in investigating the interaction between mechanic and electrical properties of cardiac muscle. To this aim, we build a Matlab graphic software (from creative commons avi player). This software is user-interactive and presents a box offering several control buttons. The main window shows an AVI video of the echographic data frame, an axis representing a multi-track of the Electrocardiographic signal over time and another axis showing the above-mentioned value of ventricular area and its related ejection fraction parameter over time expressed in seconds. The MATLAB application looks as follows.This main graphic axis shows results from the elaboration representing the main goal of this work: the trend of ventricular area over time. The max and min peak of expulsion for the diastolic cycle and the calculated Ejection Fraction are shown as well. We want to remark that a non-conventional information is provided: time needed for expulsion, which offers a possible field of investigation about internal ventricle pressure. In cardiovascular physiology, ejection fraction (E_f) is the fraction of blood pumped out of a ventricle with each heart beat. By definition, the volume of blood within a ventricle immediately before a contraction is known as the end-diastolic volume. Similarly, the volume of blood left in a ventricle at the end of contraction is end-systolic volume. The difference between end-diastolic and end-systolic volumes is the stroke volume, the volume of blood ejected with each beat. Ejection fraction (E_f) is the fraction of the end-diastolic volume that is ejected with each beat; that is, it is stroke volume (SV) divided by end-diastolic volume (EDV):

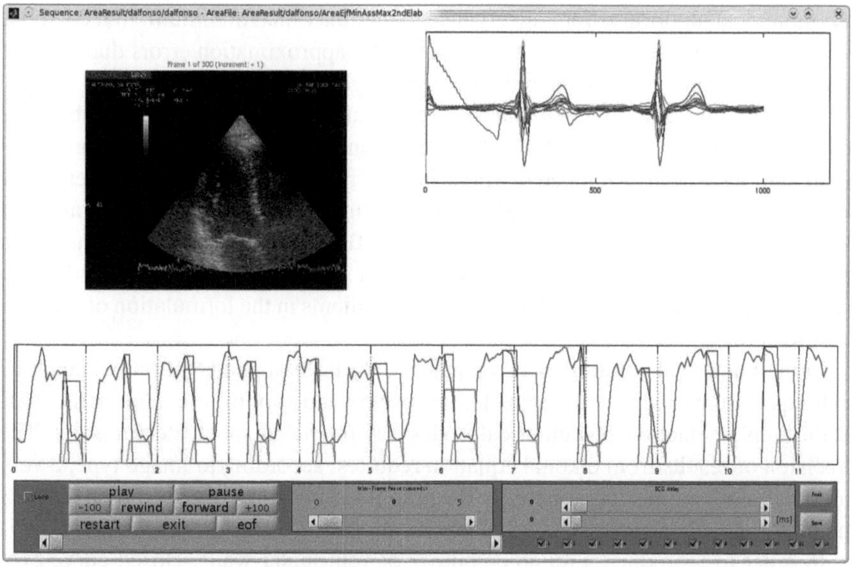

Fig. 9 Echo ECG Synchronizer application

$$E_f = \frac{SV}{EDV} = \frac{EDV - ESV}{EDV}$$

In the last figure the values of E_f is represented by the dark green line, the red one is the maximal value of EDV and the cyan one is ESV. These values are only an appraisal, because referable to an area and not to a volume information (Fig. 8).

7 Conclusions

This is a step of an extended project whose final target is the analysis of EchoCardioGraphic image sequences for non-invasive and a-posteriori medical diagnostics of heart left-ventricle diseases. The medical protocol requires the determination of local pressure and internal volume of the left ventricle during its cyclic work.

In this first step, which has many upgradable features, a specific method has been developed, based on mathematical models of image processing, for the recognition of ventricular area in different frames of EchoCardioGraphics images.

The exposed methods and their applications are an approach to answer to requests from medical diagnostics.

From the point of view of applied mathematics, numerical techniques have been used in order to obtain results which fit the problem. In echocardiographic images very ragged contours are usually available and pixel definition is low, but the described sophistication of the M-S method does not require the use of onerous numerical algorithms for convergence to the functional minimum. Indeed, those methods are typically applied in literature to skip approximation errors due to triple junctions or object occlusions in the treated images [30].

The mathematical framework has been focused on some open problems about the applicability of variational methods to time-dependent image streams. The proposed arguments have been developed in a preprint paper about segmentation and denoising of image time series by [31]. It deals with small images of biological tissues affected by cancer growth and offers a theorical study on Bounded-Variation functions which is close to our specific interest in the existence of global minima, in order to develop a theory for the dynamic contribution of time gradients in the formulation of the M-S functional.

In the numerical solution of H-J equation, we have applied "partially standard" techniques suggested by articles [17]. The approximation of front-evolution methods in the implementation of numerical codes has produced satisfactory results. The precision of results from eikonal equation requires, according to image type, a very large elaboration time, if compared to the preprocessing phase obtained with the M-S method.

In order to reproduce a reliable contour of ventricular walls, closed-curve evolution requires a processing time which is one order of magnitude larger than the preprocessing phase. A further development of H-J technique could be obtained by means of the implementation of Fast-Marching methods [13, 32]. In the preprocessing and processing phase, the direct examination of resulting images for the evolved curves and edge-enhancing allows back-regulation of parameters and verification the quality of our choices.

Various cardiologists are already trying to use our time-evolving image-processing technique by synchronization with the ECG signal in order to validate some medical hypotheses on ventricular diseases. In agreement with cardiologists involved in this project, future developments could be:

- The elaboration of ventricular areas by a ventricular "short and long side" approach, in order to obtain a better volumetric reconstruction.
- The validation of theories which allow the interpretation of correspondences between the electric signal (ECG) and ventricular volume filling (ejection fraction).
- The implementation of this protocol for an Internet service for reconstruction of the ventricular area profile, which would prove useful for modern e-healthcare.
- The study of mobility profiles of ventricular walls to draw speed vector-field curves during cardiac periodical movement; this would prove useful for the individuation of muscular portions affected by diseases.
- The possibility to model, by finite-element analysis, the ventricular pump to make internal pressure and volume fit experimental results in the comparison between real data and simulation.

References

1. Sethian JA, Vladimirsky A (2000) Fast methods for the Eikonal and related Hamilton-Jacobi equations on unstructured meshes. Proc Natl Acad Sci USA 97:5699–5703
2. Osher S, Paragios N (2003) Geometric level set methods in imaging, vision, and graphics. Springer, Berlin
3. Osher S, Sethian JA (1988) Fronts propagating with curvature-dependent speed: algorithms based on Hamilton-Jacobi formulations. J Comput Phys 79:12–49
4. Bardi M, Evans LC (1984), On Hopf's formulas for solutions of Hamilton-Jacobi equations. Nonlinear, analysis 8.
5. Camilli F (2004) An Hopf-Lax formulas for a class of measurable Hamilton-Jacobi equation. Nonlinear Anal, Elsevier 57(22):265–286
6. Camilli F, Falcone M (1997) An approximation scheme for the optimal control diffusion process Modélisation Mathématique et Analyse Numérique 29:97–122
7. Camilli F, Siconolfi A (2003) Hamilton-Jacobi Equation with a measurable dependence on the state variable. Adv Differ Equ 8(6):733–768
8. Chan TF, Shen J, Vese LA (2003) Variational PDE models in image processing. Not AMS 01, 50(1):14–26.
9. Evans LC (1998) Partial differential equations, vol 19. American Mathematical Society, Providence
10. Falcone M (1997) Numerical solution of dynamic programming equation. Appendix A in the volume M. Bardi and I. Capuzzo Dolcetta,: Optimal control and viscosity solutions of Hamilton-Jacobi-Bellman equations. Birkhäuser, Boston.
11. Falcone M, Capuzzo Dolcetta I (1997) Optimal control and viscosity solutions of Hamilton-Jacobi-Bellman equations. Birkhäuser, Boston
12. Falcone M, Ferretti R (2002) Semi-lagrangian schemes for Hamilton-Jacobi equations, discrete representation formulae and Godunov methods. J Comput Phys 175:559–575
13. Sethian JA (1999) Level set methods and fast marching methods. Cambridge University Press, Cambridge
14. Ambrosio L, Tortorelli VM (1990) Approximation of functionals depending on jumps by elliptic functionals via Γ-Convergence. Commun Pure Appl Math 43:999–1036
15. Aubert G, Kornprobst P (2002) Mathematical problems in image processing. Springer, New York
16. Morel JM, Solimini S (1995) Variational methods in image segmentation progress in nonlinear differential equations and their applications. Birkhäuser, Basel
17. Durou JD, Falcone M, Sagona M (2003) A survey of numerical methods for shape-from-shading. Kluwer Academic Publishers, Netherland
18. Pedone M, Falcone M (2003) Alcuni algoritmi per il trattamento delle immagini basati su EDP, Tesi Master Calcolo Scientifico, La Sapienza. http://pedoneweb.phys.uniroma1.it/max/master/
19. Spitaleri RM, March R, Arena D (1999) Finite difference solution of Euler equation arising in variational image segmentation. Numer Algorithms 21:353–365
20. Birindelli I, Finzi Vita S (1998) A class of quasi-linear elliptic systems arising in image segmentation. Nonlinear Differ Equ Appl NoDEA 5:445–449
21. Ambrosio L (1990) Existence theory new for class of variational problems. Arch Ration Mech Anal 111:291–322
22. Malladi R, Sethian JA, Vemuri BC (1995) Shape modeling with front propagation, a level set approach. IEEE Trans Pattern Anal Mach Intell 17:158–175
23. Chan TF, Vese LA (2001) Active contour without edges. IEEE Trans Image Process 10:266–276
24. Francfort GA, Le Q, Serfaty S (2009) Critical points of Ambrosio-Tortorelli convergence to critical points of M-S in the one dimensional Dirichlet case. ESAIM Control Optim Calc Var 15:576–598
25. Chan TF, Shen J (2005) Variational image inpainting. Commun Pure Appl Math LVIII:579–619.

26. Bourdin B, Chambolle A (2000) Implementation of an adaptive finite-element approximation of the Mumford-Shah functional. Numer Math 85:609–646
27. De Giorgi E, Carriero M, Leaci A (1989) Existence theorem for to minimum problem with free discontinuity set. Arch Rational Mech Anal 108:195–218
28. March R (1992) Visual reconstructions with discontinuities using variational methods. Image Vis Comput 10:30–38
29. Mumford D, Shah J (1989) Optimal approximation by piecewise smooth functions and associated variational problems. Commun Pure Appl Math 42:577–685
30. Ambrosio L (1989) Variational problems in SBV and image segmentation. Acta Appl Math 17:1–40
31. Barone P, Canfora MF, March R (2008) Segmentation, classification and denoising of time series of images by variational method. Preprint IAC CNR (2008).
32. Tsitsiklis JN (1995) Efficient algorithms for globally optimal trajectorie. IEEE Trans Autom Control 40(9):1528–1538

Editors Biography

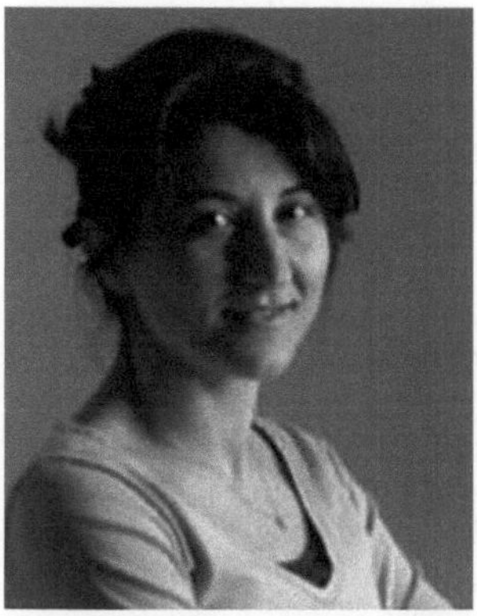

Daniela Iacoviello
Department of Computer, Control and Management Engineering Antonio Ruberti
Sapienza University of Rome
Via Ariosto 25
00185 Rome, Italy
Email: iacoviello@dis.uniroma1.it
url: http://www.dis.uniroma1.it/~iacoviel/

Daniela Iacoviello graduated in Mathematics in 1992; from 1992 to 1994 she was at the Institute of High Mathematics and in 1998 she obtained the Ph.D. in System Engineering from University of Rome "La Sapienza". Since 2002 she has been assistant professor in Automatic Control at the Department of Computer, Control and Management Engineering Antonio Ruberti of Sapienza University of Rome.

Since 2003 she has been member of the Centro Interdipartimentale di Ricerca per l'Analisi dei Modelli e dell'Informazione nei Sistemi Biomedici (CISB).

Since 2008 she has been member of the Centro Ricerche Aerospaziali Sapienza.

Since 2001 she has participated to financial programs from the Faculty and the University.

She participated to the 2005 PRIN project and to the 2009 PRIN project She was also involved in the SARFIRE project (ASI financial program 2010–2012). She is referee of many international scientific journal (Computer Methods and Programs in Biomedicine, IEEE Trans. Biomedical Engineering , International Journal of Tomography and Statistics, International Journal of Imaging, IET Image Processing, NDT and E International- Independent Nondestructive Testing and Evaluation, International Journal for Computational Vision and Biomechanics, Computer Modeling and Engineering, International Journal of Biometrics and Bioinformatics, Journal of Engineering Manufacture, Microscopy Research and Technique, Eurasip Journal on Advances in Signal Processing).

Since 2012 she has been Associate Editor of Computer Methods in Biomechanics and Biomedical Engineering : Imaging and Visualization. She is member of the Editorial Board of the Journals: International Journal of Imaging, International Journal of Computer Interaction and Information Technology; moreover she is member of the Scientific Committee of many Conferences on image analysis. Her main research interests from methodological and applicative point of view are in signal processing, image analysis, estimation theory, system identification, optimal control, neural network, bioengineering.

Since 2002 she has been Supervisor of several M.Sc. thesis.

P. Di Giamberardino et al. (eds.), *Computational Modeling of Objects Presented in Images*, 311
Lecture Notes in Computational Vision and Biomechanics 15,
DOI: 10.1007/978-3-319-04039-4, © Springer International Publishing Switzerland 2014

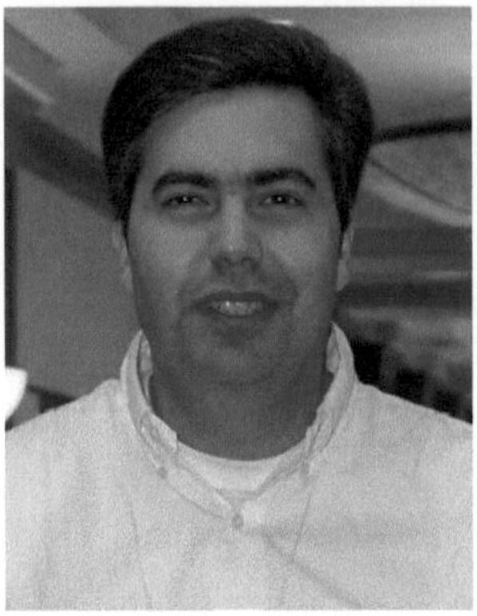

João Manuel R. S. Tavares
Faculdade de Engenharia da Universidade do Porto (FEUP)
Rua Dr. Roberto Frias, s/n
4200-465 Porto
Portugal
Email: tavares@fe.up.pt
url: www.fe.up.pt/~tavares

João Manuel R. S. Tavares is graduated in Mechanical Engineering from the University of Porto, Portugal (1992). In 1995, he obtained an M.Sc. in Electrical and Computers Engineering, in the field of Industrial Informatics, also at the University of Porto. In 2001, he obtained a Ph.D. degree in Electrical and Computers Engineering from the same University. Since 2001, he has been senior researcher and project coordinator at the Laboratory of Optical and Experimental Mechanics (LOME) of the Institute of Mechanical Engineering and Industrial Management (INEGI). He was Assistant Professor in the Department of Mechanical Engineering (DEMec) of the Faculty of Engineering of the University of Porto (FEUP) between 2001 and 2011, and since then he has been Associate Professor in the same department. He has been co-chair of several scientific national and international conferences and workshops, including CompIMAGE 2006/2010/2012, VipIMAGE 2007/2009/2011/2013, CIBEM 2011, BioDENTAL 2009/2012, TMSi 2010, IMAGAPP 2009 and EUROMEDIA 2008, founder and editor-in-chief of the Taylor and Francis international journal "Computer Methods in Biomechanics and Biomedical Engineering: Imaging and Visualization" (CMBBE: Imaging and Visualization), founder and co-editor of the Springer book series "Lecture Notes in Computational Vision and Biomechanics" (LNCV&B), editor and reviewer of several scientific journals, co-author than more of 350 scientific publications, including the co-editing of scientific books and of special issues of scientific journals, and co-author of three international patents. In the last years, he has been participating in several scientific research projects, some as coordinator, and the supervisor and co-supervisor of several M.Sc. and Ph.D. thesis. His main research areas include Computational Vision, Medical Imaging, Scientific Visualization, Biomechanics, Human-Computer Interaction and New Product Development.

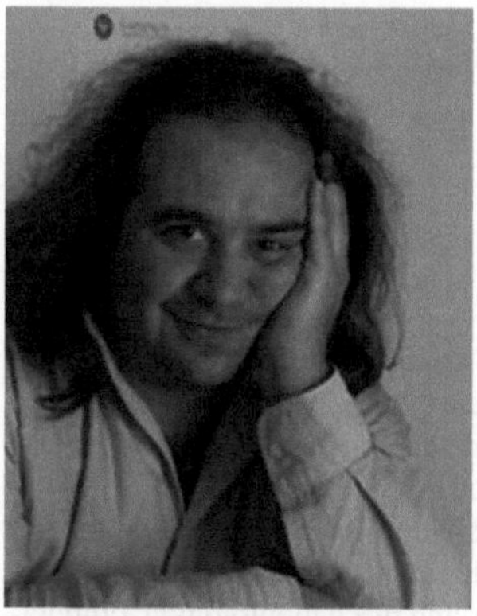

Paolo Di Giamberardino
Sapienza University of Rome
Department of Computer, Control and Management Engineering Antonio Ruberti
Via Ariosto 25
00185 Rome, Italy
Email: digiamberardino@dis.uniroma1.it; paolo.digiamberardino@uniroma1.it
url: http://www.dis.uniroma1.it/~digiamb/website

Paolo Di Giamberardino is Assistant Professor since 1996 at the Department of Computer Control and Management Engineering Antonio Ruberti of Sapienza, University of Rome. He received both the master degree (Electronic Engineering) in 1991 and the Ph.D. (Systems Engineering) in 1995 from Sapienza University of Rome.

Author or coauthor of more than 60 papers published on international journals, conference proceedings or as book chapters. Head of the Control and Systems Laboratory and co-head of The E-Learning Systems and Application Laboratory of the Department, in the last decade he has been Principal Investigator of about ten Research Projects founded by University of Rome "La Sapienza" or the Italian Ministry of Scientific Research and Technology. He also participated to several Research Projects promoted and founded by Italian and European Agencies (ESA, ASI, etc.). He is serving as reviewer for some international journals and he has been member of Scientific Committee of several International Conferences.

Since 1999 he has taught several courses at the Engineering Faculty of the University of Rome "La Sapienza", all in the field of the Automatic Control. He has been supervisor of Ph.D. students and several B.Sc. and M.Sc. students (about 15 per year).

His main research interests are in the field of nonlinear discrete time and sampled dynamical systems, in the problems of motion planning, control and coordination of mobile robots, in communication and control problems for mobile sensor networks and some aspects related to the problem of visual systems for robotic control.

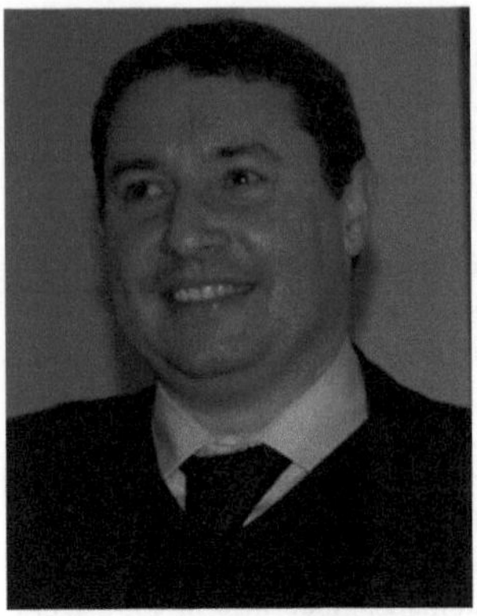

Renato Natal Jorge
IDMEC-Pole FEUP, Faculty of Engineering,
University of Porto
Rua Dr. Roberto Frias
200-465 Porto
Portugal
(rnatal@fe.up.pt)

Associate Professor at the Faculty of Engineering, University of Porto (FEUP); Mechanical Engineer from the University of Porto, 1987; M.Sc. from the University of Porto, 1991; Ph.D. from the University of Porto, 1999.

Present teaching and research interests: Computational methods in applied mechanics and engineering; New product development; Biomechanics and mechanobiology; Computational vision and medical image processing.

Between 2007 and 2011 was the Director of the "Structural Integrity Unit" research group of the Institute of Mechanical Engineering at FEUP (IDMEC—a R & D non-profit, private Research Institute). Member of the executive board of IDMEC-FEUP.

Responsible for the Supervision or Co-supervision of 12 Ph.D. students.

Co-chair of the following conferences: CompIMAGE; 14th International Product Development Management; VIPIMAGE; Fourteenth Annual Scientific Conference on WEB Technology, New Media, Communications and Telematics Theory, Methods, Tools and Applications; VIPIMAGE 2009; CompIMAGE 2010; Biodental; iDEMi'09; 6th International Conference on Technology and Medical Sciences, CIBEM 2011, VIPIMAGE 2011 and 2013; among other mini-symposia within conferences.

Founder and Editor of the International Journal for Computational Vision and Biomechanics. Guest editor of several scientific journals.

Principal Investigator for several national and European scientific projects.

Co-author of more than 100 papers in international journals and more than 300 publications in international conferences.

MIX
Papier aus verantwortungsvollen Quellen
Paper from responsible sources
FSC® C105338

If you have any concerns about our products,
you can contact us on
ProductSafety@springernature.com

In case Publisher is established outside the EU,
the EU authorized representative is:
Springer Nature Customer Service Center GmbH
Europaplatz 3, 69115 Heidelberg, Germany

Printed by Libri Plureos GmbH
in Hamburg, Germany